Epithelial Tumors of the Thymus

Pathology, Biology, Treatment

Epithelial Tumors of the Thymus

Pathology, Biology, Treatment

Edited by

Alexander Marx and
Hans Konrad Müller-Hermelink

The University of Würzburg
Würzburg, Germany

Springer Science+Business Media, LLC

Library of Congress Cataloging-in-Publication Data

Epithelial tumors of the thymus : pathology, biology, treatment / edited by Alexander Marx and Hans Konrad Müller-Hermelink.
p. cm.
"Proceedings of the First Conference on Biological and Clinical Aspects of Thymic Epithelial Tumors, held April 14-18, 1996, in Wurzburg, Germany"--T.p.verso.
Includes bibliographical references and index.

1. Thymus--Tumors--Congresses. 2. Epithelium--Tumors--Congresses. I. Marx, Alexander. II. Müller-Hermelink, Hans Konrad. III. Conference on Biological and Clinical Aspects of Thymic Epithelial Tumors (1st : 1996 : Würzburg, Germany)
[DNLM: 1. Thymoma--pathology--congresses. 2. Thymoma--therapy--congresses. 3. Thymus Neoplasms--pathology--congresses. 4. Thymus Neoplasms--therapy--congresses. WK 400 E64 1997]
RC280.T55E65 1997
616.99'443--dc21
DNLM/DLC
for Library of Congress 97-1867
CIP

DOI 10.1007/978-1-4899-0033-3

Proceedings of the First Conference on Biological and Clinical Aspects of Thymic Epithelial Tumors, held April 14 – 18, 1996, in Würzburg, Germany

Originally published by Plenum Press, New York in 1997
MyCopy version of the original edition 1997

http://www.plenum.com

10 9 8 7 6 5 4 3 2 1

www.springer.com/mycopy

PREFACE

Thymic epithelial tumors are rare and mostly malignant human neoplasms characterized by a fascinating variety of morphological features and an unrivaled frequency of associated autoimmune diseases. As a consequence, a myriad of complex diagnostic and clinical problems ensues in patients with these tumors. Since only a few specialists in each country are familiar with these problems, this volume intends to summarize the state of the art of thymic epithelial tumor pathology and biology and treatment protocols. The volume is also designed to promote the interaction between scientists from a variety of disciplines and physicians treating thymoma patients.

In the first part of the volume, morphological and immunohistological criteria are given for the various subtypes of thymic epithelial tumors. The two competing classifications and nomenclature systems existing to date are jointly considered. In addition, morphological overlaps between organotypic and nonorganotypic thymic epithelial tumors are stressed, since they may have a major bearing on diagnostic and therapeutic strategies.

The second part of the volume is devoted to recent data on normal T-cell maturation and the impact of abnormal T-cell development in thymic epithelial tumors on the development of paraneoplastic autoimmunity. Multicolor flow cytometry, the human/SCID–mouse system, transgenic mouse technology, and T-cell cloning techniques have greatly contributed to this fascinating field of research.

In the third part of the volume, the molecular, humoral, and cellular basis of paraneoplastic autoimmunity in thymic epithelial tumors is discussed. Myasthenia gravis (MG) is the most frequent and significant paraneoplastic disorder in thymoma patients. Hence, the main focus is on autoimmunity against the acetylcholine receptor striational muscle antigens, the ryanodine receptor, and neuronal structures. To shed light on pathogenetic mechanisms, MG is compared with other paraneoplastic syndromes such as acquired neuromyotonia or Stiff-Man syndrome and rippling muscle disease, which are sometimes associated with thymic epithelial tumors.

In the fourth and fifth part of the volume, the controversial fields of surgery and the management of thymectomized patients are presented. Both minimally invasive strategies and conventional thoracotomy with extended thymomectomy are compared and the role of radiotherapy and chemotherapy is discussed. Although prospective randomized studies are still missing, former retrospective trials provide the basis for the proposal of an adjuvant therapy strategy to be applied after surgery depending on the clinical stage and histology of the tumor.

This volume summarizes the results of the First Conference on Biological and Clinical Aspects of Thymic Epithelial Tumors, held April 14–18, 1996, in Würzburg, Germany. It was the first interdisciplinary meeting on this subject, bringing together leading scientists and clinicians from all over the world.

The organizers of this conference—Klaus Toyka, Thomas Kirchner, Hartmut Wekerle, and ourselves—are particularly grateful to the Deutsche Forschungsgemeinschaft and the sponsors for their financial support and wish to thank the participants of the conference for their stimulating contributions. Finally, the excellent secretarial and organizational support of Mrs. B. Goebel is gratefully acknowledged.

Alexander Marx
Hans Konrad Müller-Hermelink

CONTENTS

Part I. Histological and Immunological Characterization of Thymic Epithelial Tumors and Their Differential Diagnoses

Part III. Paraneoplastic Autoimmunity

Part V. Management of Thymectomized Patients

1

CLASSIFICATION OF THYMIC EPITHELIAL NEOPLASMS

Nancy Lee Harris*

Department of Pathology
Massachusetts General Hospital
Harvard Medical School
Boston, Massachusetts

Thymomas are tumors of thymic epithelial cells, with a variable admixture of lymphocytes. Traditional classifications have stratified thymomas by the relative proportions of lymphocytes and epithelial cells, with or without taking into account the shape of the epithelial cells (polygonal or spindle cell) (Table 1) (1–6). There are several difficulties with this approach. First, it attempts to be quantitative, yet it is in fact subjective. Second, the proportion of lymphocytes and epithelial cells often varies from one area to another in the same tumor. Finally, although some studies using these methods have shown that "epithelial-rich" tumors are more aggressive; all observers have agreed that only stage truly predicts outcome for patients with thymoma (Table 2) (7, 8, 5). Based on this experience, Levine and Rosai (4) proposed that thymomas not be classified at all based on histologic criteria, but simply stratified according to invasiveness as benign (noninvasive) and malignant (invasive). The rare cytologically malignant neoplasms of thymic origin were designated, thymic carcinomas (Table 3) (9–12).

Although this approach is eminently practical, it has two problems. First, assessment of invasion can be difficult, even in completely resected tumors, because of the lack of a true capsule in the thymus, and because of the lobulated nature of many thymomas; it is not possible at all on biopsy specimens. Second, there is a natural impulse for pathologists to classify tumors based on some morphologic principle, particularly when there is such a great spectrum of morphology and clinical behavior as there is in thymomas. In principle, tumors should be classified according to their suspected tissue of origin (histogenetic classification). The terminology used should reflect: 1. Morphology: what it looks like; 2. Histogenesis: what tissue or cell it comes from; and 3. Biology: how it will behave. Since terminology can rarely be absolutely precise, each term must be clearly defined.

* Address correspondence to Nancy Lee Harris, M.D., Department of Pathology, Warren 2, Massachusetts General Hospital, 32 Fruit Street, Boston MA 02114, USA.

Epithelial Tumors of the Thymus, edited by Marx and Müller-Hermelink.
Plenum Press, New York, 1997

Table 1. Thymic epithelial tumors: classification by % lymphoid and epithelial cells

Type	Definition
Spindle cell	>66% fusiform epithelial cells
Lymphocytic	>66% lymphs, <33% epithelial cells
Mixed	33–66% of each cell type
Epithelial	>66% polygonal epithelial cells, <33% lymphs
Thymic carcinoma	Marked atypia, necrosis, mitoses

(Lewis et al (5))

In 1985, Muller-Hermelink and his colleagues took a fresh look at the problem of thymoma classification, using insights gained from the study of the normal thymus, and proposed a histogenetic classification of thymomas, based on the morphologic resemblance of the neoplastic tissue to normal thymic compartments (13). They recognized four tumor types: cortical, predominantly cortical, medullary, and mixed (medullary and predominantly cortical); in a later publication, they recognized a subset of the cortical group with more cytologic atypia and fewer lymphocytes, which they designated well-differentiated thymic carcinoma (WDTC) (Tables 4 and 5) (14). Studies on small numbers of patients using this approach showed that the classification correlated with invasive behavior, with medullary tumors showing the least likelihood of invasion and the well-differentated thymic carcinoma the greatest invasive potential. Subsequent studies from Muller-Hermelink and others have confirmed this observation, and further demonstrated that the vast majority of relapses and death from thymoma occur in patients with either cortical thymoma or well-differentiated thymic carcinoma (15–21). Although stage remains the single most important predictor of outcome, the histologic subtype now provides important ancillary prognostic information that may permit refinement of treatment for some patients.

In studies of 122 patients with thymoma at the Massachusetts General Hospital (20–22), we reached the following conclusions. 1. The Muller-Hermelink classification can be applied to most thymic epithelial tumors. 2. Histologic subtype correlates with invasion, and is an independent predictor of outcome (Tables 6–8). 3. WDTC is an important clinicopathologic entity not previously recognized, which accounts for the majority of relapses and deaths from thymic epithelial tumors. On biopsy specimens, histologic type may be useful in guiding extent of surgery, preoperative radiation therapy, etc. Within stage II and III thymomas, histology may help in determining need for adjuvant therapy: adjuvant therapy is likely not needed for invasive medullary or mixed thymoma, but is needed for cortical thymoma and WDTC, probably regardless of extent of invasion. 4. Myasthenia gravis is associated with all types, but is most common with cortical thy-

Table 2. Thymoma: classification by % lymphocytes and epithelial cells - factors predicting outcome

Death ($p \leq 0.05$)	Recurrence ($p \leq 0.05$)
Invasion	Invasion
Size	Size
Epithelial (non-spindle)	Atypia
Multivariate analysis:	
Invasion only	

(Lewis, et al (5))

Table 3. Classification of thymomas: benign and malignant

Benign thymoma (noninvasive)
Malignant thymoma (invasive)
1. With no or minimal cytologic atypia
Locally invasive (usual)
Metastatic (rare)
2. Cytologically malignant (thymic carcinoma)
Squamous cell
Lymphoepithelioma-like
Clear cell
Sarcomatoid
Undifferentiated

(Levine and Rosai (4))

moma, and myasthenia gravis is no longer associated with a worse prognosis in thymoma. 5. The immunophenotype of the epithelial cells does not distinguish between subtypes of thymoma; this is likely due to the fact that the antigens studied may not be specific for cell types. However, the immunophenotype of the lymphoid cells does correlate with the histologic subtype in the Muller-Hermelink classification, suggesting a functional capacity of the tumor cells corresponding to normal epithelium. 6. In our studies, proliferation index (PI) as judged by Ki-67 and PCNA staining correlated with histologic type and stage, but there was too much overlap to be useful in subclassification; we were unable to assess any correlation of PI with outcome, because of small numbers of cases (Table 9). Based on our experience with this classification, we proposed some modifications to the original terminology of Kirchner and Muller-Hermelink (Table 10).

Surprisingly, given its ease of application and clinical utility, the histogenetic classification of thymoma has come under strong criticism from a number of authorities. The major criticisms are that it is: 1. unnecessary, since its categories are equivalent to earlier classifications, and it shows no better correlation with clinical features; 2. unproven, since the relationship of neoplastic to normal epithelial cells is based on morphology alone; and 3. irresponsible, since the term,WDTC may cause confusion with other thymic carcinomas, and the borderline to between WDTC and cortical thymoma is poorly defined and may not be sharp. As seen in Table 11, the categories of the Muller-Hermelink classification are not identical to those of the most commonly used prior classificaton. Furthermore, the authors of this classification freely acknowledged the lack of reproducibility of its categories and its relative insensitvity as a predictor of outcome (5). In practice, the histogenetic classification "cleans up" the categories of spindle cell and epithelial thymoma, by creating homogeneous categories of medullary thymoma and well-differentiated thymic

Table 4. Histogenetic classification of thymic epithelial tumors

Thymoma
Medullary
Mixed
Predominantly cortical
Cortical
Well-differentiated thymic carcinoma
High-grade thymic carcinomas

(Kirchner et al (14))

Table 5. Thymoma histogenetic classification: definitions

Type	Features
Medullary	Small, oval to spindle cells, no atypia, rare mitosis, few lymphocytes, no keratinization
Predominantly cortical	Organoid, lobular, resembles normal cortex with medullary differentiation and Hassal's corpuscles
Mixed	Distinct areas of medullary and predominantly cortical
Cortical	Large, plump epithelial cells with nucleoli; fewer lymphocytes than PC, lobular architecture
Well-differentiated CA	Irregular lobules, invasive growth, fewer lymphocytes, smaller epithelial cells with nuclear grooves, irregular nuclear membranes, distinct cytoplasmic borders, mitoses, focal keratinization

carcinoma. These are in fact the two most important prognostic groups, since the former has the best and the latter the worst prognosis. In addition, it "makes sense" of the morphologic heterogeneity of the former mixed and lymphocytic categories, by sorting them into organoid (predominantly cortical), composite (mixed medullary and organoid), and cortical types, all of which can be readily recognized by morphologic criteria after appropriate training. The prognostic significance of subclassification is less clear for these groups, but may become evident in larger series of patients or if new therapies become available. Even for categories without major differences in biological behavior, the establishment of well-defined morphologic categories increases the ability of pathologists to recognize the tumor as thymoma, and provides a basis for further studies of biological behavior and new therapies. Many published studies have now shown that overall the Muller-Hermelink classification is a better predictor of outcome than previous classifications (23, 15–21). Stage is still an important determinant of outcome, but invasiveness can now be predicted by histology.

The second criticism, that the relationship of the tumor subtypes to normal epithelium is unproven, is also not entirely correct (24). The vast majority of tumor classifications are based purely on a morphologic resemblance of tumor cells to normal tissues and the location of the tumor in a particular organ, not on any more sophisticated "proof," which in most cases is not available. One might as well say we cannot use the terms "ductal" or "lobular" carcinoma of the breast, or "osteo-" or "chondro-" sarcoma of bone, without "proof" of identity over and above morphology. The cells of thymomas do in fact

Table 6. Histologic classification of thymic epithelial tumors: 122 cases from Massachusetts General Hospital

		Stage			
Histology	Cases	1	2	3	4
Medullary	7%	62%	38%	0	0
Mixed	28%	72%	28%	0	0
Organoid	16%	60%	30%	10%	0
Cortical	18%	48%	33%	19%	0
WDTC	26%	0	21%	65%	14%
Hi Grade Ca	2%	0	0	100%	0
Unclass	3%	50%	25%	25%	0

(Quintanilla et al (20))

Table 7. Thymoma: correlation of size with histologic type

Subtype	Size range(cm)	Median size
Medullary	4–10	6.8
Composite	1–12	7.2
Organoid	4–28	10.1
Cortical	1–9	6.4
WDTC	5–13	8.3

(p=NS)

resemble the normal medullary or cortical epithelium, and the abundance, morphology, and immunophenotype of the lymphoid component mirrors that expected from the morphology of the epithelial cells (20). The fact that there are so far no antigenic or molecular markers for cortical or medullary thymic epithelium does not invalidate the morphologic classification, it simply means that, for now, we must rely on morphology, knowing that it has pitfalls. When specific markers become available, the classification can be refined or revised based on the new data.

Finally, the most severe criticisms of the classification relate to the term, well-differentiated thymic carcinoma (WDTC). The term, thymic carcinoma, has been used for highly malignant tumors without an organotypic pattern: squamous cell, lymphoepithelioma-like, small cell, and other types, while the tumor now called WDTC has in the past been called thymoma (25, 26). There is concern that this change in terminology could result in confusion among both pathologists and clinicians, and could lead to overtreatment of some patients with WDTC. In addition, the borderline to cortical thymoma is not clearly defined, and some cases may show both patterns in varying quantities. Both the association with cortical thymoma and the immunophenotype of the lymphoid cells in WDTC indicate a closer relationship of this tumor to thymoma than to the other tumors that have been called thymic carcinoma. Other terms could be proposed for this tumor, such as polygonal cell thymoma, atypical cortical thymoma, atypical aggressive thymoma, etc, which might convey the distinctive morphology and the aggressive behavior, while avoiding potential confusion with higher grade tumors.

However, there is no doubt that WDTC is a distinct clinicopathologic entity. In terms of its pathologic features, it is an organotypic tumor, morphologically recognizable as thymic in origin, often associated with cortical thymoma. Yet it has morphologic fea-

Table 8. Thymoma at MGH: factors predicting outcome

Freedom from relapse:
Stage (P=0.0001; hazard 5.36)
Histology (P=0.0019; hazard 8.01)
Both significant by multivariate analysis
WDTC: 59% at 5 years; 45% at 10 years
Others: 100% at 5 and 10 years
Overall survival:
Stage (P=0.0001)
Histology (P=0.0001)
WDTC: 80% at 5 years; 54% at 10 years
Others: 100% at 5 and 10 years

(Quintanilla et al (21))

Table 9. Thymoma: proliferation index and stage

Stage	# Cases	PCNA	Ki-67
I	21	3.1 (0.2–7.7)	1.5 (0.1–3.7)
II	23	4.3 (0.3–11.4)	1.6 (0.2–3.7)
III	13	6.3 (1.1–16.9)	2.9 (0.7–7.8)
IV	3	11.1 (4.7–15.1)	6.9 (2.6–10.9)

(Yang, et al (22))

tures of low-grade malignancy, including mild but definite cytologic atypia, local invasion, a relatively low proliferation fraction that is nonetheless higher than other thymomas. It also has clinical features of a low-grade carcinoma, with a propensity for local recurrence without distant metastasis. In the MGH study, all cases were invasive, compared with only 40–50% of organoid and cortical thymomas; 65% were in Stage III at diagnosis, compared with only 10–20% of organoid and cortical thymomas, and they had a relapse rate of 40% at 5 years and 60% at ten years and a mortality of 20% and 45% at 5 and 10 years, compared with virtually no relapses or deaths in other categories. Finally, even adjuvant radiation therapy in this uncontrolled study did not appear to affect the outcome in patients with WDTC (21).

Thus, the rationale for keeping the term, WDTC, is both pathological and clinical. For the pathologist, there may in fact be a continuum beween WDTC other types of thymic carcinoma, particularly the more common squamous cell and lymphoepithelioma-like types. There are rare cases that have borderline morphology, and occasional cases in which these higher grade thymic carcinomas are associated with thymoma (12). These data suggest that even high grade thymic carcinomas may be related to thymomas. Other tumor classifications include different tumor grades and combined patterns; the terms well, moderately, and poorly-differentiated can be used to denote the various grades of carcinoma, and the coexistence of different types or grades (eg cortical thymoma and WDTC) can be noted in the diagnosis. For the clinician, it is important to remember that, as rare as thymoma is, the moderately and poorly-differentiated thymic carcinomas are even more rare, and most surgeons and oncologists will never see one. Therefore, most of the aggressive thymic tumors that most clinicans will encounter are WDTC. Since WDTC may need more aggressive therapy than is currently used for thymoma, recognizing it as a form of carcinoma may provide a useful stimulus for clinicians to develop new therapies.

In summary, the following arguments are proposed for adopting the histogenetic classification of thymoma. Most tumor classifications are based on a postulated relationship to normal cell types, usually based on morphologic criteria alone. Both morphology and functional data (lymphocyte phenotype) suggest a relationsip between neoplastic and

Table 10. Modified histogenetic classification of thymic epithelial tumors

Medullary thymoma
Composite thymoma (medullary/organoid)
Organoid thymoma
Cortical thymoma
Well-differentiated thymic carcinoma
Moderately-differentiated thymic carcinoma (squamous cell)
Poorly-differentiated thymic carcinoma (lymphoepithelioma-like)

Table 11. Thymoma classifications: comparison of terms

Histogenetic (modified)	Lewis et al (5)
Medullary thymoma	Spindle cell (most) Epithelial (rare)
Organoid	Lymphocytic (most) Mixed (many)
Composite	Mixed
Cortical thymoma	Lymphocytic (many) Mixed (many) Epithelial (rare)
WDTC	Epithelial (most) Mixed (many) Spindle cell (rare)

normal thymic epithelial cell types. Even if unproven, the histogenetic approach is useful to pathologists in conceptualizing and organizing morphologic features in diagnosis, and both the concept and the terminology can be modified if new data either confirm or refute the morphologic assumptions. This classification has been shown to be usable by pathologists at a number of centers, and has clear predictive value for clinical behavior.

A consensus is needed among pathologists on a thymoma classification, if the pathologists wish to be taken seriously by their clinical colleagues. Pathologists interested in these tumors should reach a consensus on 1. the categories of thymic epithelial neoplasms that can be recognized with available techniques and that should be diagnosed; 2. the morphologic definitions and criteria for diagnosis, and 3. terminology (compromise or equivalents). Future directions for investigation should include: defining the borderline between cortical thymoma and WDTC; defining the borderline between organoid and composite thymoma; defining the sampling requirements for histologic subclassification of heterogeneous tumors; evaluation of reproducibility of the classification among pathologist; determining the existence of a medullary type of thymic carcinoma; the clinical relevance of proliferation index; finding biological markers for thymic epithelial cells; and investigating the molecular genetics of the transition from cortical thymoma to WDTC and from WDTC to higher grade thymic carcinomas. The histogenetic classification of Muller-Hermelink and associates should be recognized for what it is: a major conceptual advance in the understanding of thymomas, and a basis for further study of these rare but fascinating tumors.

REFERENCES

1. Lattes R. Thymoma and other tumors of the thymus. An analysis of 107 cases. Cancer 1962; 15:1224–1260.
2. Bernatz PE, Khonsari S, Harrison EG Jr, Taylor WF. Thymoma: Factors influencing prognosis. Surg Clin North Am 1973; 53:885–892.
3. Rosai J, Levine GD. Tumors of the thymus. Atlas of tumor pathology. 2nd series, Fasc 13. Pathology AFIo, ed. Washington, DC.: 1976.
4. Levine GD, Rosai J. Thymic hyperplasia and neoplasia: a review of current concepts. Hum Pathol 1978; 9:495–515.
5. Lewis JE, Wick MR, Scheithauer BW, Bernatz PE, Taylor WF. Thymoma. A clinicopathologic review. Cancer 1987; 60:2727–2743.

6. Rosai J. The pathology of thymic neoplasia. In: Berard C, Dorfman RF, Kaufman N ed. Malignant lymphoma. Baltimore: Williams & Wilkins, 1987. 161–183.
7. Salyer WR, Eggleston JC. Thymoma: A clincal and pathological study of 65 cases. Cancer 1976; 37:229–249.
8. Masaoka A, Monden Y, Nakahara K, Tanioka T. Follow-up study of thymomas with special reference to their clinical stages. Cancer 1981; 48:2485–2492.
9. Shimosato Y, Kameya T, Nagal K, Suemasu K. Squamous cell carcinoma of the thymus. An analysis of eight cases. Am J Surg Pathol 1977; 1:109–121.
10. Snover DC, Levine GD, Rosai J. Thymic carcinoma. Five distinctive histological variants. Am J Surg Pathol 1982; 6:451–470.
11. Wick MR, Weiland LH, Scheithauer BW, Bernatz PE. Primary thymic carcinomas. Am J Surg Pathol 1982; 6:613–630.
12. Morinaga S, Sato Y, Shimosato Y, Sinkai T, Tsychiya R. Multiple thymic squamous cell carcinomas associated with mixed type thymoma. Am J Surg Pathol 1987; 11:982–983.
13. Marino M, Müller-Hermelink HK. Thymoma and Thymic carcinoma. Relation of thymoma epithelial cells to the cortical and medullary differentiation of thymus. Virchows Arch [Pathol Anat] 1985; 407:119–149.
14. Kirchner T, Müller-Hermelink HK. New Approaches to the diagnosis of thymic epithelial tumors. Prog Surg Pathol 1989; 10:167–189.
15. Pescarmona E, Rendina EA, Venuta F, D'Arcangelo E, Pagani M, Ricci C, et al. Analysis of prognostic factors and clinicopathological staging of thymoma. Ann Thorac Surg 1990; 50:534–538.
16. Pescarmona E, Rendina EA, Venuta F, Ricci C, Ruco LP, Baroni CD. The prognostic implication of thymoma histologic subtype. A study of 80 consecutive cases. Am J Clin Pathol 1990; 93:190–195.
17. Kirchner T, Schalke B, Buchwald J, Ritter M, Marx A, Müller-Hermelink HK. Well-differentiated thymic carcinoma. An organotypical low-grade carcinoma with relationship to cortical thymoma. Am J Surg Pathol 1992; 16:1153–1169.
18. Pescarmona E, Rosati S, Rendina EA, Venuta F, Baroni CD. Well-differentiated thymic carcinoma: a clinico-pathological study. Virchows Archiv [Pathol Anat] 1992; 420:179–183.
19. Kuo, TT, Lo, SK. Thymoma: A study of the pathologic classification of 71 cases with evaluation of the Muller-Hermelink system. Human Pathol 1993; 24:766–771.
20. Quintanilla-Martinez L, Müller-Hermelink HK, Wilkins EW Jr, Ferry JA, NL, H. Thymoma: Morphologic subclassification correlates with invasiveness and immunohistologic features. A study of 122 cases.. Hum Pathol 1993; 24:958–69.
21. Quintanilla-Martinez, L, Wilkins, E, Choi, N, Efird, J, Hug, E, Harris, N. Thymoma: histologic classification predicts clinical behavior. Cancer 1994; 74:606–617.
22. Yang, W-I, Efird, J, Quintanilla-Martinez, L, Choi, N, Harris, NL. Cell kinetic study of thymic epithelial tumors using PCNA (PC10 and Ki-67 (MIB1) antibodies. Hum Pathol 1995;
23. Ricci C, Rendina EA, Pescarmona EO, Venuta F, Di Tolla R, Ruco LP, et al. Correlations between histological type, clinical behaviour, and prognosis in thymoma. Thorax 1989; 44:455–460.
24. Kornstein MJ, Curran WJ, Turrisi III AT, Brooks JJ. Cortical versus medullary thymomas: a useful morphologic distinction? Hum Pathol 1988; 19:1335–1339.
25. Wick MR. Assessing the prognosis of thymomas. Ann Thorac Surg 1990; 50:521–522.
26. Kornstein MJ. Controversies regarding the pathology of thymomas. Pathol Ann 1992; 1–15.

2

THYMIC CARCINOMA*

Yukio Shimosato

Department of Pathology
Keio University School of Medicine
Shinanomachi, Shinjukuku, Tokyo 160, Japan

1. INTRODUCTION

Existence of thymic carcinoma as an entity of mediastinal tumors has been accepted for the last 20 years or so, until when diagnosis of thymic carcinoma was almost always questioned for the presence of a primary tumor elsewhere. In fact AFIPfascicle of the second series published in 1976 by Rosa and Levine only briefly mentioned about thymic squamous cell carcinoma (1). Two years later, Levine and Rosai classified malignant thymoma into categories 1 and 2. The catagory 1 is invasive thymoma and category 2 indicated tumors showing structural and cellular atypia, which can be interpreted as carcinoma even in organs other than the thymus (2) (Table 1). A variety of subclassifications of thymic carcinoma have been proposed since then (3–5).

In 1991, Suster and Rosa after analysis of 60 cases of thymic carcinoma, divided them into low grade and high grade histology (6) (Table 2). However, as cases accumulated, some low grade tumors were found to behave as a high grade tumor, necessitating resubclassfication of the tumors. We, after review of literature and from our own experience, proposed our classification as shown in Table 3 (7). Of course, well differentiated (organotypical) thymic carcinoma of Muller-Hermelink et al (8) has been excluded from thymic carcinoma, since we consider it as atypical thymoma with aggressive behavior.

Controversies exist surrounding classification of non-invasive and invasive thymomas, but not that of thymic carcinoma. This is probably due to much lower incidence of thymic carcinoma and only a few cases were experienced by most pathologists. I myself as other pathologists have not yet experienced all the subtypes of thymic carcinoma. In this session, histological and biological characteristics of each subtype, differential diagnosis and TNM staging system of thymic carcinoma will be dealt with.

* (malignant thymoma, category 2 of Levine and Rosai; "nonorganotypical thymic carcinoma")

Epithelial Tumors of the Thymus, edited by Marx and Müller-Hermelink.
Plenum Press, New York, 1997

Table 1. Proposed classification (Levine and Rosai (1978))

Thymoma
circumscribed
malignant:
Type I (invasive thymoma with no or minimal atypia)
Type II (cytologically malignant = thymic carcinoma)
squamous cell carcinoma
lymphoepithelioma-like carcinoma
clear cell carcinoma
arcomatoid carcinoma
undifferentiated carcinoma

2. HISTOLOGICAL AND BIOLOGICAL CHARACTERISTICS

Squamous Cell Carcinoma. Histological criteria of squamous cell carcinoma is the same as that in other organs. It is divided into well, moderately and poorly differentiated squamous cell carcinoma. Grossly, it is non-encapsulated, and possesses nodular or scalloped borders with scanty necrosis if any and a tendency to become sclerotic in the central portion in well differential form, and with increased amount of coagulation necrosis in moderately to poorly differential form. Histologically, the central portion of the tumor often shows broad and sclerotic or hyalinized stroma with rare inflammatory cell response, and individual tumor cell nuclei are vesicular with prominent nucleoli. Hyaline stroma and vesicular nuclei are characteristic and important findings to exclude the possibility of a primary tumor in the lung (9). Well differentiated squamous cell carcinoma corresponds to low grade well differentiated carcinoma of Suster and Rosai (6). However, moderately to poorly differentiated squamous cell carcinoma should be placed in the high grade tumor group.

In squamous cell carcinoma, there are a few cases, histology of which suggests progression from thymoma to carcinoma. In one case we experirenced, there were multiple tumors in the thymus, pleura and lymph nodes, among which two largest tumors were squamous cell carcinoma, two showed trasition between thymoma and carcinoma and remainder contained only thymoma (10). *Adenosquamous carcinoma*: Well differentiated squamous cell carcinoma occasionally shows microcystic changes in tumor cell nests, and cystic spaces and their lining tumor cells contain Alcian blue-PAS positive mucin and im-

Table 2. Proposed classification (Suster and Rosai (1991))

Thymic carcinoma
low grade histology
well-differentiated (keratinizing) squamous cell carcinoma
well-differentiated mucoepidermoid carcinoma
basaloid carcinoma
high grade histology
lymphoepithelioma-like carcinoma
small cell/neuroendocrine carcinoma
undifferentiatedlanaplastic carcinoma
sarcomatoid carcinoma
clear cell carcinoma

Table 3. Proposed classification (Shimosato et al.)

Thymic carcinoma
squamous cell carcinoma (well, moderately, and poorly differentiated)
basaloid carcinoma
mucoepidermoid carcinoma
adenosquamous carcinoma
adenocarcinoma
small cellineuroendocrine carcinoma
lymphoepithelioma-like carcinoma
large cell carcinoma
clear cell carcinoma
sarcomatoid carcinoma

munoreactive secretory component, indicating the presence of glandular epithelial cells (11). Such a carcinoma may be called adenosquamous carcinoma. Prognosis of patients with this kind of tumor is often excellent.

Mucoepidermoid carcinoma, which was classified as a low grade tumor, is considered to be a variety of adenocarcinoma and similar to the tumor of the same name occuring in the salivary gland and bronchial gland. Recently, mucoepidermoid carcinomas of high grade malignancy have been reported (12). *Adenocarcinoma*: Although occurence of adenocarcinoma has not yet been known in the thymus, we experienced papillary adenocarcinoma with psammomatous bodies in a Japanese male, which resembles serous cyst adenocarcinoma of the ovary. This carcinoma (case #5 of Slide Workshop to be held two days later) collided with a small encapsulated thymoma composed of short spindle cells, glandular spaces and trabecular or hemangiopercytomatous features, classified as medullary thymoma by Muller-Hermelink et al. Carcinoembryonic antigen was positive in carcinoma but negative in thymoma. It invaded the lung but the patient surviving without recurrence for two years postoperatively (7). A similar case was submitted from other institution for consultation and two other cases have been seen by Dr. J. Rosai, one of which was said to have coexisted with thymoma (personal communication).

Basaloid Carcinoma. It is considered to be of low grade malignancy. It is encapsulated at least in parts, and associated with a thymic cyst in our case. Histologically, it is similar to basal cell carcinoma of the skin with solid tumor cell nests consisting of small deeply stained cells arranged haphazardly in the center and palisading at the periphery of cell nests. One case we experienced resembled grade 2 transitional cell carcinoma of the urinary bladder, in which perivascular spaces were found.

Lymphoepithelioma-like Carcinoma. It is quite similar to tumors of the same name seen in the nasopharynx. This is an highly malignant tumor. Our case was associated with EB virus, the primary tumor being positive for EBER *in situ* hybridization and DNA extracted from hepatic metastasis containing terminal repeats of EB virus DNA by southern blot analysis. No other thymic carcinoma nor thymoma so far examined by us were associated with EB virus (13).

Small Cell (Neuroendocrine) Carcinoma. It is similar to oat cell carcinoma of th lung with or without rosettes. In our consultation cases, there were glandular structures in addition to rosettes in one case, and it was a combined small cell and large cell carcinoma in another. Small cell carcinoma has been insufficiently studied so far immunohistochemically and electronmicroscopically, because of rarity of the lesion. In our cases synaptophysin was weakly positive but chromogranin A was negative. The prognosis of patients with thymic small cell carcinoma is said to be better than that of the lung.

Large Cell Carcinoma. Carcinoma without definite glandular cells or squamous features can be designated as large cell carcinoma as in the lung. A large majority of such carcinomas in the thymus appears to be of poorly differentiated squamous cell type. Clear cell carcioma is considered to be a variety of large cell carcinoma, both of which are high grade tumor.

Sarcomatoid Carcinoma. It is a very rare tumor of the thymus consisting of epithelial component, very often squamous in nature, and spindle cell mesenchymal components. Sarcomatoid carcinoma with rhabdomyosarcomatous component has been reported (3). This is of course a high grade tumor.

3. DIFFERENTIAL DIAGNOSIS

The presence of tumors in a gray zone with regard to malignancy is noted in many organs, and the thymus is not an exception. Differentiation between squamous cell carcinoma and atypical thymoma (well differentiated organotypical thymic carcinoma of Muller-Hermelink et al) may at times be difficult. However, the latter possesses features characteristics of thymoma such as perivascular spaces, lymphoid infiltrates, which contain CD1a positive immature cortical lymphocytes, and complication with myasthenia gravis, since it retains the function of the thymus. In this sense, thymoma is considered to be a functioning tumor but thymic carcinoma is not. Areas with epidermoid features in atypical thymoma possess also characteristic nuclear findings such as irregular outline with groving and often inconspicuous nucleoli.

Measurement of mean nuclear DNA contents may also be helpful in differential diagnosis of thymoma and thymic carcinoma, since a large majority of carcinoma contain aneuploid stem cell lines but rarely so in thymoma. Differential diagnoses also include metastatic carcinoma to the thymus, and malignant anterior mediastinal tumors such as carcinoid tumors, diffuse large cell lymphoma with sclerosis, and malignant germ cell tumors such as embryonal carcinoma, carcinoma arising in immature teratoma.

4. PROGNOSIS

Important factors affecting prognosis of patients are histology of the tumor and stage of the disease. Although in our cases rare high grade tumors such as small cell carcinoma, clear cell carcinoma and sarcomatoid carcinoma were not included in this study, prognosis of patients with complete surgical removal of tumors was excellent but that with incomplete removal was very poor including low grade well differentiated squamous cell carcinoma (15).

5. STAGING SYSTEM

A staging system for thymoma was reported by Masaoka et al (15), which has been used by some invesitgators. However, stage II should be revised as "microscopic invasion *not into but through* the capsule, since pathologists do not consider capsule invasion unless tumors invade through the capsule. Yamakawa, a coworker of Masaoka, recently proposed TNM classification of the thymic tumors and the staging system based on TNM classification (16) (Table 4). Again one should revise the statement in T2. In their staging system, one should note that every tumor with N+ has been placed in stage IVB. This system does not appear to be appropriate for thymic carcinoma and other malignancies of the thymus such as carcinoid tumors. Our experience indicated that thymic tumors confined to within the thymus or some of T3 invasive thymoma but with metastasis limited to anterior mediastinal lymph nodes could be cured by complete surgical removal of tumors followed by postoperative radiotherapy. Therefore, we proposed a different system (Table 5), in which N1 was included in stages II, III and IVa. Comparison of survival curves drawn by those two staging systems suggests superiority of our system (14) but which classification to be adopted must await future investigation.

Addendum

Although this is not the subject of my presentation, I should like to mention that spindle cell or medullary thymoma, particularly that with gland-like or rosette-like structures or hemangiopericytomatous features, is not a benign tumor. We have experienced three such cases with lung metastasis, although growth is rather slow (7). One illustrative case was a 59 year-old male, who underwent removal of thymoma confined to within the

Table 4. Yamakawa-Masaoka's TNM Classification and Staging (from ref. 5)

T factor
T1: Macroscopically completely encapsulated and microscopically no capsular invasion
T2: Macroscopically adhesion or invasion into surrounding tafly tissue or mediastinal pleura. or microscopic invasion *into* capsule
T3: Invasion into neighboring organs. such as pencardium, great vessels. and lung
T4: Pleural or pericardial dissemination

N factor
N0: No lymph node metastasis
N1: Metastasis to anterior mediastinal lymph nodes
N2: Metastasis to intra-thoracic lymph nodes except anterior mediastinal lymph nodes
N3: Metastasis to extrathoracic lymph nodes

M factor
M0: No hematogenous metastasis
M1: Hematogenous metastasis

Stage			
Stage I	T1	NO	MO
Stage II	T2	NO	MO
Stage III	T3	NO	MO
Stage IVa	T4	NO	MO
Stage IVb	anyT	N1,2 or 3	MO
	anyT	any N	M1

Table 5. Proposed pathological TNM and staging system of thymic epithelial tumors (National Cancer Center Hospital, Tokyo) (from ref. 14)

pT
pTl: Completely encapsulated tumor
pT2: Tumor breaking through capsule, invading thymus or tatty tissue (may be adherent to mediastinal pleura but not invading neighboring organs)
pT3: Tumor breaking through the mediastinal pleura or pericardium, or invading neighboring organs. such as great vessels and lung
pT4: Tumor with pleural or pericardial implantation

pN
pN0: No lymph node metastasis
pNl: Metastasis in anterior mediastinal lymph nodes
pN2: Metastasis in intrathoracic lymph nodes excluding anterior mediastinal lymph nodes
pN3: Metastasis in extrathoracic lymph nodes

pM
M0: No distant organ metastasis
M1: with distant organ metastasis

Pathological stage grouping

Stage I	T1, T2	N0	M0
Stage II	T1, T2	N1	M0
Stage III	T3	N0, N1	M0
Stage IVa	T4	N0, N1	M0
Stage IVb	any T	N2, N3	M0
Stage IVc	any T	any N	M1

thymus in September 1992, and developed lung metastases in April 1995 and liver metastases in October.

REFERENCES

1. Rosai R, Levine GD. Tumors of the thymus, Atlas of Tumor Pathology, Second series, Fascicle 13, Armed Forces Institute of Pathology, Washington, D.C. 1976.
2. Levine GD, Rosai J. Thymic hyperplasia and neoplasia: A review of current concepts. Hum Pathol, 1978; 9:495–515
3. Snover DC, Levine GD, Rosai J. Thymic carcinoma. Five distinctive histological variants. Am J Surg Pathol. 1982; 6: 451–470.
4. Wick, MR, Weiland LH, Scheithauer BW, Bernatz PE. Primary thymic carcinoma, Am J Surg Pathol, 1982; 6: 613–630.
5. Truong LD, Mody DR, Cagle Pt Jackson-York GL, Schwartz MR, Wheeler TM. Thymic carcinoma. A clinicopathologic study of 13 cases. Am J Surg Pathol, 1990; 14:151–166.
6. Suster S, Rosai J. Thymic carcinoma: A clinicopathologic study of 60 cases. Cancer 1991; 67:1025–1032.
7. Shimosato Y Mukai K. Tumors of the mediastinum, Atlas of Tumor Pathology, Third series, Armed Forces Institute of Pathology. Washington. D.C. (in press).
8. Kirchner T, Schalke R, Buchwald J, Ritter M, Marx A, Muller-Hermelink HK. Well-differentiated thymic carcinoma: An organotypical low-grade carcinoma with relationship to cortical thymoma. Am J Surg Pathol 1992;16: 1153–1169.
9. Shimosato Y Kameya T, Nagai K, Suemasu K. Squamous cell carcinoma of the thymus. An analysis of eight cases. Am J Surg Pathol. 1977; 1:109–121.
10. Morinaga S, Sato Y Shimosato y Shinkai T Tsuchiya R. Multiple thymic squamous cell carcinomas associated with mixed type thymoma. Am J Surg Pathol, 1987; 11:982–988.

11. Matsuno Y Mukai K, Noguchi M, Sato Y Shimosato Y Histochemical and immunohistochemical differentiation in thymic carcinoma. Acta Pathol Jpn. 1989; 39: 433–438.
12. Moran AC, Suster S. Mucoepidermoid carcinomas of the thymus. A clinicopathologic study of six cases. Am J Surg Pathol. 1995; 19: 826–834.
13. Matsuno Y Mukai K, Uhara H, Akao I, Furuya S, Sato Y Hirohashi S, Shimosato Y Detection of Epstein-Barr virus DNA in a Japanese Case of lymphoepithelioma-like thymic carcinoma. Jpn J Cancer Res. 1992; 83:127–130.
14. Tsuchiya R, Koga K, Matsuno ;Y Mukai K, Shimosato Y Thymic carcinoma: Proposal for pathological TNM and staging. Pathol Internatl, 1994; 4: 505–512.
15. Masaoka A, Monden Y Nakahara K, Tanioka T. Follow-up study of thymomas with special reference to their clinical stage. Cancer 1981; 48: 2485–2492.
16. Yamakawa Y Masaoka A, Hashimoto T, Niwa H, Mizuno T, Fujii Y, Nakahara K. A tentative tumor-node-metastasis classfication of thymoma, Cancer 1991; 68: 1984–1987.

3

THYMOMA/THYMIC CARCINOMA

A Distinctive, Unusual Morphologic Entity

Cesar A. Moran*†

Department of Pulmonary and Mediastinal Pathology
Armed Forces Insitute of Pathology
Washington, D.C. 20306-6000

ABSTRACT

Primary epithelial neoplasms, namely thymomas, comprise the bulk of epithelial thymic tumors in the anterior mediastinum. However, thymic carcinomas are also well known to occur as primary thymic epithelial tumors. These two neoplasms appear to arise de novo and have been regarded as two entirely separate entities. Nevertheless, in unusual circumstances it is possible to observe the occurrence of these two well known histopathologic patterns in the same tumor. Whether one neoplasm—thymoma—gives rise to another more aggressive tumor—carcinoma—remains an unresolved puzzle. However, it is logical to assume that since the two tumors are observed in continuity, this particular phenomenon may represent a spectrum of lesions that go from the conventional thymoma to another more aggressive neoplasm such as thymic carcinoma. Our experience with such cases highlights the importance of proper sampling when dealing with thymic epithelial neoplasms and the risk of attempting to asses such tumors with a limited biopsy or aspiration cytology specimens.

INTRODUCTION

Thymic epithelial tumors, namely thymomas are neoplasms that are currently under scrutiny regarding their classification and behavior. It has been stated by some authors that morphologic analysis of these tumors correlates well with prognosis while others have

* The opinions herein contained are the private views of the author and are not to be construed as the official views of the department of the Air Force or the Department of Defense.

† Address for correspondence: Cesar A. Moran, M.D., Associate Chairman & Chief Mediastinal Pathology, Dept. Pulmonary & Mediastinal Pathology, Armed Forces Institute of Pathology, Washington, D.C. 20306-6000. Phone: (202) 782-783; fax: (202) 782-5017.

Epithelial Tumors of the Thymus, edited by Marx and Müller-Hermelink.
Plenum Press, New York, 1997

followed a more conventional approach using encapsulation as a predictor of behavior. Whether one classification is better that the other is under study. However, one aspect that is of utmost importance is the fact that a good sampling of epithelial thymic neoplasms must be done. This sampling will be of help not only to properly subclassify any thymoma but also to avoid missing a more aggressive neoplasm, namely thymic carcinoma.

We have been able to examine numerous cases in which a thymoma was in close association with a thymic carcinoma. This latter association, although unusual, has rarely been reported in the literature. This phenomenon may occur more often than has previously been realized. Therefore, it becomes crucial to properly asses thymic epithelial neoplasms.

CLINICAL FEATURES

Clinically, these patients are not any different from other patients in which thymomas are found. The median age in which these tumors are found is in individuals in the sixth decade of life. However, younger or older individual may be affected. We have not found any evidence of sex predilection. The symptomatology presented by these patients is also varied. Some patients may present completely asymptomatic and their tumors are evidenced after a routine radiographic study. On the other hand, some patients may present with symptoms of shortness of breath, chest pain, etc., symptoms more likely related to the size of the anterior mediastinal tumor. Interestingly, a small number of patients may present with myasthenia gravis as an associated condition.

MORPHOLOGIC FEATURES

Gross Features

The gross appearance of these tumors do not allow separation from thymomas. They can reach a large size of more than 15 cm in greatest dimension. The tumors may appear well-encapsulated and well-circumscribed without evidence of invasion into adjacent structures. Some tumors may show at cut surface prominent cystic changes. However, most of the time, they will have a soft, tan, homogeneous, slightly nodular surface. Focal necrosis and hemorrhage may be seen.

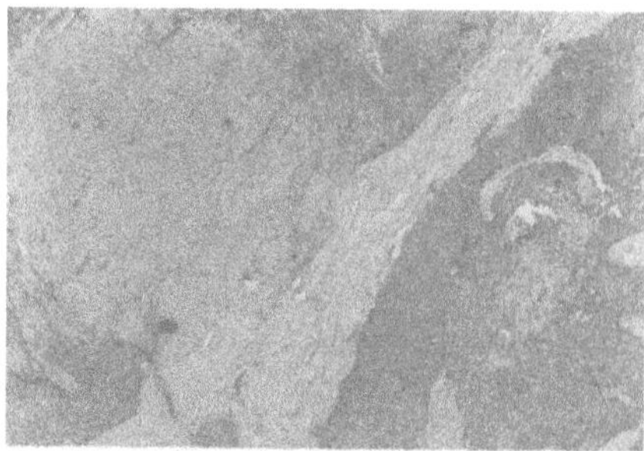

Figure 1. Low power view of a carcinoma with clear cell features arising from a conventional thymoma (epithelial rich thymoma).

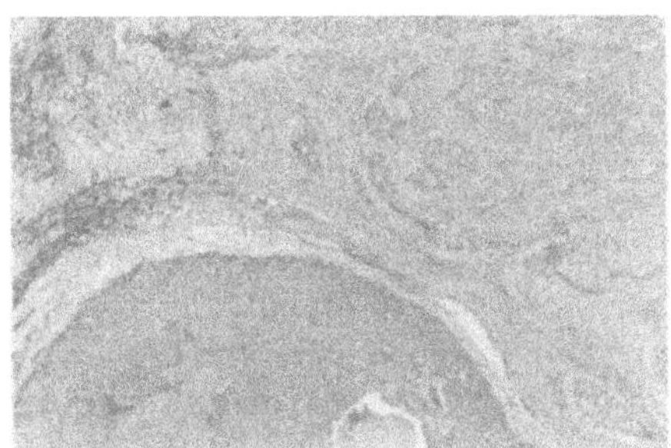

Figure 2. Low power view of a thymic epithelial neoplasm showing features of conventional thymoma and thymic carcinoma.

Histologic Features

The main histopathologic features of these tumors are the presence of a conventional type of thymoma, using any of the existing classifications, and the presence of areas of frank carcinoma. Even though, in our experience, most of the known subtypes of thymoma were observed, it is important to note that some of the conventional areas of thymoma were represented by tumors with histopathologic features of neoplasms considered less aggressive such as the spindle cell thymoma. In many of these cases there were areas of transition between a conventional thymoma and a thymic carcinoma (Figs. 1–3). The carcinomas associated with thymomas include the spectrum of well to poorly differentiated squamous cell carcinomas.

In our experience, we were not able to determine any specific association of a carcinoma with any specific subtype of thymoma, clinical setting, sex or age. Therefore, we consider that these cases represent a possible spectrum of differentiation of thymic epithelial neoplasms.

COMMENT

Thymomas in general are unusual neoplasms that in the last years have been the center of much study. Conventional approach to their classification has been questioned and new approaches towards their classification have been presented. Unfortunately, new modalities have also clouded a clear understanding of these tumors with the logical confusion among pathologists as to their proper assessment. In addition, the use of a relatively new term, such as "well-differentiated thymic carcinoma," have made classification of thymic epithelial neoplasms much more confusing since, for the majority of pathologists, the term "well-differentiated carcinoma" shows features which in the past have been linked to a

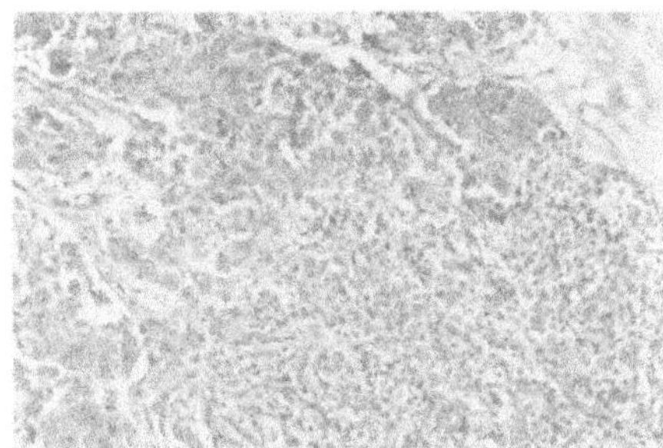

Figure 3. High power view of a transition between conventional thymoma and a thymic carcinoma (well-differentiated squamous cell carcinoma).

conventional thymoma. This latter term remains nebulous for some authors and still awaits a better and clearer definition. We consider that it is possible that such description is perhaps an intermediate step between thymoma and thymic carcinoma and have regarded similar cases under the designation of "atypical thymoma," acknowledging the presence of more cellular atypia. In our view, such a term clearly defines an entity by acknowledging the presence of cytologic atypia while it is not yet the one observed in overtly malignant lesions such as thymic carcinoma.

On the other hand, we have been able to study numerous cases in which mediastinal tumors have shown features of a conventional thymoma and a thymic carcinoma. This latter phenomenon clearly illustrates the issue of a possible continuum in these tumors and raises the issue that these two hitherto separate entities may represent a spectrum of differentiation. In addition, it highlights the issue of predicting behavior of thymomas on morphologic features. We were able to see cases in which the thymoma showed features which have been regarded as non-aggressive histology (spindle cell thymoma). The latter feature in thymomas has been regarded as a feature equated to indolent behavior. We, on the other hand, believe that such assessment may prove risky when dealing with these neoplasms and believe that even if this type of histology is present, a reasonable number of sections must be taken in order to avoid missing a hidden, more aggressive tumor.

In our experience, the behavior followed by these tumors with combine features of thymoma and thymic carcinoma, is mainly related to the degree of differentiation exhibited by the carcinomatous component. Those tumors that show a less differentiated carcinoma have a more guarded prognosis than those with better differentiated carcinomas.

In synthesis, the phenomenon herein described raises the possibility that thymomas and thymic carcinomas merely represent a spectrum of differentiation. On the other hand, it also highlights the notion that lesions that are supposed to be indolent, such as the case of spindle cell thymoma, may be associated with more aggressive neoplasms such as carcinoma, therefore casting some doubts as to the true significance of histologic subtyping in the assessment of behavior for thymomas. We also consider that the term "well-differentiated carcinoma" is still not a well defined term. Features listed under such designation are also observed in thymomas. Therefore, we prefer the term "atypical thymomas," acknowledging the presence of cytologic atypia. This term, in addition, may represent an intermediate step of differentiation between thymoma and thymic carcinoma. Lastly, the generous sampling that must be undertaken to assess thymic epithelial neoplasms can not be overemphasized. This may prove beneficial in the assessment of these lesions in order to avoid missing a hidden more aggressive neoplasm.

REFERENCES

1. Kirchner T, Muller-Hermelink HK: New approaches in the diagnosis of thymic epithelial tumors. Prog Surg Pathol 1989; 10:167–189.
2. Kirchner T, Schalke B, Buchwald J, et al: Well-differentiated thymic carcinoma. An organotypical low-grade carcinoma with relationship to cortical thymoma. Am J Surg Pathol 1992; 16:1153–1169.
3. Kuo T-T, Lo S-K: Thymoma: A study of the pathologic classification of 71 cases with evaluation of the Muller-Hermelink system. Hum Pathol 1993; 24:766–771.
4. Marino M, Muller-Hermelink HK: Thymoma and thymic carcinoma: relation of thymoma epithelial cells to the cortical and medullary differentiation of thymus. Virchows Arch [A] 1985; 407:119–149.
5. Masaoka A, Monden Y, Nakakara T, Tanioka T: Follow-up studies of thymoma with special reference to their clinical stages. Cancer 1981; 48:2485–2492.
6. Moran CA, Suster S: Current status of the histologic classification of thymoma. Int J Surg Pathol 1995; 3:67–72.

7. Morinaga S, Sato Y, Shimosato Y, Sinkai T, Tsuchiya R: Multiple thymic squamous cell carcinomas associated with mixed type thymoma. Am J Surg Pathol 1987; 11:982–988.
8. Pescarmona E, Rendina EA, Venuta F, Ricci C, Baroni CD: Recurrent thymoma: evidence for histological progression. Histopathology 1995; 27:445–449.
9. Shimosato Y: Controversies surrounding the classification of thymoma. Cancer 1994; 74:542–544.
10. Suster S, Moran CA: Primary thymic epithelial neoplasms showing combined features of thymoma and thymic carcinoma: A clinicopathologic study of 22 cases. Am J Surg Pathol 1996 (In press).

4

A CLINICOPATHOLOGICAL STUDY OF THYMOMAS IN SINGAPORE

Ivy Sng and Puay Hoon Tan

Department of Pathology
Singapore General Hospital
Outram Road, Singapore 169601

1. AIMS

The aims of this study are two-fold. Firstly, to study the clinicopathological features of thymic epithelial tumours accessioned in the Department of Pathology of the Singapore General Hospital over a five-year period of 1988–1992, and secondly to assess the predictive utility of the Muller-Hermelink system of classification of thymic epithelial tumours.

Singapore is a small island republic state with a population of three million persons. It is a multiracial country and the ethnic distribution is according to the following proportion: Chinese 77%, Malay 15%, Indian 7% and others 1%. The Department of Pathology of the Singapore General Hospital is the main centre receiving pathological specimens from all government hospitals of the republic. We were therefore able to study thymic epithelial tumours operated on by the cardio-thoracic surgeons of the two major hospitals, the Singapore General Hospital and Tan Tock Seng Hospital in Singapore.

2. MATERIALS AND METHODS

The records of all thymic surgical specimens accessioned at the Department of Pathology over a five year period between 1988 and 1992 (inclusive) were retrieved. There were seventy three cases and the slides of all the cases were available for histological review on haematoxylin and eosin stained slides by both authors. Thirteen cases were diagnosed as non-neoplastic or reactive thymic lesions and were hence not included in the main study. There were thus sixty cases of thymic epithelial tumours, fifty-seven of which were surgical excision specimens, two were fine needle aspiration cytology specimens and one case was a core needle biopsy. The cases were classified into histologic subtypes according to the Muller-Hermelink system. [1,2] and would now be categorised as the organotypic thymic epithelial tumours. These are a separate category from the non-organotypic high grade thymic carcinomas. The presence of lymphoid follicular hyperplasia either

Epithelial Tumors of the Thymus, edited by Marx and Müller-Hermelink.
Plenum Press, New York, 1997

Table 1. Staging system of Masaoka et al.

Stage I	Microscopically completely encapsulated and microscopically no capsular invasion
Stage II	Macroscopic invasion into surrounding fatty tissue or mediastinal pleura, or microscopic invasion into capsule
Stage III	Macroscopic invasion into neighbouring organs i.e. pericardium, great vessels or lung
Stage IVa	Pleural or pericardial dissemination
Stage IVb	Lymphogenous or haematogenous metastasis

within the tumour substance or in adjacent residual non-neoplastic thymic tissue was noted. Relevant clinical data were obtained from the patient's medical records, the Singapore Cancer Registry and the Singapore Registry of Births and Deaths. All the tumours were staged according to the system of Masaoka et al.[3] (Table 1) The presence of myasthenia gravis and patient outcome were studied.

3. RESULTS

3.1. Patient Data

There were 26 males (43%) and 34 females (57%). Forty-nine patients were ethnic Chinese (82%), eight were Malays (13%), one was an Indian (2%) and two were Indonesians (3%). These paralleled roughly the racial distribution of the population of Singapore. The age ranged from 22 to 69 years with a median of 46 years. Seventeen patients (28%) had myasthenia gravis of which there was a female preponderance with 12 females (71%) against 5 males (29%). In twenty three patients the tumours were discovered incidentially on chest radiographs. The presenting symptoms in the others were persistent cough in eight patients, chest pain in eight and palpitation in two. Two patients had signs of superior vena caval obstruction. In the follow-up of disease outcome, information was available in 54 cases. Ten patients (19%) died between 0.5 to 55 months from the time of diagnosis, with a median of six months. Eight patients died from the thymic tumour, one from myasthenia gravis and the other patient from bronchopneumonia.

3.2. Pathological Features

Macroscopic Findings. The tumours ranged in size from 2 cm to 21 cm with a median of 8 cm. The macroscopic appearance was generally that of an encapsulated and lobulated tumour with greyish-tan cut surface.

Microscopic Findings. In 58 cases, the sections from the 57 surgically excised specimens and a core-needle biopsy specimen were studied and subtyped according to the Muller-Hermelink classification. One fine-needle aspirate specimen was also classified when a subsequent biopsy was obtained. The distribution of the histological subtypes is illustrated in Table 2.

Table 2. Type of thymoma versus stage

Type	Stage				
	I	II	III	IV	Total
Cortical	2	7	11	0	20 (33.8%)
Predominantly cortical	1	4	1	0	6 (10.1%)
Medullary	2	0	1	0	3 (5.1%)
Mixed	11	1	0	0	12 (20.3%)
Well differentiated thymic carcinoma	0	2	6	4	12 (20.3%)
Other thymic carcinomas/unclassified	1	0	4	1	6 (10.1%)
Total	17	14	23	5	59 (100%)

Detailed microscopic findings are according to a published report.[4]

4. CLINICOPATHOLOGICAL CORRELATION

4.1. Histological Subtype and Stage of Thymomas

The histological subtype and stage were studied. Table 2 illustrates the distribution of the stage of the various types of thymic epithelial tumours. The largest number, 23 cases, accounting for 38% of the total were in Stage III and these demonstrated gross invasion of neighbouring organs at surgery and this was confirmed histologically. Twelve of the 29 patients where the thymoma was thought to be grossly encapsulated during surgery (clinical stage I) showed microscopic evidence of capsular penetration and this, according to the Masaoka system of staging upgraded them to stage II. These were five cortical, four predominantly cortical and one mixed thymoma and two well differentiated thymic carcinomas.

The percentage distribution of the number of cases within each histological subtype according to the stage was analysed. The medullary and mixed thymomas fared more favourably with the greater proportion of cases being in early stage i.e. stage I. (Fig 1) The only exception was the case of medullary thymoma who presented at surgery in Stage III with lung infiltration and involvement of the superior vena cava, although it was questioned whether the lung involvement was a distinct infiltration or fibrous adhesions with a pushing tumour front. The patient succumbed to the disease 17 months post surgery. Most of the cortical thymomas and well differentiated thymic carcinomas were in Stages III and IV (Fig 2). The association between histological subtype and invasive behaviour as evidenced by the Masaoka staging system was statistically significant using the chi-square test ($p<0.0005$). These findings are in general agreement with other series as that of Quintanilla-Martinez et al [5] and the Asian series of Ho et al [6] and Kuo et al [7].

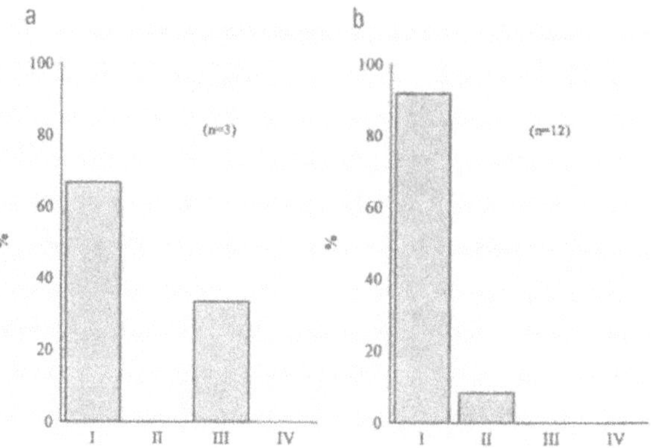

Figure 1. Stage of thyoma: (a) medullary; (b) mixed.

4.2. Myasthenia Gravis

Seventeen patients had myasthenia gravis. Of these eleven (64%) had cortical thymomas, two (12%) predominantly cortical thymoma, one (6%) mixed thymoma and three (18%) well differentiated thymic carcinoma. There was significant correlation between the histological subtype and the occurrence of myasthenia gravis ($p<0.05$). There was no correlation between myasthenia gravis and the stage of the thymoma ($p>0.05$). The presence of lymphoid follicular hyperplasia in 12 of 17 cases (71%) of thymomas from patients with myasthenia gravis substantiates the observation of others that thymuses in the vicinity of myasthenia gravis associated thymomas demonstrate germinal centre formation more frequently than thymuses from non-myasthenic controls [5,8,9].

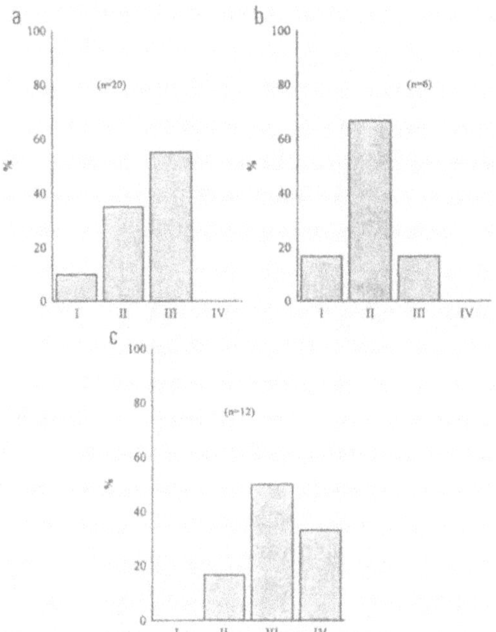

Figure 2. Stage of thyoma: (a) cortical; (b) predominantly cortical; (c) well-differentiated thymic carcinoma.

4.3. High Grade Thymic Carcinomas

There were five (8%) cases of thymic carcinoma which were distinguished from the other thymic epithelial tumours by clear-cut cytologic atypia and lack of organoid features. Two were squamous cell carcinomas, and one each of an undifferentiated carcinoma, clear cell carcinoma and a neuroendocrine carcinoma. They were devoid of organoid features, not associated with myasthenia gravis and except for one case, all were in advanced stage of Stage III or IV. These tumours would be classified as category II malignant thymoma.

5. CONCLUSION

Of the sixty cases of thymic epithelial tumours studied, we were able to classify them into sub-types according to the Muller-Hermelink classification. There was occasional difficulty in distinguishing cortical thymoma and well differentiated thymic carcinoma, however this has been addressed by others who have demonstrated some sharing of histological and clinical features in both these subtypes [6,10.] Invasive behaviour as evidenced by advanced stages is seen in cortical thymomas, predominantly cortical thymomas, well-differentiated thymic carcinomas and other high grade carcinomas. The association between thymoma and myasthenia gravis was seen in the subtypes of cortical and predominantly cortical thymomas and well-differentiated thymic carcinomas.

6. ACKNOWLEDGMENTS

We would like to express our appreciation to our surgical colleagues of Singapore General Hospital and Tan Tock Seng Hospital for providing the material, to Professor Muller-Hermelink for reviewing some of the cases, to Miss S Fook-Chong for the statistical analysis and to Dr K L Chuah and Mdm G Ng for assistance in graphic preparations and typing.

REFERENCES

1. Muller-Hermelink HK, Marino M, Palestro G. Pathology of thymic epithelial tumour. In The Human Thymus, Histopathology and Pathology. Ed. Muller-Hermelink. Berlin: Springer Verlag, 1986: 207–268.
2. Kirchner T, Muller-Hermelink HK. New approaches to the diagnosis of thymic epithelial tumours Progress in Surg. Pathol. 1989: 10; 167–189.
3. Masaoka A, Monden Y, Nakahara K, Tanioka T. Follow-up study of thymomas with special reference to their clinical stages. Cancer 1981: 48; 2485–2492.
4. Tan PH, Sng ITY. Thymoma - a study of 60 cases in Singapore. Histopathology 1995: 26; 509–518.
5. Quintanilla-Martinez L, Wilkins EW Jr, Ferry JA, Harris NL. Thymoma - morphologic subclassification correlates with invasiveness and immunohistologic features: a study of 122 cases. Hum Pathol 1993: 24; 958–969.
6. Ho FSC, Fu KH, Lam SY, Chiu SW, Chan ALC, Muller-Hermelink HK. Evaluation of a histogenetic classification for thymic epithelial tumours. Histopathology 1994: 25; 21–29.
7. Kuo TT, Lo SK. Thymoma. A study of pathologic classification of 71 cases with evaluation of the Muller-Hermelink system. Hum Pathol 1993: 24; 766–771.
8. Rosai J, Levine GD. Tumours of thymus, In Atlas of Tumour Pathology, Sec Ser, Fasc 13: Armed Forces Institute of Pathology, Washington DC 1976.

9. Fujii Y, Monden Y, Nakahara K et al. Antibody to acetylocholine receptor in myasthenia gravis: Production by lymphocytes from thymus and thymoma, Neurology 1984: 34; 1182–1186.
10. Kirchner T, Schalke B, Buchwald J, Ritter M, Marx A, Muller-Hermelink HK. Well-differentiated thymic carcinoma. An organotypical low-grade carcinoma with relationship to cortical thymoma. Am J Surg Pathol 1992: 16; 1153–1169.

5

THYMOMA

A Clinicopathologic Study of 60 Cases

Alessandra Cancellieri,[1] Alberto Cavazza,[2] Giorgio Gardini,[2]
Maurizio Boaron,[3] Nicola Santelmo,[3] and Giuseppe Baruzzi[1]

[1]Department of Pathology
Ospedale Maggiore
Bologna, Italy
[2]Department of Pathology
Arcispedale S. Maria Nuova
Reggio Emilia, Italy
[3]Department of Thoracic Surgery
Ospedale Maggiore
Bologna, Italy

INTRODUCTION

The classification of thymomas has often represented a troublesome topic for the pathologist. In the attempt to correlate the various histologic subtypes with the clinical behaviour and the prognosis of the tumors, Marino and Müller-Hermelink[5] and Kirchner et al.[2] proposed a new histogenetic classification of thymomas based on the similarities between neoplastic epithelial cells and normal thymic components. In the present study, 60 thymomas were reclassified according to the histogenetic classification and their clinicopathological data were evaluated in order to assess if any histological features could correlate with the stage of the tumor, therefore being worth reporting in the histopathologic diagnosis. Besides, we performed an immunocytochemical study, to assess whether the positivity to the Ki-67 antigen, as evaluated by the monoclonal antibody MIB-1, could add any remarkable data about the proliferation rate of the neoplastic cells.

MATERIALS AND METHODS

Sixty cases of thymomas surgically resected between 1978 and 1996 were retrieved from the files of Ospedale Maggiore, Bologna (41 cases) and Arcispedale S.Maria Nuova, Reggio Emilia (19 cases). All the cases were benign or malignant, type 1 thymomas, that

Epithelial Tumors of the Thymus, edited by Marx and Müller-Hermelink.
Plenum Press, New York, 1997

is, thymic carcinomas were excluded from the study. They were all classified according to Marino and Müller-Hermelink[5] and Kirchner et al.[2] in medullary, mixed, organoid and cortical thymomas and well differentiated thymic carcinomas (WDTC) and staged on the staging system of Masaoka et al.[6]. Follow up data were available for 19 patients.

Immunohistochemistry was performed on representative blocks using MIB-1 antibody against Ki-67 nuclear antigen (Immunotech) and avidin-biotin-peroxidase complex (ABC) method[1]. After a pre-treatment in a microwave oven, sections were incubated for 1 hour at room temperature with a dilution 1:50. The MIB-1 labeling index was evaluated by light microscopy with a 40x and an oil-immersion 100x objectives. At least two series of 200–500 epithelial cells each were counted and the results expressed in percentage of positive nuclei. When a double component was present (e.g., cortical thymoma with WDTC, mixed predominantly cortical or medullary thymoma), the prevailing one was evaluated.

Statistical analysis was performed by chi square test.

RESULTS

Patients' age ranged between 22 and 80, the average age being 56 years. Thirty-six patients were females, 24 males, with a female to male ratio of 1.5:1. Myasthenia gravis was present in 13 patients, 6 of which were cortical thymomas, 2 were WDTC, 3 organoid thymomas and 2 were mixed predominantly medullary thymomas. Seventeen cases (28%) were in stage I, 36 (60%) in stage II, 6 (10%) in stage III and only one patient (2%) had a stage IV tumor. The size of the tumors ranged between 2 and 20 cm, with the average size of 7.7 cm; its distribution through the different histotypes and stages is reported in Tables 1 and 2. No statistically significant correlation was noted between the size of the tumors and the histotypes, or between size and stages; nevertheless a trend toward finding larger tumors in advanced stages can be suggested.

With regard to pathological features, the 60 cases included 1 medullary thymoma, 12 mixed predominantly medullary thymomas, 13 organoid (mixed predominantly cortical) thymomas, 23 cortical thymomas and 11 well differentiated thymic carcinomas. Medullary thymoma and mixed, predominantly medullary thymomas were grouped together on the base of their similarities. Foci of necrosis were present in higher percentages as the stage increased (Table 3), the difference being statistically significant ($p>0.05$). Among cortical thymomas, squamoid areas reminiscent of WDTC prevailed in higher stages (Table 4), although without statistical significance, perhaps due to the limited number of cases.

Follow up data with a minimal interval of 3 years were available for 19 patients: 14 of them are alive and well, 3 died of unrelated causes, and only in 2 patients the tumor relapsed, the first recurrence occurring after 2 and 4 years, respectively.

The results of the MIB-1 study, as evaluated in 52 cases, are reported in Table 5. No prevalence seems to emerge among the different histotypes, the organoid thymoma accounting for the highest values. However, regarding the stage, stage III and IV exhibit higher values than stages I and II, and, if we deal with the different histotypes as separate groups, we can see that cortical thymomas and WDTC exhibit higher values in higher stages. The same trend is not identifiable in medullary/mixed and organoid thymomas and between stages I and II.

Table 1. Average size (cm ± SD) and histotype

Medullary/mixed	7.88 ± 1.79
Organoid	9.11 ± 5.25
Cortical	6.74 ± 2.72
WDTC	7.08 ± 2.46

Table 2. Average size (cm ± SD) and stage

Stage I	7.5 ± 3.54
Stage II	7.3 ± 2.64
Stage III	8.9 ± 2.71
Stage IV	11

Table 3. Distribution of necrosis in the different stages (N° of cases)

	Stage I	Stage II	Stage III	Stage IV
necrosis-	15	23	2	0
necrosis+	2	13	4	1

Table 4. Distribution of squamoid areas (WDTC) of cortical thymomas in the different stages (N° of cases)

	Stage I	Stage II	Stage III	Stage IV
cort.	3	14	0	0
cort+WDTC	0	4	2	0

Table 5. Average MIB-1 values (% ± SD) and histotypes

Medullary/mixed	1.2 ± 0.61
Organoid	2.9 ± 1.65
Cortical	1.9 ± 0.5
WDTC	1.0 ± 1.22

DISCUSSION

In the present study, we tried to cross correlate all the clinico-pathological data of the tumors with stage and histotype.

Quite predictably, we found a statistically significant correlation between stage and histotype both in the histopathological, American classification[4] ($p<0.05$) and in the histogenetic, European classification ($p<0.01$), as evaluated by chi square statistical analysis. This is widely reported in the literature and does not need any further comment.

The age distribution of the different histotypes shows a prevalence of the medullary/composite group in the elders: this is consistent with the data found in the literature and with Rosai's remarkable intuition[9] about the similarities between the spindle cells of medullary thymomas and the atrophic epithelial islands that can be found in involuted, post-mature thymuses.

The size of the tumors does not seem to correlate either with the histotype or with the stage. As a matter of fact and according to the literature, the first two largest tumors in our series (20 and 19 cm in their greatest axis) belong to the organoid category, that is almost always benign or minimally invasive, whilst the two smallest ones, 2 and 2.9 cm, represent examples of cortical thymomas with squamoid areas and WDTC, respectively, and both presented in stage II. A trend towards finding larger tumors in advanced stages can be suggested, but the differences are not statistically significant.

Myasthenia gravis (MG) was present in 13 cases, 6 of which were cortical thymomas, 2 were WDTC, 3 were organoid thymomas and 2 were mixed predominantly medullary thymomas, cortical thymomas and WDTC therefore accounting for the 61.5% of all cases with MG. No particular relationship was found between the size of the tumor, age and sex of the patients and the presence of MG.

Besides clinical data, we tried to investigate the existence of any pathological features possibly correlating with the stage of the tumors. Remarkable data about the presence of necrosis seemed to emerge. Indeed, the presence of microscopic foci or grossly visible areas of coagulative necrosis seems to prevail in higher stages, as shown in Table 2. This correlation is statistically significant ($p<0.05$). On the contrary, no correlation was found between necrosis and histotype, probably because of the smaller number of cases in each group. This can be particularly interesting if a small biopsy is performed for diagnostic purposes, e.g. core needle biopsy. In the presence of necrosis, if a preoperatory diagnosis of thymoma is given, we can expect to have to face a tumor in advanced stages.

Another feature worth noting is the relationship between the stage and the presence of solid nests of epithelial squamoid cells resembling WDTC in cortical thymomas. According to the criteria of Kirchner[2], we classified our cases as WDTC when squamoid areas represented >50% on histological sections. However, in many cases of cortical thymoma, significant (i.e., easily appreciable) squamoid areas were present, in a percentage between 1 and 50% of the whole specimen. Not surprisingly, the presence of squamoid areas is noted in an increasing percentage of tumors in higher stages. There is no statistical significance of the distribution, probably due to the limited number of cases, but these data seem to confirm that cortical thymoma and WDTC are the benign and malignant counterparts of a whole spectrum of tumors, which includes various combinations of the two components. The same considerations drawn regarding the presence of necrosis on small biopsies are also applicable to the presence of squamoid areas; the same can be said about the advice to report the presence of such features in the histopathologic diagnosis.

With regard to the follow up, we have data with an interval longer than 3 years in 19 cases out of 47 (13 cases are very recent). Among the patients, only 2 women experienced recurrences after 2 and 4,8,10 years, respectively. The 2-year relapsed case was a cortical thymoma with significant areas of WDTC which presented in stage III and was not completely resectable at the time of the first surgical procedure. She has now (after 3 years) experienced an unresectable recurrence around the great vessels, so that no material from the recurrent tumor is available. The other patient was the only one who died of the disease 12 years after the first excision with distant (brain) metastases. It is worth noting that over the course of the years the tumor changed slightly from a cortical thymoma with minimal squamoid areas (stage II1) to a tumor predominantly composed of squamoid areas, i.e., an actual WDTC. This can be therefore considered a further example of the phenomenon of histological progression described by Pescarmona et al.[7] in 9 cases of thymoma with cortical features, some of which displayed a WDTC pattern in the recurrences, according to the theory that WDTC is the malignant counterpart of cortical thymoma.

Besides the analysis of clinico-pathological data, a proliferation study was performed using the MIB-1 antibody against Ki-67 nuclear antigen. Few studies about proliferation rate of thymomas are reported in the literature: two of them, using AgNORs[10] and DNA flow cytometry[3], showed a statistically significant difference between thymomas (benign and malignant, that is, invasive thymomas) and thymic carcinomas, but failed to obtain the same difference in the first category. That is to say that these studies fail in differentiating benign from invasive thymomas and can only help in distinguishing entities that are very different on histological ground. Furthermore, another work was published in 1995[8], by a group who performed a manual count of AgNOR values, as we did, to avoid the masquerading effect of lymphocytes. In this work, several hints are given: firstly, they exclude thymic carcinomas from the count so that they deal only with thymomas, that is one of our goals. Secondly, they found out a different AgNOR and DNA flow cytometry count in stage I (non invasive) and in stage II, III and IV (invasive) tumors. Thirdly, they established that the prognosis of encapsulated tumors is not modified in microinvasive tumors but is very different in frankly invasive ones. It is worth noting that they report a 50% survival at 10 years for the 8 cases of medullary (spindle cell) thymomas: moreover, the 2 patients who died at less than 2 years displayed a high proliferative activity, suggesting that the prognosis of thymoma can be poor even with a "benign" histology, when the proliferative rate is high. At last, 3 months ago another work was published[11], using PCNA and MIB-1, on 62 cases of thymic epithelial tumors, including 2 poorly differentiated carcinomas. The Authors managed to find a statistically significant difference in MIB-1 score - evaluated by manual count - between stage IV tumors and all the other lower staged ones. They also report an increase of value with the increase of histological grade, with medullary thymomas accounting for the lowest values and WDTC for the highest, however reaching a statistical significance only between WDTC and medullary thymoma.

In our series, if the average value of MIB-1 labeling index in the different histotypes is evaluated, no particular prevalence seems to emerge. Actually, it is the organoid category (that comprehends the largest tumors but is almost always benign or minimally invasive) to exhibit the higher proliferative rate. Moreover, the lowest rate belongs to the WDTC group whilst the medullary/composite category also exhibit a brisk proliferation rate, in spite of the almost always benign nature of the tumor. However, if we consider the different histotypes as different groups, a trend towards a linear relationship between average MIB-1 value and stage seems to emerge for cortical thymoma and WDTC. The difference is not statistically significant, but this trend is worth being further investigated in a higher number of cases. It is also quite remarkable that, in the WDTC group, the highest values are exhibited by two quite curious cases, both of which show, in addition to typical features of WDTC such as perivascular spaces, epithelial palisading, lymphocytic infiltrate, an evident atypia of the neoplastic cells, and, most interesting of all, a clear-cut keratinization of the epithelial cells. This is in contrast with what is reported in the first description of the tumor by Kirchner. A fascinating interpretation of this feature could be that these two tumors represent some sort of linkage between benign and invasive thymomas as a group and thymic carcinomas.

In conclusion, our data indicate that there are two pathological features that deserve to be reported in the diagnosis. The first one is the presence of necrosis which shows a statistically significant correlation with the stage of the tumor. The second one is the presence of foci of WDTC in cortical thymomas, which prevails in higher stages. With regard to the proliferation study, MIB-1 does not seem to correlate with the increasing grade of malignancy through the different histotypes. However, if we distribute the cases in the different histological categories and separately evaluate MIB-1 index, we can notice a trend towards a linear relationship in 2 of the 4 groups. A larger number of cases is needed so as to verify whether a statistical significance can be achieved.

REFERENCES

1. Hsu SM, Raine L, Fanger H. Use of avidin-biotin peroxidase complex (ABC) in immunoperoxidase technique: a comparison between ABC and unlabelled antibody (PAP) procedures. J Histochem Cytochem 1981;29:577–580.
2. Kirchner T, Schalke B, Buchwald J, Ritter M, Marx A, Müller-Hermelink HK. Well-differentiated thymic carcinoma. An organotypical low-grade carcinoma with relationship to cortical thymoma. Am J Surg Pathol 1992;16:1153–1169.
3. Kuo T, Lo S. DNA flow cytometry study of thymic epithelial tumors with evaluation of its usefulness in the pathologic classification. Hum Pathol 1993;24:746–749.
4. Lewis JE, Wick MR, Scheithauer BW, Bernatz PE, Taylor WF. Thymoma. A clinicopathologic review. Cancer 1987;60:2727–2743.
5. Marino M, Müller-Hermelink HK. Thymoma and thymic carcinoma. Relation of thymoma epithelial cells to the cortical and medullary differentiation of thymus. Virchows Arch [A] 1985;407:119–149.
6. Masaoka A, Monden Y, Nakahara K, Tanioka T. Follow-up study of thymomas with special reference to their clinical stage. Cancer 1981;48:2485–2492.
7. Pescarmona E, Rendina EA, Venuta F, Ricci C, Baroni CD. Recurrent thymoma: evidence for histological progression. Histopathology 1995;27:445–449.
8. Pich A, Chiarle R, Chiusa L, Ponti R, Geuna M, Casadio C, Maggi G, Palestro G. Long-term survival of thymoma patients by histologic pattern and proliferative activity. Am J Surg Pathol 1995; 19:918–926.
9. Rosai J. Mediastinum. In: Rosai J. Ackerman's surgical pathology, 8th edition, volume 1. Mosby eds. St. Louis, Missouri, 1996, p. 450.
10. Tateyama H, Mizuno T, Tada T, Eimoto T, Hashimoto T, Masaoka A. Thymic epithelial tumours: evaluation of malignant grade by quantification of proliferating cell nuclear antigen and nucleolar organizer regions. Virchows Arch [A] 1993;422:265–269.
11. Yang W, Efird JT, Quintanilla-Matinez L, Choi N, Harris N. Cell kinetic study of thymic epithelial tumors using PCNA (PC 10) and Ki-67 (MIB-1) antibodies. Hum Pathol 1996;27:70–76.

6

p53-ALTERATIONS IN THYMIC EPITHELIAL TUMORS

G. Weirich,[1] P. Schneider,[2] C. Fellbaum,[1] H. Brauch,[1] W. Nathrath,[1] M. Scholz,[3] H. Präuer,[2] and H. Höfler[1]

[1]Institute of Pathology
[2]Department of Thoracic Surgery
[3]Institute for Medical Statistics and Epidemiology
School of Medicine
Technical University Munich
Munich, Germany

1. SUMMARY

On the basis of histopathology thymic epithelial tumors are subdivided into organotypic thymomas and non-organotypic thymic carcinomas. Although thymomas do not exhibit gross cellular atypia they may behave clinically malignant. To warrant the pathologic detection of malignancy in thymic epithelial tumors the tumor suppressor *p53* was analysed whose alterations are known to be a common event during carcinogenesis. The analysis of the *p53*-protein was carried out by immunohistochemistry using a monoclonal (*D0–1*) and a polyclonal antibody (*CM-1*). The *p53*-gene was analysed by PCR-SSCP of the exons 5–8 and DNA-sequencing. In thymomas including well-differentiated thymic carcinomas *p53*-protein alterations were detected with the polyclonal antibody *CM-1* but not with the monoclonal antibody *D0–1,* and no mutations were found in exons 5–8 of the *p53*-gene. In contrast, in non-organotypic thymic carcinomas mutant *p53*-protein was detected with both the monoclonal and the polyclonal antibodies. The integration of morphological, clinical and *p53*-analysis data identified three major groups of thymic epithelial tumors: (1) benign thymomas with a low incidence of *p53*-protein alterations; (2) malignant thymomas (including well-differentiated thymic carcinomas) with a high incidence of *p53*-protein alterations; in both thymoma groups no *p53*-gene mutations were found at the genetic level (exons 5–8); (3) non-organotypic thymic carcinomas with a high incidence of *p53*-protein alteration, simultaneous occurrence of *p53*-gene mutations and 17p LOH. We consider the immunohistochemical analysis of the *p53*-protein not only a new useful tool in the pathological evaluation of thymic epithelial tumors. *p53*-protein alterations are also correlated with shortened survival times and their detection can therefore be used for prognostical judgement. The failure of the monoclonal antibody *D0–1* to detect altered

Epithelial Tumors of the Thymus, edited by Marx and Müller-Hermelink.
Plenum Press, New York, 1997

p53-protein in thymomas points to an epitope concealing event of the *D0–1* binding site in these tumors.

2. INTRODUCTION

The histopathological analysis of thymic epithelial tumors aims mainly at the judgement of tumor dignity and survival prognosis. Two competitive pathological classifications currently claim to fulfill these requirements: (1) the revised classification of Rosai and Levine[1] and the updated histogenetic classification of Marino, Müller-Hermelink and Kirchner[2,3,4]. The classification of Rosai and Levine defines three different types of thymic epithelial tumors according to their non-invasive/invasive growth pattern: benign non-invasive thymomas, malignant invasive thymomas and invasive thymic carcinomas with gross cellular atypia. The histogenetic classification of Müller-Hermelink and collegues (MMHK) defines six different subtypes of thymic epithelial tumors according to their histo-cytological appearance: benign medullary and mixed-type thymomas, low malignant predominantly cortical, cortical thymomas and well-differentiated thymic carcinomas (these five tumor types are further called thymomas), and high malignant non-organotypic thymic carcinomas. Both classifications are prognostically relevant[5,6,7] but there are several drawbacks that point to the need of supplementary parameters of dignity judgement in these tumors. (1) Invasive behavior is a late event in carcinogenesis and consequently this parameter is not suitable for the early detection of malignancy; (2) Minimal invasive behavior can only be judged by extensive sampling of the tumor's capsule environment. (3) In biopsies the histologic distinction between different subtypes of thymic epithelial tumors (i.e. spindle-shaped medullary thymomas and spindle-shaped subtypes of well-differentiated thymic carcinomas) may be difficult. This study aimed at characterizing thymic epithelial tumors on the basis of molecular events that could help to overcome these drawbacks. The target molecule of this study was *p53*, a well characterized tumor suppressor that is involved in a large variety of human malignancies[8]. *p53* is integrated in the complex autoregulatory feedback system of the cell cycle, the motor of proliferation[9]. Many tumors were shown to harbor mutated *p53*, that either lost its function in growth control or even promotes cellular growth due to a dominant gain of function. Most mutations hit the conserved regions between exon 5–8 of the *p53*-gene[8]. Due to the fact that mutated *p53*-proteins tend to exhibit a prolonged biological half-life they accumulate in the cell nucleus and can be detected by immunohistochemistry[10].

3. MATERIAL AND METHODS

Briefly, 44 archival samples of thymic epithelial tumors were typed according to the updated pathological classification of Marino, Müller-Hermelink and Kirchner and consisted of: three medullary thymomas, 14 mixed-type thymomas, four predominantly cortical thymomas, seven cortical thymomas, seven well-differentiated thymic carcinomas, and nine non-organotypic thymic carcinomas (one squamous, two lymphepithelial, one neuroendocrine, one sarcomatoid, two not further classifiable, one undifferentiated carcinoma). 42 patients were controlled in post-operative follow-up. 18 patients suffered from myasthenia gravis.

For immunohistochemistry, sections were taken from representative blocks of each tumor and dewaxed according to routine procedures. Treatment for antigen retrieval (microwave, lead thiocyananate) preceded an overnight incubation with the anti-*p53*-antibodies *D0–1* (monoclonal) that recognizes the N-terminal aminoacids 19–25 of the *p53*-protein[11] and *CM-1* (polyclonal) that recognizes the entire protein[12] (both antibodies were kindly provided by Lane DP, Dundee, Scotland). Reaction intensitiy was enhanced using the double-bridge- and APAAP methods[13,14]. Reactions were estimated to be informative when at least 10% of tumor cells showed intranuclear staining.

Statistical analysis was performed by correlation of immunohistochemical data with histopathology, clinical stages and the occurrence of myasthenia gravis using Fisher's exact test. The effect of *p53*-alterations on survival times was determined by Kaplan-Meier survival curve estimates and Log-rank test.

DNA was extracted by standard procedures from the same tumor blocks used for immunohistochemistry[15]. The *p53*-exons 5–8 were amplified by single-round PCRs using intronic primer pairs[16]. PCR-products were further analysed by SSCP using discontinuous eletric and density gradients (DISK-SSCP). Direct sequencing of PCR-products was used in cases informative in SSCP.

4. RESULTS

Intranuclear immunoreactivity was observed in epithelial cells but not in thymocytes or stromal cells. In thymomas, immunoreaction with the polyclonal antibody *CM-1* was observed in 5/7 well-differentiated thymic carcinomas, 4/7 cortical thymomas, 2/4 predominantly cortical thymomas, 2/14 mixed-type thymomas and none of the medullary thymomas. In contrast, immunoreactivity with the monoclonal antibody *D0–1* was not observed in these tumors. Among non-organoid thymic carcinomas 7/9 were reactive with polyclonal antibody *CM-1* and among these 4 with monoclonal antibody *D0 1*. Staining was uniformly intense with both antibodies (> 80 % cells reactive). Statistical analysis revealed a significant correlation between the above described incidence of *CM-1*-based anti-*p53* immunoreaction and histological parameters ($p < 0.01$, Fisher's exact test): immunoreaction was strongly evident in non-organoid thymic carcinomas, and to a lower extent in well-differentiated thymic carcinomas, cortical thymomas and predominantly cortical thymomas, whereas mixed-type thymomas and medullary thymomas exhibited a low incidence of immunoreaction. Further, *CM-1* immunoreactivity correlated significantly with clinical stages ($p < 0.01$, Fisher's exact test). This finding indicates that immunohistochemical detection of *p53*-protein parallels tumor invasiveness. Kaplan-Meier survival curve estimates revealed a substantially lower survival in patients with immunoreactive thymic epithelial tumors than those with non-reactive tumors ($p < 0.05$, Log-rank test). No significant correlation was detected between *p53*-alteration and the occurrence of myasthenia gravis.

Among amplifiable 42 cases exon-specific PCR products were obtained and analysed by SSCP. Three tumors showed band shifts. In a non-organoid thymic carcinomas with neuroendocrine differentiation a loss of heterozygosity (LOH) and a point mutation in the remaining allele at codon 242 (exon 7) were detected. The mutation consisted in a G→C transversion that leads to a aminoacid change (ser→cys). Another non–organoid thymic carcinomas with sarcomatoid differentiation equally showed a showed LOH and a point mutation at the hot spot codon 273 which is located in exon 8[8]. This mutation consisted in a G→A transition that is responsible for a aminoacid change in the p53–protein (arg«his). Both cases were immunoreactive for polyclonal antibody CM–1 AND monoclonal antibody D0–1. Further, in one cortical thymoma a point mutation hit codon 213 and consisted of a A→G transition in one gene with conservation of the wild–type sequence on the second allele.This mutation was a silent germline mutation of the p53–gene. No immunoreaction was observed in this case neither with CM–1 nor with D0–1 antibodies. Wild type band patterns in exons 5–8 were observed in all residual immunoreactive and non-reactive cases.

5. DISCUSSION

In past decades cytologically benign but invasive thymomas prompted a bewildering variety of pathological classifications that were mostly irrelevant to prognosis. Currently, two prognostically relevant competitive classification systems are in use: the classification of Rosai and Levine and the classification of Müller-Hermelink and colleagues (MMHK). The revised classification of Rosai and Levine[1] is mainly based on tumor invasion of the thymus' capsule whereas the MMHK classification circumvents the exclusive need for the capsule's invasion assessment by applying cyto-histologic parameters for dignity judgment.

In the present study the tumor suppressor *p53* appeared distinctly different in thymomas, well-differentiated thymic carcinomas inclusive, and non-organotypic thymic carcinomas. The immunohistochemical detection of *p53*-protein correlated with main histologic tumor types according to the MMHK system, clinical stages (Masaoka's system) and the patients' survival times. Our data imply that *p53*-alterations are not involved in clinically benign thymomas (medullary and mixed-type thymomas). In the majority of potentially malignant thymomas (predominatly cortical, cortical thymomas, and well-differentiated thymic carcinomas), altered *p53*-protein was monitored by immunohistochemistry — no mutations of the *p53*-gene exons 5–8 were found. There are two possible explanations for these findings: (1) In such tumors, *p53*-gene mutations might be located up- or downstream of the exons 5–8. However, mutations in *p53* exons 1–4 and 9–11 and in introns seem to be rare events[8,9]; (2) In potentially malignant thymomas, detectable amounts of wildtype *p53*-protein might reflect the augmented proliferation rate of the tumors, as *p53* transcription is also activated during cell proliferation. If this were the case, one would expect a random distribution of immunoreactive cases. In contrast, the immunohistological detection of *p53*-protein in this study correlated with clinical stages, and survival times.

There was a strikingly divergent immunoreactivity pattern in thymomas: the polyclonal antibody *CM-1* detected *p53* in 62% of thymomas and in most non-organotypic thymic carcinomas, but only in the latter tumor group *p53*-protein was also detected with the monoclonal antibody *D0–1*. This divergence might be due to the differing *p53*-recognition by these antibodies. The polyclonal antibody *CM-1* recognizes the entire *p53*-protein by binding to many different epitopes[12], whereas the monoclonal antibody *D0–1* specifically binds to the N-terminal aminoacids 19–25 of the *p53*-protein[11]. Several proteins are known to interact with *p53*. Out of these, *E1B* and *MDM2* bind to the N-terminal region of the *p53*-protein[17,18]. The *MDM2* binding site maps to the N-terminal aminoacids 1–52 of the *p53*-protein, the *E1B* binding site being located between aminoacids 1 and 123. The *MDM2-p53* and *E1B-p53* interactions can therefore interfere with binding of the monclonal antibody *D0–1* and specifically hamper the immunoreaction with this antibody. The *MDM2-p53* and *E1B-p53* interactions can both stabilze the *p53*-protein which consequently accumulates in the cellular nucleus. *MDM2-p53* or *E1B-p53* interactions could therefore explain two main findings in thymomas: (1) the absence of *D0–1* immunoreactivity in cases reactive with *CM-1*; (2) the lack of *p53*-gene mutations. We therefore consider the *MDM2* or *E1B* to be involved in the pathogenesis of thymomas.

In contrast to thymomas, non-organotypic thymic carcinomas were partly reactive with both antibodies and in 50% of these cases *p53*-gene mutations were detected. One missense point mutation found in a sarcomatoid thymic carcinoma hit codon 273 (exon 8), a hot spot site involved in many different human malignancies[8]. The other missense point mutation hit a neuroendocrine thymic carcinoma at codon 242 (exon 7). Both mutation events are not linked to any specific causative agent[19]. A third silent point mutation was identified as a heterozygous germline mutation — identical base transitions were found in this patients' cortical thymoma and peripheral blood lymphocytes. The mutation was located in codon 213 (exon 6). The patient's cortical thymoma was not immunoreactive. This finding was further evidence for the antibodies' specificity to detect altered *p53*. Our results further imply that the immunoreaction with the polyclonal antibody *CM-1* is not specifically related to *p53*-mutations in the exons 5–8, whereas the monoclonal antibody *D0–1* reliably seems to indicate mutated *p53*-proteins.

By histology, clinical data, immunohistochemistry and DNA-analysis we could identify three major entities of thymic epithelial tumors: (1) benign thymomas with rare occurrence of detectable amounts of *p53*-protein and no *p53*-gene mutations in exons 5–8; (2) low malignant thymomas with frequent occurrence of detectable amounts of *p53*-protein and no *p53*-gene mutations in exons 5–8; (3) high malignant non-organotypic thymic carcinomas with frequent occurrence of detectable amounts of *p53*-protein and the simultaneous occurrence of *p53*-gene mutations and 17p LOH. *p53*-alteration was not linked to the occurrence of *myasthenia gravis*.

CM-1-based immunohistochemical detection of *p53*-protein corroborates the MMHK classification of thymomas and points to a biological relationship between the thymoma subtypes. Therefore, *CM-1*-based immunohistochemical detection of *p53*-protein is considered a useful tool in the evaluation of thymomas' dignity and it futher appears to be an independent prognostic marker.

Details of this study were recently submitted to the American Journal of Pathology.

REFERENCES

1. Wick MR, Scheithauer BW, Weiland LH, Bernatz PE Primary thymic carcinomas Am J Surg Pathol 6: 1982; 451-470
2. Marino M, Müller-Hermelink HK Thymoma and thymic carcinoma. Relation of thymoma epithelial cells to the cortical and medullary differentiation of thymus Virchows Arch [Pathol Anat] 407: 1985; 119-149
3. Kirchner T, Müller-Hermelink HK New approaches to the diagnosis of thymic epithelial tumors Prog Surg Pathol 10: 1989; 167-189
4. Kirchner T, Schalke B, Buchwald J, Ritter M, Marx A, Müller-Hermelink HK Well-differentiated thymic carcinoma. An organotypical low-grade carcinoma with realtionship to cortical thymoma Am J Surg Pathol 16(12): 1992; 1153-1169
5. Rosai J, Levine GD Tumors of the thymus Second series, fascicle 13; Washington, USA; Armed Forces Institute of Pathology; 1976
6. Quintanilla-Martinez L, Wilkins EW, Choi N, Efird J, Hug E, Harris NL Thymoma. Histologic subclassification is an independent prognostic factor Cancer 74(2): 1994; 606-617
7. Schneider PM, Fellbaum C, Rex A von, Bollschweiler E, Fink U, Präuer HW Epithelial thymic tumors: histological subclassification, staging and residual tumor category are independent prognostic factors Annals Surg Oncol, 1996, in press
8. Hollstein M, Sidransky D, Vogelstein B, Harris CC p53 mutations in human cancers Science 253: 1991; 4953
9. Levine AJ, Momand J, Finlay CA The p53 tumor suppressor gene Nature 351: 1991; 453-456

10. Friend S p53: a glimpse at the puppet behind the shadow play Science 265: 1994; 334-335
11. Vojtesek B, Bártek J, Midgley CA, Lane DP An immunohistochemical analysis of the human nuclear phosphprotein p53. New monoclonal antibodies and epitope mapping using recombinant p53 J Immunol Meth 151: 1992; 237-244
12. Midgley CA, Fisher CJ, Bártek J, Vojtesek B, Lane D, Barnes DM Analysis of p53 expression in human tumours: an antibody raised against human p53 expressed in Escherichia coli J Cell Sci 101: 1992; 183-189
13. Vacca LL "Double bridge" techniques of immunocytochemistry. In: Techniques in immunocytochemistry. Bullock GR, Petrusz P (Hrsg.) Academic Press, New York USA, 1: 1982, p 155
14. Cordell JL, Falini B, Erber WN, Ghosh AK, Abdulaziz Z, MacDonald S, Pulford KAF, Stein H, Mason DY Immunoenzymatic labeling of monoclonal antibodies using immune complexes of alkaline phosphatase and monoclonal anti-alkaline phosphatase (APAAP complexes) J Histochem Cytochem 32(2): 1984; 219-229
15. Wright DK, Manos MM Sample preparation from paraffin-embedded tissues. In: PCR protocols: A guide to methods an applications. Innis MA, Gelfand DH, Sninsky JJ, White TJ (Hrsg) Academic Press, San Diego, USA; 1st ed, 1990, pp 153-158
16. Lohmann D, Pütz B, Reich U, Böhm J, Präuer H, Höfler H Mutational spectrum of the p53 gene in human small-cell lung cancer and relationship to clinico-pathological data Am J Pathol 142: 1993; 907-915
17. Picksley SM, Vojtesek B, Sparks A, Lane DP Immunochemical analysis of the interaction of p53 with MDM2; — fine mapping of the MDM2 binding site on p53 using synthetic peptides Oncogene 9: 1994; 2523-2529
18. Chen J, Marechal V, Levine AJ Mapping of the p53 and mdm-2 interaction domains Mol&Cell Biol 13 (7): 1993; 4107-4114
19. Chang F, Syrjänen S, Tervahauta A, Syrjänen K Tumourigenesis associated with the p53 tumour suppressor gene Br J Cancer 68: 1993; 653-661

7

p53 PROTEIN EXPRESSION IN THYMIC EPITHELIAL TUMORS

Naoki Hino,* Kazuya Kondo, Takanori Miyoshi, Tadashi Uyama, and Yasumasa Monden

Second Department of Surgery
School of Medicine
University of Tokushima
Kuramoto-cho, Tokushima 770, Japan

ABSTRACT

We investigated the expression of p53 protein by immunohistochemical analysis using the anti-p53 polyclonal antibody (CM-1) in 12 thymomas and 13 thymic carcinomas.

All 6 noninvasive thymomas showed an absence of nuclear staining, and one of the 7 invasive thymomas (14%) showed nuclear staining focally. Eight of the 12 thymic carcinomas (67%) showed nuclear staining. Three of 8 cases showed nuclear staining in more than 50% of the tumor cells.

p53 protein accumulation is highly frequent in thymic carcinomas, but not in thymomas. The accumulation of p53 protein seems to play an important role in the carcinogenesis of thymic carcinomas.

INTRODUCTION

Thymic epithelial tumors are broadly classified into thymomas and thymic carcinomas. Thymomas exhibit cytologically bland neoplastic epithelial cells and a variable number of non-neoplastic T lymphocytes. Thymomas show zonal differentiation, i.e. cortex and medulla elements, which is similar to the normal thymus to some extent[1 2 3]. Thymomas occasionally show invasive growth and pleural seeding, but lymphogenous or hematogenous metastasis is rare. In contrast, thymic carcinomas do not show zonal differentiation, and their epithelial cells show obvious cytological atypia, and are not able to at-

* Correspondence: Naoki Hino, Second Department of Surgery, School of Medicine, The University of Tokushima, Kuramoto-cho, Tokushima 770, Japan. Tel +81-886-33-7143; fax +81-886-33-7144.

tract and retain immature T lymphocytes[1 2 3]. Thymic carcinomas grow invasively and frequent show lymphogenous or hematogenous metastasis.

It may be interesting to investigate the genetic events in tumorgenesis of these tumors. In human cancers, many kinds of oncogene and antioncogene has been reporeted recently, and alteration of the p53 gene is probably the most common abnormality[4].

To clarify the relationship between the tumor suppressor gene p53 and thymic epithelial tumors, we investigated the expression of p53 protein in thymomas and thymic carcinomas.

MATERIALS AND METHODS

Materials

Tumor tissues were obtained from 13 thymoma and 12 thymic carcinoma patients who had undergone surgery or taken biopsy at the Second Department of Surgery, School of Medicine, the University of Tokushima from 1980 to 1994. All tissues were fixed in formalin, and embedded in paraffin wax.

The patients with thymoma included 2 males and 11 females, whose ages ranged from 29 to 80 years (average 51.7 years). Two patients had myasthenia gravis. The clinical stage of thymoma was determined according to the criteria of Masaoka et al.[5] Six of the 13 thymomas were noninvasive tumors, clinical Stage I. The other 7 thymomas were invasive tumors, clinical Stage II, III, or IV (Table 1).

The patients with thymic carcinoma included 8 males and 4 females, whose ages ranged from 47 to 86 years (average 60.5 years). They showed no complications, such as myasthenia gravis (Table 1). The clinical stage of thymic carcinoma was determined according to the criteria of Masaoka et al.[5]

Table 1. Clinical findings in 25 thymic epithelial tumors

		thymic carcinoma (n=12)		thymoma (n=13)	
Age			60.5±10.21 (47~86)		51.7±16.54 (29~80)
Sex	Male		8		2
	Female		4		11
Histology		Sq	8	Lym	2
		Sp	1	Mix	6
		Ud	1	Ep	5
		Sm	1		
		Ad	1		
Disease stage		I	0		6
		II	2		2
		III	3		3
		IVa	1		1
		IVb	6		1

Sq: squamous cell carcinoma; Sp: spindle cell carcinoma; Ud: undifferentiated carcinoma; Sm: small cell carcinoma; Ad: adenosquamous cell carcinoma;
Lym: Lymphocyte predominant type; Mix: Mixed type; Ep: Epithelial predominant type.

Five normal lung and 17 lung carcinoma tissues (7 lung carcinoma tissues with missense mutation in the p53 gene, one with nonsense mutation, and 9 with wild-type p53 gene, which were previously reported[6]) were used as a control in immunohistochemical staining for p53 protein.

Immunohistochemical Staining for p53

Five-micron thick paraffin-embedded section of each thymoma and thymic carcinoma was cut, deparaffinized, and rehydrated through xylene and graded alcohols. For antigen retrieval, the sections were placed in a Coplin jar containing 0.01M citrate buffer (pH 6.0) and microwaved at 5-min intervals for a total 15 min at maximal level in a household microwave oven[7]. Endogenous peroxidase was inhibited with 3% hydrogren peroxide and nonspecific binding was blocked with bovine serum albumin. Sections were incubated with anti-p53 polyclonal antibody, CM-1 (Novocastra Laboratories Ltd., Newcastle, UK) diluted 1:1500 at room temperature for 60 min . After washing with tris-buffered saline (TBS, pH7.6), the sections were incubated for 15 min with biotinylated anti-rabbit and anti-mouse immunoglobulins and incubated with streptavidin conjugated to horseradish peroxidase for 15 min using an LSAB kit (DAKO Corp., CA). The peroxidase reaction was developed with a 0.05% solution of diaminobenzidine tetrahydrochloride. Sections were counterstained with hematoxylin.

When under the light microscopic study the nuclei of tumor cells were observed to be stained focally or diffusely by the polyclonal antibody, the tumor was classified as "positive" for p53 protein. A tumor in which nuclei were not stained, or only a few nuclei stained in some microscopic fields (X200), as "negative".

RESULT

Normal Lungs and Lung Carcinomas

Three of the 9 lung carcinomas with wild-type p53 (33%) and all 7 lung carcinomas with p53 missense mutation (100%) stained positively. The p53 expression in lung carcinomas by immunohistochemical analysis with microwave treatment was significantly correlated with the p53 gene missense mutation ($P<0.05$) by Fisher's exact probability test.

The one lung carcinoma with p53 nonsense mutation and all 5 normal lungs showed an absence of nuclear staining in immunohistochemical analysis.

Thymomas

Only one of 13 thymomas was positive for p53 expression. p53 was focally stained on the border of the tumor(Fig. 1a). This case was diagnosed as "invasive thymoma, atypia type combined thymic carcinoma".

Thymic Carcinomas

The number of p53 positive cases in 12 thymic carcinoma was 8 (67%) (Fig. 1b).

The positive rate of staining in individual was 100% (2/2) in Stage II, 67% (2/3) in Stage III, and 57% (4/7) in Stage IV. The expression of p53 protein in the thymic carci-

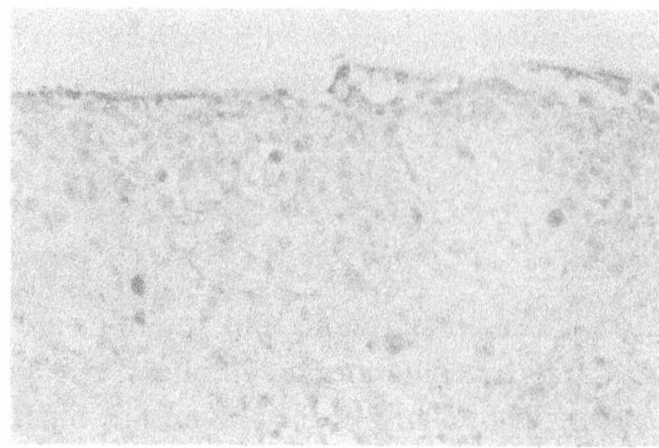
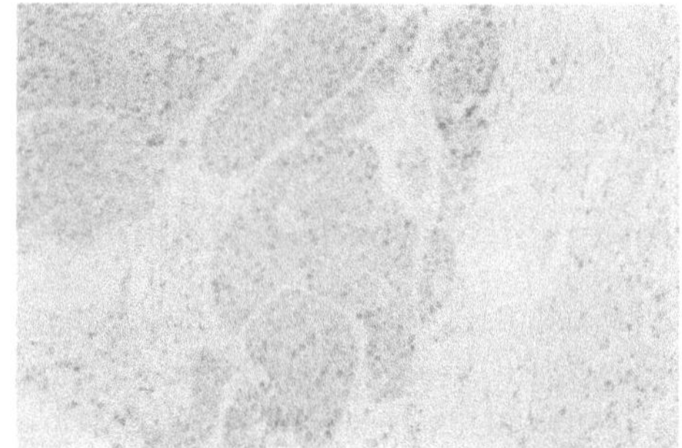

Figure 1. The staining patterns in p53 immunohistochemistry with antibody CM-1. *Left:* Invasive thymoma with atypia shows expression of p53 protein on the border of tumor. *Right:* Nuclear staining of a majority of nuclei is present in thymic carcinoma.

noma tissues was not correlated with clinical stage. Three cases showed nuclear positive staining in more than 50% of the tumor cells.

DISCUSSION

Thymic carcinoma has long been the source of controversy due to the lack of agreement regarding its definition and proper criteria for diagnosis. Since Shimosato et al. reported eight cases of primary squamous cell carcinoma of the thymus[8], there have been many reports on thymic carcinoma[9 10 11]. Thymic epithelial tumors are broadly classified into thymomas and thymic carcinomas. We define thymic carcinoma as a neoplasm of thymic epithelial cells that exhibits cytological atypia and is not associated with nonneoplastic immature T lymphocytes, in accord with Shimosato[12].

We examined p53 protein expression in thymic epithelial tumors by immunohistochemical analysis using polyclonal antibody (CM-1) with antigen retrieval by microwave. Only one of the 13 thymomas (8%) was stained positively by p53 antibody. In contrast, 8 of the 12 thymic carcinomas (67%) were stained positively (Fig. 2). These results indicate that p53 protein accumulates frequently in thymic carcinomas, but not in thymomas. The p53 protein accumulation interferes with the ability of wild-type p53 to inhibit tumor growth[6 13]. According to this principle, thymic carcinomas have a tendency to proliferation compared with thymomas.

It is very interesting that the single thymoma case positive for p53 protein showed both characteristics of thymoma and thymic carcinoma. The tumor showed marked nuclear atypia accompanying with immature T lymphocytic infiltration. Similar cases were reported by Shimosato et al. and Müller-Hermelink et al. Shimosato diagnosed these tumors as "invasive thymoma, atypical type"[12], and Müller-Hermelink diagnosed them as "well differentiated thymic carcinoma"[14].

It has been reported that p53 protein accumulation is caused by missense mutation of the p53 gene or by interaction of p53 protein with some oncoproteins. The overexpression of the p53 protein in lung cancer in the present study was correlated with the missense mutations of p53 gene. p53 protein expression in thymic carcinoma may be correlated with the p53 gene mutation.

In conclusion, p53 protein accumulation was highly frequent in the thymic carcinomas, but not in the thymomas. We suggest that thymoma and thymic carcinoma may pro-

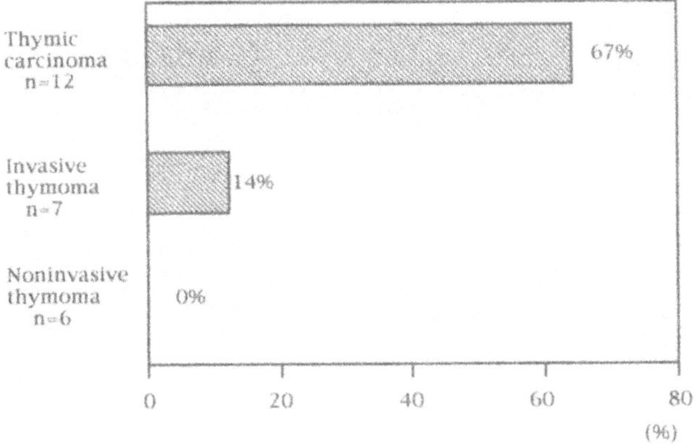

Figure 2.

gress through different pathways from the thymic epithelial cells, and that accumulation of p53 protein may be an important step in the complicated process of carcinogenesis in thymic carcinoma.

REFERENCES

1. Kodama T, Watanabe S, Sato Y, Shimosato Y, Miyazawa N. An immunohistochemical study of thymic epithelial tumors I. Epithelial component. Am J Surg Pathol 1986;10:26–33.
2. Sato Y, Watanabe S, Mukai K, Kodama T, Upton MP, Goto M, et al. An immunohistochemical study of thymic epithelial tumors II. Lymphoid Component. Am J Surg Pathol 1986;10:862–70.
3. Kondo K, Mukai K, Sato Y, Matsuno Y, Shimosato Y, Monden Y. An immunohistochemical study of thymic epithelial tumors III. The distribution of interdigitating reticulum cells and S-100b-positive small lymphocytes. Am J Surg Pathol 1990;14:1139–47.
4. Bartek J, Bartkova J, Vojtesek B, Staskova Z, Lukas J, Rejthar A, et al. Aberrant expression of the p53 oncoprotein is a common feature of a wide spectrum of human malignancies. Oncogene 1991;6:1699–703.
5. Masaoka A, Monden Y, Nakahara K, Tanioka T. Follow-up study of thymomas with special reference to their clinical stages. Cancer 1981;48:2485–92.
6. Kondo K, Umemoto A, Akimoto S, Uyama T, Hayashi K, Ohnishi Y, et al. Mutations in the P53 tumour suppressor gene in primary lung cancer in Japan. Biochem Biophys Res Commun 1992;183:1139–46.
7. Shi SR, Key ME, Kalra KL. Antigen retrieval in formalin-fixed, paraffin-embedded tissues: an enhancement method for immunohistochemical staining based on microwave oven heating of tissue sections. J Histochem Cytochem 1991;39:741–8.
8. Shimosato Y, Kameya T, Nagai K, Suemasu K. Squamous cell carcinoma of the thymus. An analysis of eight cases. Am J Surg Pathol 1977;1:109–21.
9. Wick MR, Scheithauer BW, Weiland LH, Bernatz PE. Primary thymic carcinomas. Am J Surg Pathol 1982;6:613–30.
10. Truong LD, Mody DR, Cagle PT, Jackson YG, Schwartz MR, Wheeler TM. Thymic carcinoma. A clinicopathologic study of 13 cases. Am J Surg Pathol 1990;14:151–66.
11. Suster S, Rosai J. Thymic carcinoma. A clinicopathologic study of 60 cases. Cancer 1991;67:1025–32.
12. Shimosato Y. Controversies surrounding the subclassification of thymoma. Cancer 1994;74:542–44.
13. Hayashi K. PCR-SSCP: a method for detection of mutations. Genet Anal Tech Appl 1992;9:73–9.
14. Kirchner T, Schalke B, Buchwald J, Ritter M, Marx A, Müller HH. Well-differentiated thymic carcinoma. An organotypical low-grade carcinoma with relationship to cortical thymoma. Am J Surg Pathol 1992;16:1153–69.

8

p53 OVEREXPRESSION AND THYMOMA PROGNOSIS

Achille Pich, Roberto Chiarle, Luigi Chiusa, Manuela Motta, and Giorgio Palestro

Department of Biomedical Sciences and Human Oncology
Section of Pathology
University of Turin
Via Santena 7, 10126 Torino, Italy

1. SUMMARY

Overexpression of the p53 protein has been retrospectively investigated in 90 surgically resected thymomas at diagnosis, using the monoclonal antibody DO7 on routinely processed specimens. p53 accumulation was compared with tumour clinicopathological features, DNA flow cytometry content and cell proliferative activity, assessed by the counts of the argyrophilic nucleolar organizer regions (AgNORs). The purpose was to verify whether the overexpression of the p53 protein could offer additional prognostic information. p53 accumulation was detected in 48 cases (53.4%). No association was found between p53 overexpression and thymoma clinicopathologic features, although p53 protein tended to be more frequently expressed in invasive (61.4%) than noninvasive cases (45.7%, $p=0.19$) and in DNA aneuploid (71.4%) than diploid cases (48.7%, $p=0.15$). A strong association was found between p53 immunostaining and AgNOR counts: p53 positive cases had higher AgNOR counts (6.34) than p53 negative thymomas (5.36, $p=0.012$). In univariate analysis, the 10 year survival rates were significantly higher (83%) for p53 negative than for p53 positive patients (52%, $p=0.019$). AgNOR counts, tumour DNA content, histological subtypes of the American classification, clinical stage and invasion were also strongly associated with survival. In the multivariate analysis, only tumour stage ($p<0.001$) and AgNOR counts ($p=0.009$) retained an independent prognostic significance. Our results indicate that tumour invasion and cell proliferative activity are the most significant parameters predicting survival in thymoma. p53 overexpression is directly correlated to cell proliferative activity and may be regarded as an additional, although not independent, prognostic factor.

Epithelial Tumors of the Thymus, edited by Marx and Müller-Hermelink.
Plenum Press, New York, 1997

2. INTRODUCTION

The prognosis of thymoma is still a matter of debate. While tumour invasiveness is a prognostic factor widely recognized [1–7], controversies exist for other parameters, clinical or morphological. Myasthenia gravis has been reported to be an indicator of poor prognosis [2]; however this was not subsequently confirmed [4]. The histological pattern is significant in some studies [1,4,6–9], but not in others [2,5]. Recently, the DNA content of thymoma cells, evaluated by flow cytometry [7,10], and the cell proliferative activity, as expressed by the counts of the argyrophilic proteins associated with the nucleolar organizer regions (AgNORs) [6,7], have been proposed as new prognostic indicators in thymoma.

In the last years, mutations of the p53 tumour suppressor gene have been detected in several neoplasias. The majority of p53 mutations produces proteins with altered conformation and prolonged half-life [11], which may accumulate in the nucleus, can be immunohistochemically detected in formalin-fixed, paraffin-embedded tissues, and appear to be involved in the development, progression and prognosis of many human tumours [12–15]. p53 accumulation is directly correlated to the cell proliferative activity, as indicated by the association with S-phase fraction [14,15]. Little is known about the role of p53 overexpression in thymoma, although higher rates of p53 accumulation have been detected in invasive thymomas and thymic carcinomas than in noninvasive thymomas [16].

In this work we have retrospectively investigated p53 overexpression in 90 surgically resected thymomas at diagnosis, using an immunohistochemical method on routinely processed specimens. We compared p53 accumulation with tumour clinicopathological features, DNA content and cell proliferative activity. The aim was to assess whether the overexpression of the p53 protein could offer additional prognostic information.

3. MATERIAL AND METHODS

Ninety thymomas were collected from the files of the Pathology Section of the Department of Biomedical Sciences and Human Oncology, University of Turin, Italy, from the period 1979 to 1987. Patients included 50 females and 40 males whose ages ranged from 14 to 76 years (mean, 49 years); 55 had associated myasthenia gravis. All patients received surgery: 72 radical and 18 partial tumour resection; 27 had also adjuvant post-operative radiotherapy, 5 chemotherapy and 3 chemotherapy plus radiation therapy. A minimum follow-up of 5 years for censored patients or to death was available for all the cases; the length of follow-up ranged from 1 to 161 months (mean, 72 months). Multiple samples were collected from each case, fixed in 10% formalin for 24 h and embedded in paraffin. Serial sections from the same tissue blocks were used for histological typing, p53 immunostaining, AgNOR staining and DNA flow cytometry. According to the American classification system [1,4], 11 cases were spindle cell (S), 35 predominantly lymphocytic (PL), 22 mixed lymphoepithelial (MLE) and 22 predominantly epithelial (PE) thymomas. According to the European scheme [17], 11 cases were medullary (MT), 53 mixed cortico-medullary (MixT), 7 predominantly cortical (PCT) and 19 cortical (CT) thymomas. No evidence of malignant cytology could be observed in the multiple samples examined for each case. Staging was assessed according to the criteria of Masaoka et al. [3]; 46 were stage I, 19 stage II, 13 stage III and 12 stage IVa thymomas. Forty-six were noninvasive and 44 were invasive thymomas.

3.1. p53 Staining and Scoring

Four µm thick dewaxed sections were placed in a glass box filled with 10mM, pH 6.0 citrate buffer and subjected to microwave irradiation at 750 W for two periods of 5 min each. They were stained with the p53 specific monoclonal antibody DO7 (Oncogene Science, Inc., Uniondale, N.Y., U.S.A.), which reacts with both wild and mutant types of p53 proteins, at 1:75 dilution for 2 h at room temperature, using the Labelled Streptavidin Biotin (LSAB) method (Dakopatts, Glostrup, Dk) and diaminobenzidine as chromogen. p53 scoring was independently performed by three pathologists (A.P., R.C. and L.C.) using a standard light microscope equipped with an ocular reticle (x15) and a x40 objective. In each case, at least 1.000 tumour cells were counted from 10 selected areas, ensuring that the whole section was scanned. Only nuclear staining was evaluated. All the reactive nuclei were considered positive, regardless of the intensity of the staining, and the fraction of the stained nuclei was determined. Cases with more than 10% stained nuclei were scored as positive. The interobserver variation was less than 5%. Tumours of known p53 overexpression (i.e. high grade mammary carcinomas) were used as positive controls. Normal mouse serum was substituted for primary antibody as a negative control.

3.2. DNA Flow Cytometry

One hundred µm thick sections from paraffin embedded tissues were treated with propidium iodide according to Hedley et al. [(18)]. Twenty thousand events were acquired using a FACScan flow cytometer (Becton Dickinson Immunocytometry Systems, San Jose, CA, U.S.A.) with a 488 nm Argon ion laser, equipped with a doublet discrimination module and the Cell Fit program, version 2.0 (Becton Dickinson Immunocytometry Systems). Histograms were grouped as diploid and aneuploid according to the criteria previously reported [(7)].

3.3. AgNOR Staining and Scoring

Three µm thick sections from formalin fixed, paraffin embedded tissues were stained with the AgNOR method as previously described [(6)]. Random fields were independently examined by two pathologists (A.P. and R.C.), using a x100 oil immersion lens. At least 100 tumour epithelial cells were counted in each case, trying to separate individual NORs within clumps by optical sectioning, and the mean number of AgNORs per nucleus was calculated. The interobserver variation was less than 5%. An effective internal control was provided by the intermingling lymphocytes that on average have one single silver stained dot.

3.4. Statistical Analysis

Associations between p53 overexpression and thymoma clinicopathologic characteristics or DNA content were estimated by the Yates corrected chi-square. Association between p53 overexpression and AgNOR counts was assessed by one way analysis of variance (ANOVA). Univariate survival analysis were based on the Kaplan-Meier product-limit estimates of survival distribution. Differences between survival distributions were tested using the generalized Wilcoxon test. The relative importance of multiple prognostic factors on survival was estimated using the Cox proportional hazards regression model. All data were processed with BMDP statistical software (BMDP Statistical Software, Los Angeles, CA., U.S.A.). As a level of significance, P less than 0.05 was taken.

4. RESULTS

4.1. Distribution of p53 Immunoreactivity in Thymomas

p53 overexpression was detected in 48 cases (53.4%). The positivity of the DO7 monoclonal antibody was strictly confined to the nucleus of thymoma epithelial cells, in proportion that varied from case to case (Figs. 1 and 2), and between different areas within the same section. The staining showed some gradation in the intensity from nucleus to nucleus. Lymphocytes and stromal cells were unstained.

No association was found between p53 overexpression and thymoma clinicopathologic features, although p53 protein tended to be more frequently expressed in invasive (61.4%) than noninvasive cases (45.7%, p=0.19) and in DNA aneuploid (71.4%) than diploid cases (48.7%, p=0.15). A strong association was found between p53 immunostaining and AgNOR counts: p53 positive cases had higher AgNOR counts (6.34) than p53 negative thymomas (5.36, p=0.012). The results are summarized in Table 1.

4.2. Survival Analysis

At the time of analysis 27 (30%) patients had died of disease, and 63 (70%) were censored, with a mean follow-up for censored patients of 89 months. The overall 5 and 10 year survival rates were 75% and 67%, respectively. p53 overexpression was highly associated with prognosis: the 10 year survival rates were 83% for p53 negative vs. 52% for p53 positive cases (p=0.019) (Table 2 and Fig. 3). Significant association was also found between prognosis and AgNOR counts, DNA content, histological subtypes of the American classification, clinical stage and invasion, as previously reported [6,7].

The 10 year survival rates were 90% for cases with ≤5.58 AgNOR/cell vs. 44% for cases with >5.58 AgNOR/cell (p<0.0001); 73% for diploid vs. 38% for aneuploid cases (p=0.005); 87% for PL, 69% for MLE, 68% for S and 34% for PE thymomas (p=0.0006); 87% for stage I, 78% for stage II, 25% for stage III-IVa patients (p<0.0001); 87% for noninvasive vs. 44% for invasive cases (p=0.0001). A trend towards significance was found for the histological subtypes of the European classification: the 10 year survival rates were 72% for MixT, 68% for MT, 57% for PC and CT thymomas (p=0.13). Sex, age and myasthenia gravis were not associated with survival.

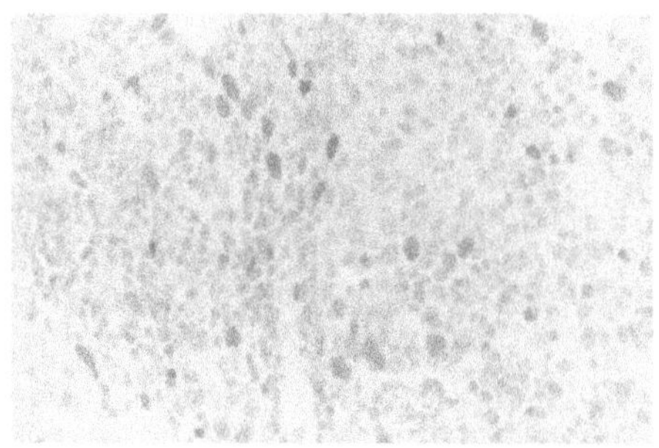

Figure 1. Predominantly cortical thymoma showing p53 expression in more than 10% neoplastic cells (positive case). LSAB immunoperoxidase method with light haematoxylin counterstain. Original magnification, x350.

Table 1. p53 expression and clinicopathologic features, DNA content, and AgNOR counts in thymoma

Variable	N	Positive cases (%)	Negative cases (%)	p
All series	90	48 (53.4)	42 (46.6)	
Sex				
M	40	23 (57.5)	17 (42.5)	
F	50	25 (50)	25 (50)	0.62
Age (yr)				
≤48.5	45	25 (55.6)	20 (44.4)	
>48.5	45	23 (51.1)	22 (48.9)	0.8
Histological type (American classification)				
S	11	4 (36.4)	7 (63.6)	
PL	35	17 (48.6)	18 (51.4)	0.31
MLE	22	12 (54.5)	10 (45.5)	
PE	22	15 (68.2)	7 (31.8)	
Histological type (European classification)				
MT	11	4 (36.4)	7 (63.6)	
MixT	53	26 (49.1)	27 (50.9)	0.22
PCT	7	5 (71.4)	2 (28.6)	
CT	19	13 (68.4)	6 (31.6)	
Clinical stage				
I	46	21 (45.7)	25 (54.3)	
II	19	11 (57.9)	8 (42.1)	0.48
III	13	8 (61.5)	5 (38.5)	
IVa	12	8 (66.7)	4 (33.3)	
Invasion				
Noninvasive	46	21 (45.7)	25 (54.3)	
Invasive	44	27 (61.4)	17 (38.6)	0.19
Myasthenia gravis				
Present	55	27 (49.1)	28 (50.9)	
Absent	35	21 (60)	14 (40)	0.42
DNA content				
Diploid	39	19 (48.7)	20 (51.3)	
Aneuploid	21	15 (71.4)	6 (28.6)	0.15
AgNOR counts				
mean ± SD	5.88±1.8	6.34±1.9	5.36±1.6	0.012*

S: spindle cell thymoma; PL: predominantly lymphocytic thymoma; MLE: mixed lymphoepithelial thymoma; PE: predominantly epithelial thymoma; MT: medullary thymoma; MixT: mixed corticomedullary thymoma; PCT: predominantly cortical thymoma; CT: cortical thymoma.

* One way analysis of variance (ANOVA)

Figure 2. Predominantly lymphocytic thymoma showing p53 expression in only two nuclei (negative case). LSAB immunoperoxidase method with light haematoxylin counterstain. Original magnification, x350.

Table 2. Correlation between p53 expression and survival in thymoma

Variable	N	5 year survival rates (%)	10 year survival rates (%)	p
All series	90	75	67	
p53 expression				
negative	42	86	83	0.019
positive	48	66	52	

When all the variables significant in the univariate analysis were introduced in the Cox model, only tumour stage (chi-square 22.8; $p<0.001$) and AgNOR counts (chi-square 6.8; $p=0.009$) retained independent prognostic significance (Table 3).

5. DISCUSSION

The main purpose of this work was to verify if p53 overexpression had a prognostic significance in thymoma. Indeed p53 overexpression was associated with a poor survival. This is in line with the findings reported for lung [13], gastric [12] and mammary carcinomas [14,15]. p53 accumulation was also related to cell proliferative activity in thymoma: indeed p53 positive cases had a very high AgNOR counts (6.34) as compared to the negative cases (5.36, $p=0.012$), in line with the reported association between p53 accumulation and S phase fraction [14,15]. Therefore, the combination of the loss of the cell-cycle regulatory function of the p53 protein (as indicated by p53 accumulation) and a rapid growth rate of tumour cells (as indicated by high AgNOR counts) may result in an aggressive thymoma phenotype with a poor survival. Surprisingly, a large number of p53 positive cases (21/46) was found in noninvasive stage I thymomas: this is in line with the high rate of p53 accumulation detected in mammary carcinoma in situ [19] and cervical intraepithelial neoplasia [20]. Hayashi et al [16] also found an elevated p53 overexpression in stage I-II thymomas. This suggests that in thymoma p53 mutations may occur early in the neoplastic process and may precede the development of tumours with a fully malignant and invasive phenotype. However, one must be aware that calculation of p53 overexpression by immunohistochemical means is far from being standardized, with variation in the antibodies used (CM-1, Pab 1801, Pab 421, Pab 240, DO7) which recognize various epitopes of p53 protein, and in criteria for calculating positive p53 staining, which may be based on the number of stained cells [20], the intensity of the positive nuclei [15] or the combination of number and intensity [14]. Furthermore, a wide intratumour heterogeneity of p53 expression was also detected in breast carcinomas [15]: however our counting system is highly representative, because it is based on a quantitative evaluation of p53 immunostaining in the whole specimen, regardless of the intensity of the staining.

The present study also confirms the role of traditional parameters, such as tumour invasion, clinical stage and histological pattern, in the assessment of prognosis in thy-

Table 3. Results of effective variables in multivariate analysis of thymomas. Cox model

Variable	Improvement chi-square	p value	R.R.
Clinical stage	22.8	<0.001	1.88
AgNOR counts	6.8	0.009	6.39

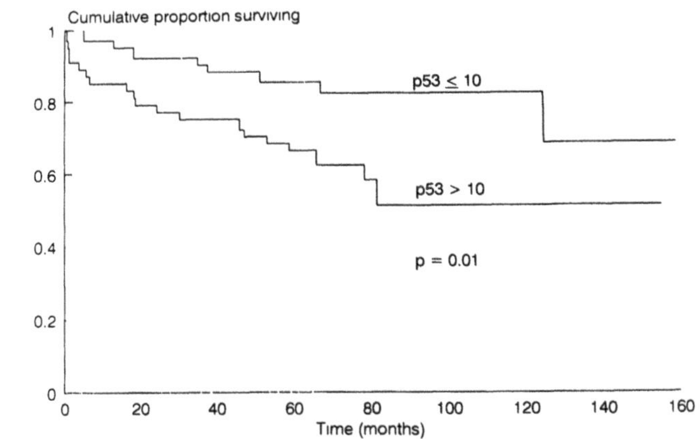

Figure 3. Kaplan-Meier survival curves for thymomas categorized according to the expression of p53 protein.

moma patients. In particular, tumour invasion was the most significant and independent prognostic factor, like in other large series [1–5]. We also found a prognostic relevance for the histological pattern, when the American classification system was applied, in line with the results of some investigators [1,4]. However, when the European classification was utilized, we only found a borderline significance. This is in contrast with Pescarmona et al. [8] and Quintanilla Martinez et al. [9] but in accordance with Dawson et al. [5]. The difference may depend on the low number of medullary types (11/90) and the high number (53/90) of mixed cortico-medullary thymomas in our series, or, more likely, on the intratumoural heterogeneity of thymoma histological pattern. This may account for the interobserver variation in tumour typing reported by Dawson et al. [5], and also suggests that a correct histological typing requires a careful and complete sampling of each resected specimen, the evaluation of numerous sections and precise criteria for the diagnosis.

Our study, which is based on the analysis of multiple parameters, also confirms the prognostic role of new factors, such as the tumour DNA content and cell proliferative activity. Aneuploid tumours had a shorter survival than diploid cases, in accordance with Davies et al. [10]. In particular, AgNOR counts, which are related to the cell proliferative and duplication activity [21], were the only independent prognostic factor in the multivariate analysis, besides tumour invasion . This is in line with the correlation between AgNOR counts and survival that has been reported in several human tumours [21]. Furthermore, AgNOR counts may be regarded as one of the best procedures for assessing the cell proliferative activity in lymphocyte rich tumours such as thymomas: in fact flow cytometry cannot reliably discriminate between proliferating epithelial cells and lymphocytes in paraffin embedded tissues, and the immunostaining of PCNA or MIB-1 reveals all the proliferative cells in thymoma, both reactive lymphocytes and tumour epithelial cells, which may be similar in size.

In conclusion, a traditional parameter (tumour invasion) and a more recent one (cell proliferative activity) appear the most significant and independent prognostic factors in thymoma. Tumour histology may have a prognostic role, provided that a complete sampling and a careful examination of each resected specimen is performed, and clearly established criteria are utilized for the diagnosis. p53 overexpression is associated with cell proliferative activity and patients survival, although it is not an independent prognostic factor. p53 overexpression occurs early in the neoplastic process and may be considered as an indicator of potential aggressiveness of the thymoma.

6. ACKNOWLEDGMENTS

This work was supported by grants from the Italian Ministero dell'Università e Ricerca Scientifica e Tecnologica (MURST 40% and 60%).

7. REFERENCES

1. Bernatz PE, Harrison EG, Clagett O: Thymoma: a clinicopathological study. J Thorac Cardiovasc Surg 42:424–44, 1961
2. Rosai J, Levine GD: Tumors of the thymus. In Atlas of Tumor Pathology, series 2, fascicle 13. Firminger HI (ed). Washington DC, Armed Forces Institute of Pathology, 1976
3. Masaoka A, Monden Y, Nakahara K, Tanioka T: Follow-up study of thymomas with special reference to their clinical stages. Cancer 48:2485–2492, 1981
4. Lewis JE, Wick MR, Scheithauer BW, Bernatz PE, Taylor WF: Thymoma. A clinicopathologic review. Cancer 60:2727–2743, 1987
5. Dawson A, Ibrahim NBN, Gibbs AR: Observer variation in the histopathological classification of thymoma: correlation with prognosis. J Clin Pathol 47:519–523, 1994
6. Pich A, Chiarle R, Chiusa L, Palestro G: Argyrophilic nucleolar organizer region counts predict survival in thymoma. Cancer 74:1568–1574, 1994
7. Pich A, Chiarle R, Chiusa L, Ponti R, Geuna M, Casadio C, Maggi G, Palestro G: Long-term survival of thymoma patients by histologic pattern and proliferative activity. Am J Surg Pathol 19:918–926, 1995
8. Pescarmona E, Rendina EA, Ricci C, Venuta F, Ruco LP, Baroni CD: The prognostic implication of thymoma histologic subtyping: a study of 80 cases. Am J Clin Pathol 93:190–195, 1990
9. Quintanilla-Martinez L, Wilkins EW, Choi N, Efird J, Hug E, Harris NL: Thymoma. Histologic Subclassification is an independent prognostic factor. Cancer 74:606–617, 1994
10. Davies SE, Macartney JC, Camplejohn RS, Morris RW, Ring NP, Corrin B: DNA flow cytometry of thymomas. Histopathology 15:77–83, 1989
11. Levine AJ, Momand J, Finlay CA: The p53 tumour suppressor gene. Nature 351:453–455, 1991
12. Martin HM, Filipe MI, Morris RW, Lane D, Silvestre F: p53 expression and prognosis in gastric carcinoma. Int J Cancer 50:859–862, 1992
13. Quinlan DC, Davidson AG, Summers CL, Warden HE, Doshi HM: Accumulation of p53 protein correlates with a poor prognosis in human lung cancer. Cancer Res 52:4828–4831, 1992
14. Allred DC, Clark GM, Elledge R, Fuqua SA, Brown RW, Chamness GC, Osborne CK, McGuire WL: Association of p53 protein expression with tumor cell proliferation rate and clinical outcome in node-negative breast cancer. J Natl Cancer Inst 85:200–206, 1993
15. Lipponen P, Ji H, Aaltomaa S, Syrjänen S, Syrjänen K: p53 protein expression in breast cancer as related to histopathological characteristics and prognosis. Int J Cancer 55:51–56, 1993
16. Hayashi Y, Ishii N, Obayashi C, Jinnai K, Hanioka K, Imai Y, Itoh H: Thymoma: tumour type related to expression of epidermal growth factor (EGF), EGF-receptor, p53, v-erb B and ras p21. Virchows Arch 426:43–50, 1995
17. Müller-Hermelink HK, Marino M, Palestro G. Pathology of thymic epithelial tumors. In The human thymus. Histophisiology and pathology. Current topics in pathology, Müller-Hermelink HK (ed). Berlin, Heidelberg, New York, Tokio, Springer-Verlag, 1986, vol 75: pp 207–268
18. Hedley DW, Friedlander ML, Taylor IW, Rugg CA, Musgrove EA: Method for analysis of cellular DNA content of paraffin-embedded pathologic material using flow cytometry. J Histochem Cytochem 31:1333–1335, 1983
19. Poller DN, Roberts EC, Bell JA, Elston CW, Blamey RW, Ellis IO: p53 protein expression in mammary ductal carcinoma in situ: relationship to immunohistochemical expression of estrogen receptor and c-erbB-2 protein. Hum Pathol 24:463–468, 1993
20. Bosari S, Roncalli M, Viale G, Bossi P, Coggi G: p53 immunoreactivity in inflammatory and neoplastic diseases of the uterine cervix. J Pathol 169:425–430, 1993
21. Derenzini M, Sirri V, Trerè D: Nucleolar organizer regions in tumor cells. Cancer J 7:71–77, 1994

9

METALLOTHIONEIN EXPRESSION IN THYMOMAS

A Tumor Marker for Spindle and Squamoid Thymoma Cells

Tseng-tong Kuo and Sin-Kai Lo

Departments of Pathology and Public Health
Chang Gung College of Medicine and Technology and Chang Gung Memorial Hospital
Kwei San, Tao Yuan, Taiwan

INTRODUCTION

Metallothioneins (MTs) are a group of low molecular weight and cysteine-rich intracellular proteins involved in metal homeostasis and detoxication.[1] Immunohistochemical expression of MT have been observed in certain normal tissues[1,2] and tumors with more aggressive clinical course and poor outcome.[1,3,4] MT expression in thymomas was studied to see if it can be used as a marker of the invasive potential of the thymomas.

MATERIALS AND METHODS

Immunohistochemical study of MT expression was performed on 27 noninvasive thymomas, 20 microinvasive thymomas, and 23 macroinvasive thymomas with formalin-fixed and paraffin-embedded tissues using avidin-biotin-peroxidase complex method with antibody E9 (Dako).

RESULTS AND DISCUSSION

Statistically significant difference in MT expression was found among the three groups of thymomas (p=0.020). However, MT expression was observed in both noninvasive and invasive thymomas. Analysis of MT expression according to the histologic types revealed that 8 of 9 spindle cell thymomas (medullary thymoma[5]), 1 of 11 small polygonal cell thymoma (predominantly cortical thymoma[5]), 3 of 13 mixed thymomas, 7 of 29 large polygonal cell thymomas (cortical thymoma[5]), and 7 of 8 squamoid thymomas (so-called

Epithelial Tumors of the Thymus, edited by Marx and Müller-Hermelink.
Plenum Press, New York, 1997

well differentiated thymic carcinoma[6]) significantly overexpressed MT. The strongest MT expression was observed in 6 spindle cell thymomas and 6 squamoid thymomas. The positive staining in other types of thymomas was mainly due to sporadic presence of spindle or squamoid thymoma cells or focal staining of marginal cells of the tumor nodules. Therefore, MT was overexpressed in both the least aggressive spindle cell thymoma and the aggressive squamoid thymoma. MT expression can not be used to distinguish invasive thymomas from noninvasive thymomas. Nevertheless, MT expression appears to be a tumor marker for the spindle and squamoid thymoma cells and can be helpful in the study of the classification of thymomas.

ACKNOWLEDGMENT

Supported by Grant NSC84–2331-B-182–089 from the National Science Council of the Republic of China and Chang Gung Medical Research Fund NMRP495.

REFERENCES

1. Cherian MG. The significance of the nuclear and cytoplasmic localization of metallothionein in human liver and tumor cells. Environ Health Perspect 1944; 102 suppl 3:131–135.
2. Danielson KG, Obi S, Huang PC. Immunochemical detection of metallothionein in specific epithelial cells of rat organs. Proc Natl Acad Sci (USA) 1982; 79:2301–2304.
3. Schmid KW, Ellis IO, Gee JMW, et al. Presence and possible significance of immunocytochemiscally demonstrable metallothionein over-expression in primary invasive ductal carcinoma of the breast. Virchows Arch A Pathol Anat 1993; 422:153–159.
4. Zelger B, Hittmair A, Schir M, et al. Immunohistochemically demonstrated metallothionein expression in malignant melanoma. Histopathol 1993; 23:257–264.
5. Marino M, Muller-Hermelink HK. Thymoma and thymic carcinoma. Relation of thymoma epithelial cells to the cortical and medullary differentiation of thymus. Virchows Arch A Pathol Anat Histopathol 1985; 407:119–149.
6. Kirchner T, Schalk B, Buchwald J, Ritter M, Marx A, Muller-Hermelink HK. Well differentiated thymic carcinoma: an organotypical low-grade carcinoma with relationship to cortical thymoma. Am J Surg Pathol 1992; 16:1153–1169.

10

CYTOKERATIN (CK) PROFILE IN THYMOMAS

CK 10 Is a Marker for Cortical Thymomas and CK 20 a Marker for Medullary Thymomas

J. P. Enoksson,[1] M. Albertsson,[2] A. Cervin,[2] K. Friström,[2] and L. Johansson[1]

[1]Department of Pathology
[2]Department of Oncology
Lund University Hospital, Sweden

1. ABSTRACT

Background

Thymomas are epithelial tumors that have a strong correlation to autoimmune disease. A classification that correlates with prognosis has been proposed. We classified 79 thymoma specimens and identified the CK immunophenotypes of these tumors.

Methods: 79 thymoma specimens from 64 patients were classified and studied immunohistologically using monoclonal antibodies for CK 7, 8, 10, 10/13, 17, 18, 19, 20 and CAM5.2 and MNF 116.

Results

There were 17 well differentiated carcinomas, 39 cortical thymomas, 7 predominantly cortical thymomas, 11 mixed thymomas and 5 medullary thymomas. All cases were immunoreactive with MNF 116, CAM5.2, CK 8 and 19 and most cases with CK 17 and 18. Most thymomas stained focally with CK 7, usually within perivascular cells or microcysts. CK 10 was almost exclusively found in Hassall's corpuscles in the well differentiated carcinomas and cortical thymomas but not in the other types. CK 20 was immunoreactive in singular cells in all medullary thymomas, but rarely in other types.

Epithelial Tumors of the Thymus, edited by Marx and Müller-Hermelink.
Plenum Press, New York, 1997

Conclusion

CK 10 is an excellent marker for Hassall's corpuscles and therefore also for cortical thymomas and well differentiated carcinomas. CK 20 seems to be a good marker for small cells, primarily in the medullary thymomas. CK 7 is primarily found in perivascular cells, and can be of use in future studies on the blood-thymus barrier. CAM5.2, MNF 116, CK 8 and CK 19 are excellent markers for the epithelial cells of all subtypes of thymomas.

2. INTRODUCTION

The most common epithelial tumors of the thymus - thymomas - have a strong correlation with autoimmune disease, i.e. myasthenia gravis. Histopathological classification of thymomas has long been based on the relation between the epithelial and the lymphoid components of the tumors[1]. However, correlation between this classification and clinical outcome as well as grade of malignancy has been difficult to obtain[2] and thus many researchers have suggested that the only prognostic factor of importance is invasion of the capsule[3].

At least six types of epithelial cells have been described in the thymus, of which three types are cortical and two medullary[4]. There is also a spindled epithelial cell, present in the perivascular spaces where it is thought to take part in the so-called blood-thymus barrier[5]. Cortical and medullary types are said to be of importance in the histogenesis of thymomas[6,7]. A classification based on these two types of epithelial cells has been proposed[7,8]. By separating thymomas into six different types, cortical, medullary, mixed common, predominantly cortical, predominantly medullary and well differentiated carcinoma, a better correlation with capsular invasion, metastasizing potential and autoimmune disease has been achieved[2,9].

Immunohistochemical methods are useful in a number of diagnostic situations, e.g. to differentiate epithelia from mesenchyme and classify hematological disorders. As for thymomas, antibodies to subset of lymphocytes (CD antibodies) and CK have been used in several studies[10,11]. There are 20 different CK:s[12], whereof CK 20 recently was identified[13,14]. In this study we report the cytokeratin phenotype of 79 thymomas classified according to Marino and Müller-Hermelink and Kirchner and Müller-Hermelink. We utilized monospecific antibodies to CK 7, 8, 10, 10/13, 17, 18, 19 and 20 and the widely used CK antibodies MNF 116 and CAM5.2.

3. MATERIAL AND METHODS

The material consists of 79 histological specimens from 64 patients with thymomas operated, usually with total thymectomy, at the University Hospital in Lund, Sweden, during the period 1980–1994. Slides were cut from formaline-fixed and paraffin-embedded blocks and stained with hematoxylin-eosin. The tumors were classified as medullary thymoma, predominantly medullary thymoma, cortical thymoma, predominantly cortical thymoma, mixed thymoma and well-differentiated carcinoma.

For the immunohistochemical examination slides were cut from formaline-fixed and paraffin-embedded blocks. All slides were stained in an automatic immunostainer TechMate 500 with DAKO ChemMate Detection Kit peroxidase/DAB (antibodies and dilu-

Table 1. Antibodies and dilutions

Antibody	Dilution	Enzyme	Manufacturer
CAM5.2	1:10	Yes	Becton & Dickinson
MNF 166	1:100	Yes	DAKO A/S, Copenhagen
CK 7	1:50	Yes	DAKO A/S, Copenhagen
CK 8	1:50	Yes	DAKO A/S, Copenhagen
CK 10	1:50	No	DAKO A/S, Copenhagen
CK 10/13	1:100	No	DAKO A/S, Copenhagen
CK 17	1:5	Yes	DAKO A/S, Copenhagen
CK 18	1:2	Yes	DAKO A/S, Copenhagen
CK 19	1:50	Yes	DAKO A/S, Copenhagen
CK 20	1:20	Yes	DAKO A/S, Copenhagen

tions are given in table 1). As enzyme was used ChemMate Proteinase K (intended for use with TechMate 500). The staining was scored 0–3 (absent, weak, moderate, strong). It was noted whether the staining was general or focal (< 50 % tumor cells positive), confined to cells within specific regions (in Hassall's corpuscles, in cells lining microcysts or vessels) or to singular cells.

The antibody for CK 10/13 gave unreproducable results and it was thus omitted from the study.

4. RESULTS

4.1. Well-Differentiated Carcinomas

There were 17 well-differentiated carcinoma, composed of almost exclusively large, irregular epithelial cells with bloated nuclei with coarse chromatin structure and prominent nucleoli. Mitoses were easily seen. The epithelial cells regularly palisaded around perivascular spaces and microcysts. Lymphocytes were sparse or totally absent. Occasionally, Hassall's corpuscles were seen. The result of the immunohistochemical examination is given in table 2.

Table 2. Well-differentiated carcinomas

	n pos	%	~/N	~/pos	F	S	C	H	PC
MNF 116	17	100	3	3					
CAM5.2	17	100	2,7	2,7	1				
CK 7	16	94	2,8	3	8	1	3	1	5
CK 8	17	100	2,3	2,3	1				
CK 10	9	53	1,6	3	2	2		5	
CK 17	17	100	2,5	2,4	7	2	3	2	4
CK 18	16	94	1,7	1,8	3		2		3
CK 19	17	100	2,8	2,8	1				
CK 20	5	29	0,5	1,8	1	4			

Notes: ~/N = Average staining intensity of all tumors; ~/pos = Average staining intensity of all positive tumors; F=Focal < 50% positive tumor cells; H = Hassall's corpuscle; S = Staining in singular cells; C = Cells lining cystic spaces within the tumor; PC = Perivascular cells.

Table 3. Cortical thymomas

	n pos	%	~/N	~/pos	F	S	C	H	PC
MNF 116	39	100	2,8	2,8					1
CAM5.2	39	100	2,5	2,4	2			1	2
CK 7	35	90	2,1	2,3	14	1	2	5	4
CK 8	39	100	2,2	2,2	1				2
CK 10	17	44	1,2	2,8	1	4		11	1
CK 17	36	92	2,3	2,5	18	4	2	5	4
CK 18	31	79	1,6	2	11	8		2	5
CK 19	39	100	2,7	2,7				1	1
CK 20	10	26	0,5	1,9		8		2	

Notes: ~/N=Average staining intensity of all tumors; ~/pos=Average staining intensity of all positive tumors; F=Focal < 50% positive tumor cells; H=Hassall's corpuscle; S=Staining in singular cells; C=Cells lining cystic spaces within the tumor; PC=Perivascular cells.

4.2. Cortical Thymomas

There were 39 cortical thymomas, composed of large, oval cells with pale cytoplasm and large, oval nuclei with one prominent nucleolus. The histology ranged from a starry-sky pattern, with cortical cells dispersed on a dense background of lymphocytes, to a pattern with clusters of epithelial cells and less lymphocytes. A lobular growth with interspersing fibrous septa were regularly seen. Hassall's corpuscles were often seen in small areas of medullary differentiation in conjunction with remnants of normal thymus. The result of the immunohistochemical examination is given in table 3.

4.3. Predominantly Cortical Thymomas

There were 7 predominantly cortical thymomas. Histologically these tumors showed large areas of widely dispersed cortical cells, reminiscent of the normal thymic cortex, and areas of cells assuming the characteristics of cortical, medullary or intermediate cell types. The cortical cells had pale cytoplasm and round to oval-shaped nuclei with a prominent nucleolus. To be designated as a predominantly cortical thymoma the tumor had to be composed of at least 50% of the component reminiscent of normal thymus. The result of the immunohistochemical examination is given in table 4.

Table 4. Predominantly cortical thymomas

	n pos	%	~/N	~/pos	F	S	C	H	PC
MNF 116	7	100	3	3					
CAM5.2	7	100	2,7	2,7	2				1
CK 7	6	71	1,7	2,4	1				1
CK 8	7	100	1,7	1,7	1				
CK 10	0	0	0	0					
CK 17	7	100	2,3	2,3	4				1
CK 18	7	100	2,4	2,4	1	2			1
CK 19	7	100	2,7	2,7					
CK 20	2	29	2	2		2			

Notes: ~/N = Average staining intensity of all tumors; ~/pos = Average staining intensity of all positive tumors; F=Focal < 50% positive tumor cells; H = Hassall's corpuscle; S = Staining in singular cells; C = Cells lining cystic spaces within the tumor; PC = Perivascular cells.

Table 5. Mixed thymomas

	n pos	%	~/N	~/pos	F	S	C	H	PC
MNF 116	11	100	3	3					
CAM5.2	11	100	2,6	2,6	1				
CK 7	9	82	2,2	2,7	2	1	2		2
CK 8	11	100	2,5	2,5	2				
CK 10	1	9	0,2	2		1			
CK 17	11	100	2,2	2	5	1	1		1
CK 18	11	100	2,5	2,2	3	1	2		2
CK 19	11	100	3	3					
CK 20	0	0	0	0					

Notes: ~/N=Average staining intensity of all tumors; ~/pos=Average staining intensity of all positive tumors; F=Focal < 50% positive tumor cells; H=Hassall's corpuscle; S=Staining in singular cells; C=Cells lining cystic spaces within the tumor; PC=Perivascular cells.

4.4. Mixed Thymomas

There were 11 mixed thymomas. They could generally be divided into two groups: one with separate areas of differentiation, cortical or medullary, and one with cells assuming characteristics of both medullary, cortical and intermediate types. In the cortical areas of some tumors, delicate fibrous septa were seen. The result of the immunohistochemical examination is given in table 5.

4.5. Medullary Thymomas

There were 2 medullary thymomas, mainly composed of spindleshaped cells arranged in a storiform pattern with nuclei showing homogeneous chromatin and inconspicuous nucleoli. Few lymphocytes were seen. Hassall's corpuscles were absent and cortical differentiation was not seen. There were 3 predominantly medullary thymomas. In these tumors there were scattered areas with cortical differentiation in a mainly medullary cell population. The cortical areas often resembled the benign cortex of the thymus; no mitoses were seen.

As there were few cases of medullary and predominantly medullary thymomas they were all classified as medullary thymomas. The result of the immunohistochemical examination is given in table 6.

Table 6. Medullary thymomas

	n pos	%	~/N	~/pos	F	S	C	H	PC
MNF 116	5	100	3	3					
CAM5.2	5	100	3	3					
CK 7	5	100	3	3					2
CK 8	5	100	2,4	2,4					
CK 10	1	20	0,6	3		1			
CK 17	5	100	2	2	2				
CK 18	5	100	2,4	2,4					
CK 19	5	100	2,6	2,6					
CK 20	5	100	2	2		5			

Notes: ~/N = Average staining intensity of all tumors; ~/pos = Average staining intensity of all positive tumors; F=Focal < 50% positive tumor cells; H=Hassle's corpuscle; S=Staining in singular cells; C=Cells lining cystic spaces within the tumor; PC=Perivascular cells.

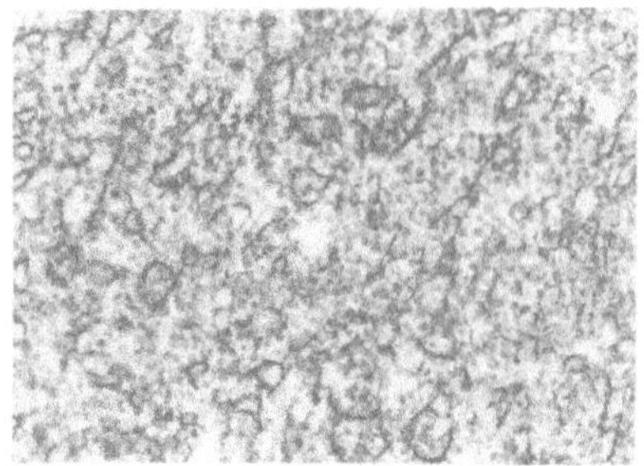

Figure 1. Photomicrograph showing general staining with MNF 116 in a cortical thymoma. X400.

5. DISCUSSION

Reports of CK:s in thymomas and in normal thymus are relatively sparse. Two studies of rat thymus[15,16] have identified several cytokeratin phenotypes. Cortical cells were immunoreactive only with CK 8 and 18 while subcapsular/perivascular cells, together with a subset of medullary cells, were immunoreactive with CK 7, 8 and 19. In the medullary cells four different subsets were identified showing various combinations of CK 8, 10, 18 and 19. In postnatal human thymus, KB-37, a marker of squamous basal cells, as well as CK 13, 14 and 19, stained the subcapsular epithelium[17]. CK 8, 18 and 19 stained cortical cells while CK 19 also stained stellate medullary cells. Most medullary cells were also positive with CK 13, 14 and 17. In singular and in groups of cells around the Hassall's corpuscles immunoreactivity for CK 8 and 18 was found. The outermost cells of Hassall's corpuscles reacted with CK 19 and KB-37. Peripherally in Hassall's corpuscles simple epithelium CK:s (7, 8, 18) and stratified nonkeratinizing epithelia CK:s (4, 13, 14, 17) were co-expressed with CK 10/11. The central parts of Hassall's corpuscles, however, were almost exclusively positive with CK 10/11.

In our study the routinely used CK antibodies CAM5.2 and MNF 116 (Fig 1), and the monospecific antibodies for CK 8 and 19 (Fig 2), were immunoreactive with the epithelial cells of all thymomas as well as all normal thymus tissue.

Antibodies to CK 7 stained the majority of the tumors (Fig 3), mainly in a focal pattern. The immunoreactivity was found in perivascular cells and in microcysts, but also in occasional Hassall's corpuscles. Immunoreactivity for CK 7 has also been described in cells lining perivascular spaces in rat thymus[15]. Perivascular cells ensheathe vessels in a way analogous to the oligodendroglia of the nervous system and hypothetically form part of the blood-thymus barrier[5].

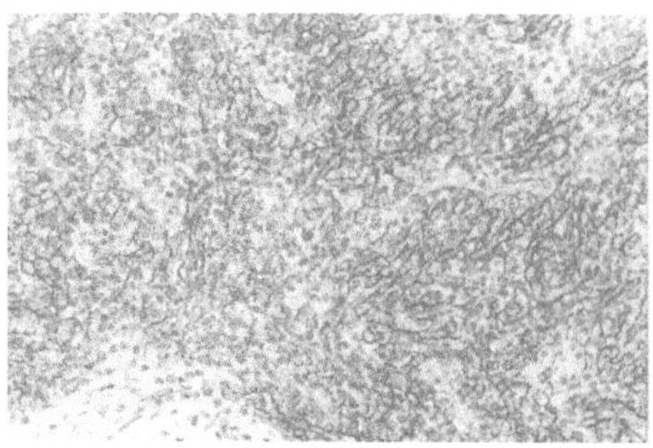

Figure 2. Photomicrograph showing mixed thymoma immunoreactive with CK 19. X400.

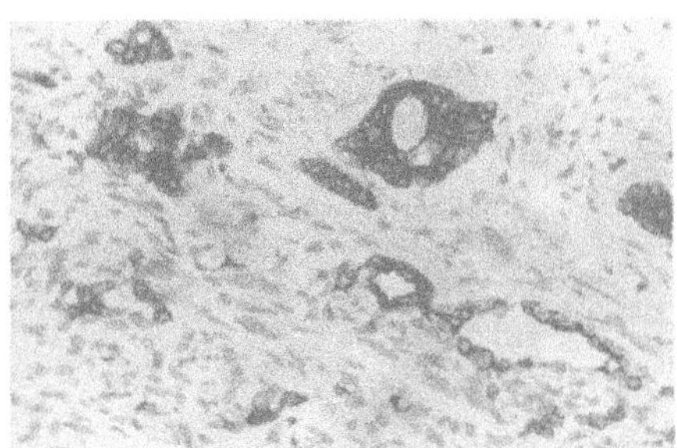

Figure 3. Photomicrograph. Perivascular cells immunoreactive with CK 7 in a medullary thymoma. X400.

CK 17 and 18 stained virtually all tumors, however usually in a focal pattern. In the well differentiated carcinomas, CK 17 and CK 18 were identified in singular cells, microcysts and Hassall's corpuscles. As the distribution of CK 17 and 18 was highly variable no general conclusions can be drawn.

In our study the antibody for CK 10, a highly specialized CK normally found in keratinized epithelia, showed a remarkable affinity for the epithelial cells of Hassall's corpuscles (Fig 4). It thus stained 11 of the cortical thymomas and 5 of the well differentiated carcinomas. Hassall's corpuscles were absent in the predominantly cortical thymomas, the mixed thymomas and the medullary thymomas, and staining for CK 10 was only found in scattered, singular cells. CK 10 has previously been found in epithelial cells of the thymus[15] and in Hassall's corpuscles[16,17]. Since Hassall's corpuscles are highly specialized medullary structures, our results suggest that Hassall's corpuscles are present in cortical thymomas and well differentiated carcinomas because they are not a part of the neoplastic process in these tumors. This supports the theory of different embryological origins for cortical and medullary cells[4].

CK 20, mainly found in intestinal epithelium, gastric foveolar epithelium, the urothelium and Merkel cells, was recently identified[13,14]. It is not only found in carcinomas derived from these locals, but also in carcinomas of the bile duct, gall bladder, hepar and pancreatic ducts, where CK 20 normally is not found. CK 20 was also identified in reticulum cells of the thymus[14]. However, these data were only presented in a table, but not commented upon in the text. We found CK 20 in small, singular cells (Fig 5) in all the medullary thymomas, but only in about 30% of the other types.

It has been shown that the normal epithelium of the oral cavity and the bronchial epithelium, both foregut-derived, lack CK 20 expression, but that taste buds and Merkel cells of the oral cavity show strong expression of CK 20[14]. This suggests that the thymic cells reacting with CK 20 may not be derived from the normal epithelial cells of the

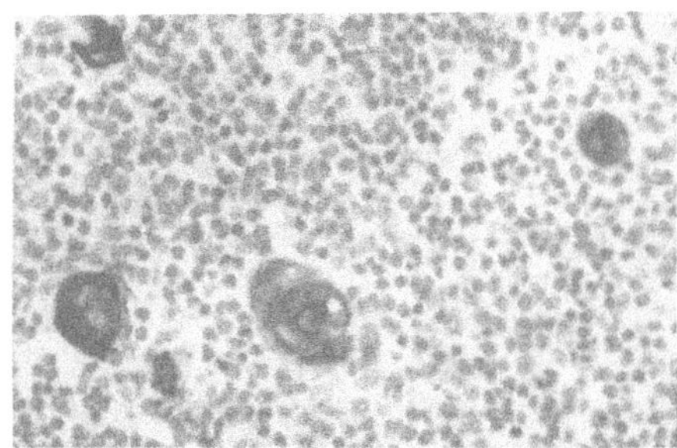

Figure 4. Photomicrograph showing staining for CK 10 in Hassall's corpuscles in a cortical thymoma. X400.

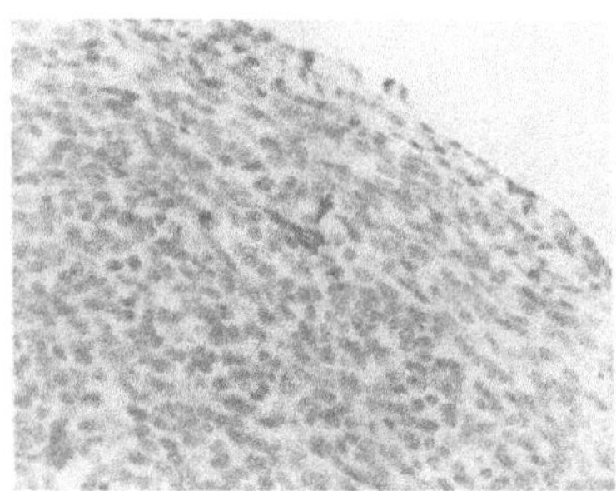

Figure 5. Photomicrograph. Staining for CK 20 in a singular, dendritic cell (arrow) in a medullary thymoma. X 1000.

foregut, but indeed from Merkel cells. A few studies have proposed the neuroectoderm as a contributor to the thymus anlage[18], making it possible for the thymic cells to be neuroectodermal in origin. However, most authors think the embryological origin of cortical and medullary cells to be separate[4]. As the CK 20 positive cells mainly are found in medullary thymomas, the cells may be derived from a distinct region of the third or fourth pharyngeal pouches.

Conclusively, CK 10 was identified in Hassall's corpuscles in cortical thymomas and well differentiated carcinomas. CK 20 was identified in small, singular cells in all the medullary thymomas. CK 7 was mainly distributed in perivascular cells. The cytokeratin antibodies CAM5.2 and MNF 116, as well as CK 8 and 19, are all excellent markers for the eptithelial cells of the thymomas and the normal thymus.

REFERENCES

1. Rosai J, Levine GD. Tumors of the thymus. In: Atlas of tumor pathology, 2nd series, fascicle 13. Armed Forces Institute of Pathology, 1976. Washington.
2. Pescarmona E. Rendina EA, Venuta F, Ricci C, Ruco LP, Baroni CD. The prognostic implication of thymoma histologic subtyping: A study of 80 consecutive cases. Am J Clin Pathol. 1990:93(2):190–195.
3. Lewis JE, Wick MR, Scheithauer BW et al. Thymoma: A clinicopathological review. Cancer. 1987;60:2727–2743.
4. Kornstein MJ. Pathology of the thymus and mediastinum. Vol 33 in the series Major Problems in Pathology. WB Saunders, Philadelphia 1995.
5. Kendall MD. The morphology of perivascular spaces in the thymus. Thymus. 1989;13:157–164.
6. Müller-Hermelink HK, Marino M, Palestro G, Schumacher U, Kirchner T. Immunohistological evidence of cortical and medullary differentiation in thymoma. Virchows Arch A Pathol Anat Histopathol. 1985;408:143–161
7. Marino M, Müller-Hermelink HK. Thymoma and thymic carcinoma. Relation of thymoma epithelial cells to the cortical and medullary differentiation of the thymus. Virchows Arch A Pathol Anat Histopathol. 1985;407:119–49.
8. Kirchner T, Müller-Hermelink HK. New approaches to the diagnosis of thymic epithelial tumors. Prog Surg Pathol. 1989;10:167–189.
9. Quintanilla-Martinez L, Wilkins EW Jr, Choi N, Efird J, Hug E, Harris NL. Thymoma. Histologic subclassification is an independent prognostic factor. Cancer. 1994;74:606–617.
10. Kirchner T, Schalke B, Buchwald J, Ritter M, Marx A, Müller-Hermelink HK. Well differentiated thymic carcinoma: an organotypical low-grade carcinoma with relationship to cortical thymoma. Am J Surg Pathol. 1992:16;1153–1169.
11. Fukai L, Masaoka A, Hashimoto T, Yamakawa Y, Mizuno T, Tanamura O. Cytokeratins in normal thymus and thymic epithelial tumors. Cancer. 1993;71:99–105.
12. Moll R. Molecular diversity of cytokeratins: significance for cell and tumor differentiation. Acta Histochem Suppl. 1991;41:117–127.

13. Moll R, Schiller DL, Franke WW. Identification of protein IT of the intestinal cytoskeleton as a novel type I cytokeratin with unusual properties and expression pattern. J Cell Biol. 1990;111:567 580.
14. Moll R, Löwe A, Laufer J, Franke WW. Cytokeratin 20 in human carcinomas: a new histodiagnostic marker detected by monoclonal antibodies. Am J Pathol. 1992;140:427–447.
15. Colic M, Jovanovic S, Mitrovic S, Dujic A. Immunohistochemical identification of six cytokeratin-defined subsets of the rat thymic epithelial cells. Thymus. 1989;13:175–85.
16. Colic M, Jovanovic S, Vasiljevski M, Dujic A. Ontogeny of thymic epithelium defined by monoclonal anti-cytokeratin antibodies. Dev Comp Immunol. 1990;1:67–75.
17. Shezen E, Okon E, Ben Hur H, Abramsky O. Cytokeratin expression in human thymus: Immunohistochemical mapping. Cell Tissue Res. 1995 ;279:221–231.
18. Kuratani S, Bockman DE. Impaired development of the thymic primordium after neural crest ablation. Anat Rec. 1990;228:185–190.

11

NEUROENDOCRINE DIFFERENTIATION IN THYMIC EPITHELIAL TUMORS

Immunohistochemical Studies

Tsunekazu Hishima,[1*] Masashi Fukayama,[2] Yukiko Hayashi,[1] Takeshi Fujii,[2] Katsumi Arai,[1] Yumiko Shiozawa,[1] Nobuaki Funata,[1] and Morio Koike[1]

[1]Department of Pathology
Tokyo Metropolitan Komagome Hospital
[2]Department of Pathology
Jichi Medical School
Tochigi, Japan

The classification of thymic epithelial tumors is an issue of some controversy[1]. Müller-Helmelink et al. proposed a scheme based on the morphological differences of normal thymic epithelial cells: i.e., cortical or medullary[2]. While their proposed classification is theoretical, it has been successfully applied to thymic epithelial tumors without cellular atypia. However, the morphology of thymic epithelial tumors with cellular atypia is considerably different than that of their normal counterparts. Recently we found that the CD5 molecule, which is authentically expressed in T-lymphocytes and some B-lymphocytes, is expressed in thymic carcinoma and atypical thymoma[3].

In the present study, we extended our observation to neuroendocrine (NE) tumor of the thymus, and also evaluated the range of neuroendocrine differentiation in non-NE CD5(+) and CD5(-) thymic tumors by immunohistochemical and ultrastructural techniques.

I. HISTOLOGICAL CLASSIFICATION (TABLE 1)

Thirty-three cases of thymic epithelial tumors were tentatively divided into four groups based on the histological diagnoses of three pathologists: thymic carcinoid (n=8), thymic carcinoma (n=8), thymoma (n=12), and atypical thymoma (n=5).

* Correspondence: Tsunekazu Hishima, Department of Pathology, Tokyo Metropolitan Komagome Hospital, 3-18-22 Honkomagome, Bunkyo-ku, Tokyo 113, Japan.

Epithelial Tumors of the Thymus, edited by Marx and Müller-Hermelink.
Plenum Press, New York, 1997

Table 1. 33 cases of thymic epithelial tumors

	Subtype	Number of Cases
Thymic carcinoid		8
Thymic carcinoma	SCC [1]	8
Atypical thymoma		5
Thymoma	Ep [2]	5
	Mx [3]	7

[1] SCC: Squamous cell carcinoma
[2] Ep: Predominantly epithelial thymoma
[3] Mx: Mixed epithelial-lymphocytic thymoma

Atypical thymoma, which we used in this study to describe tumors of intermediate morphology, was defined, when the diagnoses were different among three pathologists, or when it was difficult to determine whether the tumor was thymic carcinoma or thymoma.

All of the thymic carcinomas were squamous cell carcinoma with moderate to poor differentiation. Twelve thymomas consisted of 5 predominantly epithelial thymomas and 7 mixed epithelial-lymphocytic thymomas.

II. CD5 EXPRESSION (TABLE 2)

To determine the differences between the cellular phenotypic characteristics of thymic epithelial tumors, immunohistochemical analysis with lymphocyte markers (CD1a, 3, 4, 5, 8, 10, 20, 21, 25, 30, 57 and 72) was performed. Among the surface-antigens examined, lymphocyte markers expressed in the epithelial cells of the thymus were CD10 (J5), CD57 (Leu7) and CD5 (Leu1 and UCHT2). CD10 was detected in epithelial cells in 2 of 8 thymic carcinomas, 2 of 5 atypical thymomas, and 2 of 12 thymomas. Immunostaining with anti-CD 57 MAb showed intense positivity only in one case of thymoma. On the

Table 2. Expression of lymphocyte markers

	Epithelial component	Lymphoid component	
	CD5	TdT	OKT6
Thymic carcinoid	0/3	0/1	0/1
Thymic carcinoma	8/8	0/8	1/8
Atypical thymoma	2/5	2/5	3/5
Thymoma	0/12	9/12	8/12

Number of positive cases / number of examined cases

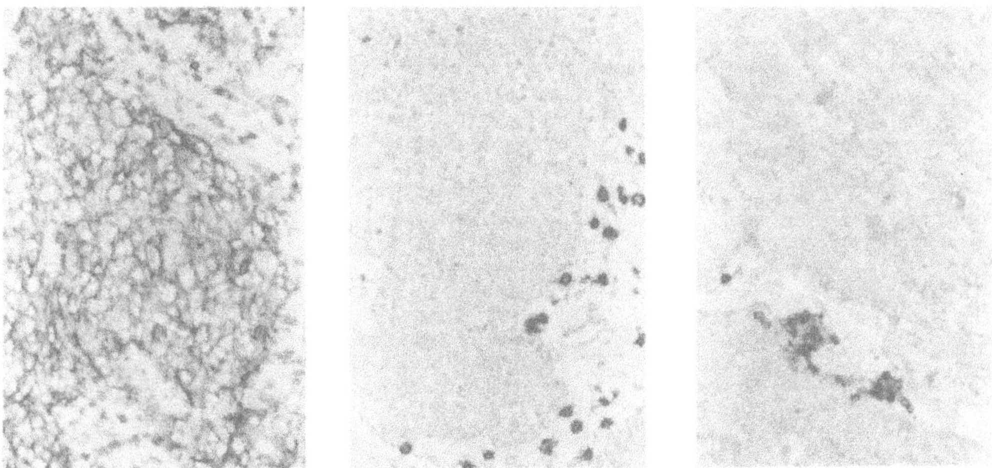

Figure 1. Immunostaining for CD5 (Leu1). The vast majority of epithelial cells and infiltrating lymphocytes were immunostained for CD5 in thymic carcinoma (*left*). CD5 is identified in infiltrating lymphocytes, but not in epithelial cells of thymic carcinoid (*center*) or thymoma (*right*).

other hand, CD5, a type of receptor molecule that signals cell growth in T-cells, was expressed in neoplastic epithelial cells of the thymus, in thymic carcinoma (8 of 8) and atypical thymoma(2 of 5), but not in thymoma (none of 12) and thymic carcinoid (none of 4) (Figure 1). Positive staining appeared diffusely at the cell membrane. Pan B-cell marker CD72, which is the ligands for CD5, was not found in the epithelial cells.

As previous reported5, infiltrating lymphocytes in thymic carcinoma and thymic carcinoid showed a CD1a (OKT6) (-) and TdT (-) mature T-cell phenotype, whereas there was an infiltration of CD1a (OKT6) (+) and TdT (+) immature T-cells in thymoma.

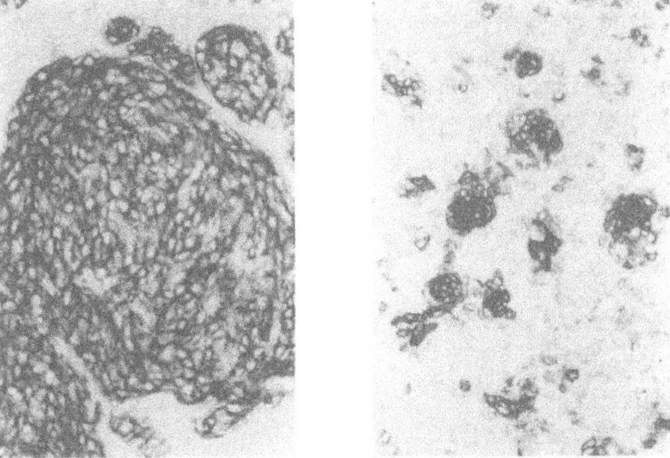

Figure 2. Immunostaining for Goa. Diffuse surface reactivity for Goa is found in thymic carcinoid (*left*) and cells positive for Goa is also detected in CD5(+) tumor (atypical thymoma) (*right*), but moderate in number.

Table 3. Antibody reagents

Antibody	Clonality	Source
Neuroendocrine markers		
Synaptophysin	monoclonal	Boehringer Mannheim
Synaptophysin	polyclonal	DAKO
Goα [1]	polyclonal	MBL
BASCA [2](NCAM)	monoclonal	Dr Kameya T
Hormonal markers		
hCGα [3]	polyclonal	Dr Okumura H
hCGβ [4]	polyclonal	Dr Okumura H
ACTH [5]	polyclonal	DAKO
Calcitonin	polyclonal	DAKO
CGRP [6]	polyclonal	MILAB
GRP [7]	polyclonal	Dr Yanaihara N
Serotonin	polyclonal	Immunonuclear Corporation
Somatostatin	polyclonal	DAKO

[1] Goα: GTP binding protein Goα subunit
[2] BASCA: brain-associated small-cell lung cancer antigen
[3] hCGα: human chorionic gonadotropin α–subunit
[4] hCGβ: human chorionic gonadotropin β–subunit
[5] ACTH: adrenocorticotropic hormone
[6] CGRP: calcitonin gene-related peptide
[7] GRP: gastrin-releasing peptide

III. NEUROENDOCRINE DIFFERENTIATION

In this study, we reclassified 33 thymic epithelial tumors into 8 thymic carinoids, 10 CD5(+) tumors, and 15 CD5(-) tumors, and evaluated neuroendocrine features by immunohistochemistry. Table 3 lists the antibodies for NE cells (synaptophysin, GTP binding protein Goa subunit; Goa, and neuronal adhesion molecule; NCAM) and against various hormonal substances. Immunohistochemical results are summarised in Table 4. All of the thymic carcinoids showed diffuse and intense immunoreacrivity for the three NE markers. Most tumor cells exhibited cytoplasmic staining for synaptophysin, with either monoclonal or polyclonal antibodies, and staining on their surface membrane for Goa and NCAM (Fig. 2A). In other thymic tumors, cells that were positive for NE cell markers were much more frequently detected in CD5(+) tumors than in CD5(-) tumors, but small to moderate in number (Fig. 2B). Immunoreactivity for at least one of the three NE markers was observed in 8 of 10 CD5(+) tu-

Table 4. Expression of neuroendocrine markers

	Synaptphysin	Go α	NCAM	Total #
Thymic carcinoid	8/ 8(100)	8/ 8(100)	3/ 3(100)	8/ 8(100)
CD5(+) tumor	7/10 (70)	6/10 (60)	6/10 (60)	8/10 (80)
CD5(-) tumor	2/15 (13)	1/15 (8)	1/ 8 (13)	2/15 (13)

Number of positive cases / number of examined cases (%)
#Total: at least one of three neuroendocrine markers is positive

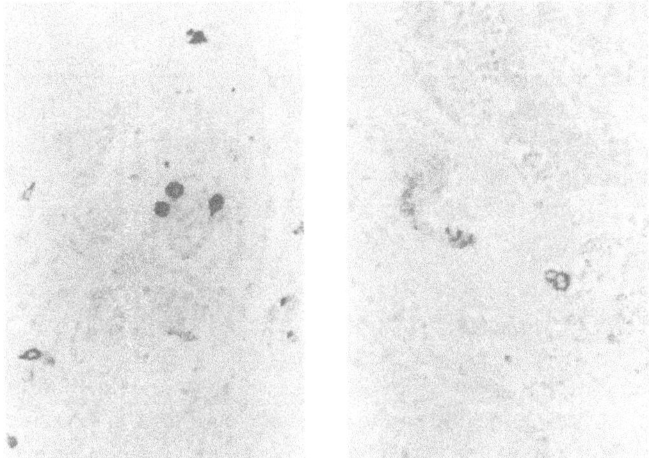

Figure 3. Immunostaining hormonal markers. Scattered cells positive for hCGa in thymic carcinoid (*left*) and a few cells positive for ACTH in CD5(+) tumor (thymic carcinoma) (*right*) are identified.

mors (80%; 6 thymic carcinomas and 2 atypical thymomas), but in only 2 of 15 CD5(-) tumors (13%; one atypical thymoma and one thymoma). The frequencies of positivity for synaptophysin, Goa, and NCAM were significantly different between CD5(+) tumors and CD5(-) tumors ($p<0.01$, $p<0.01$, and $p<0.05$, respectively).

IV. EXPRESSION OF HORMONAL MARKERS (TABLE 5)

Immunohistochemical analysis of 8 thymic carcinoids disclosed the intracytoplasmic presence of human chorionic gonadotropin a-subunit (hCGa) in all cases, human chorionic gonadotropin b-subunit (hCGb) in 3 cases, adrenocorticotropic hormone (ACTH) in 3 cases, calcitonin in 2 cases, calcitonin gene- related peptide (CGRP) in 2 cases, and serotonin in one case (Figure 3A). Cells positive for these hormonal products were few in number, but scattered throughout the tumor.

In CD5(+) tumors in which cells positive for synaptophysin and Goa were identified, only a few ACTH- or hCGa-positive cells were identified in one case and 3 cases, respectively (Figure 3B). None of the cells in any of the CD5(-) tumors were positive for any hormonal substance, including two cases with cells positive for general NE markers.

Table 5. Expression of hormonal markers

	hCGα	hCGβ	ACTH	Calcitonin	CGRP	Serotonin
Thymic carcinoid	8/ 8	3/ 8	3/ 8	2/ 8	2/ 8	1/ 8
CD5(+) tumor	3/10	0/10	1/10	0/10	0/10	0/10
CD5(-) tumor	0/15	0/15	0/15	0/15	0/15	0/15

Number of positive cases / number of examined cases

All the other markers examined were negative.

V. DENSE-CORE GRANULES

Ultrastructurally, numerous dense-core granules (DCG) from 90 to 300 nm in diameter were found within the cytoplasm of all 4 thymic carcinoids. In non-NE tumors, rare DCG from 120 to 400 nm in diameter were sparsely distributed throughout 12 of the 13 tumors examined, including 5 cases which did not contain NE cells immunohistochemically. It was difficult to determine whether these DCG were secretory granules or small lysosomes by routine electrone microscopy.

VI. MULTIDIRECTIONAL DIFFERENTIATION

While investigating the phenotypic differences in thymic epithelial tumors, we found that CD5, a type of receptor molecule on the lymphocyte surface, is expressed by neoplastic epithelial cells of thymic carcinoma and some thymoma with cellular atypia[3]. In the present study, we sought to extend this observation to tumor with NE differentiation (i.e., thymic carcinoid). CD5 expression is not observed in thymic carcinoid or typical thymoma, which is also a differentiated tumor in which normal thymic epithelial cells can induce the infiltration of immature T-lymphocytes within the tumor[5]. In a preliminary study, we found that some epithelial cells in the fetal thymus showed CD5-immunoreactivity by immunoelectron-microscopy (unpublished observation). Therefore, CD5 in neoplastic thymic epithelial cells might be a fetal phenotype, which is mostly expressed in the immature form. The phenomenon known as a multidirectional differentiation is based on the capability of neoplastic cells to follow various lines of differentiation which reflect those of the normal counterpart, e.g., epithelial stem cells from which the carcinoma is derived[6]. NE differentiation is considered as a good example of this phenomenon and has been reported in various non-NE carcinomas of many organs. In the present study using immunohistochemical tequniques, NE differentiation occurred frequently in CD5(+) tumors, but not in CD5(-) tumors. Furthermore, the strong correlations among CD5-expression, cellular atypism, and multidirectional differentiation suggest that CD5(+) thymic tumor may be derived from totipotential stem cells of thymic epithelium, whereas other differentiated CD5(-) tumors may be derived from more specifically committed cells to either NE cells or functional epithelial cells of the thymus (Figure 4).

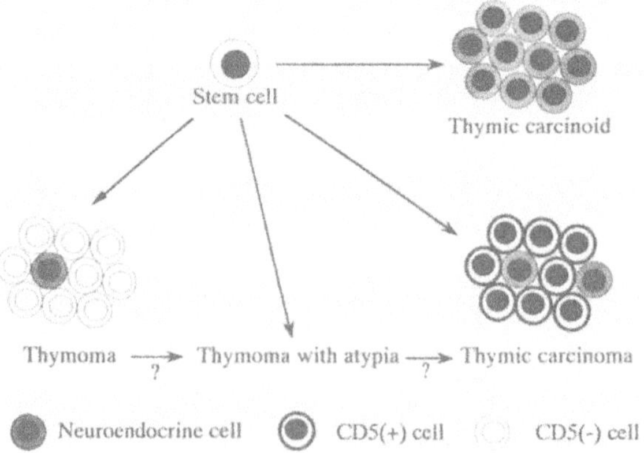

Figure 4. Schematic diagram of the various lines of differentiation in thymic epithelial tumors. Thymic carcinoma may originate from totipotential stem cells which have the capability to differentiate into CD5(+) cells and NE cells. In contrast, thymic carcinoid and thymoma may be derived from more specifically committed cells and functional CD5(-) cells, respectively.

VII. CONCLUSION

We demonstrated strong correlations among CD5-expression, cellular atypism, and NE differentiation in a distinct type of thymic epithelial tumor. It is unclear whether CD5 is merely a marker for other characteristics of the tumor or whether it plays an important role in the development of thymic tumors. CD5 is a receptor-type molecule expressed by T-lymphocytes and some B-lymphocytes which signals growth activity through interaction with a ligand, e.g., CD72 on B-lymphocyte[5]. Although we favor the latter possibility, further study is required to disclose the molecular mechanism and biological significance of CD5 expression in thymic epithelial cells, which may lead to a better understanding of tumorigenesis of the thymic gland.

REFERENCES

1. Shimosato Y: Controversies surrounding the subclassification of thymoma. Cancer 1994, 74: 542–544
2. Müller-Hermelink HK, Marks A, Kirchner TH: Advances in the diagnosis and classification of thymic epithelial tumours. Recent advances in histopathology. Edited by Anthony PP and MacSween RM. Churchill Livingstone, 1994: pp49–72
3. Hishima T, Fukayama M, Fujisawa M, Hayashi Y, Arai K, Funata N, Koike M: CD5 expression in thymic carinoma. Am J Pathol 1994, 145: 268–275
4. Van de Velde H, Von Hoegen I, Luo W, Parness JR, Thielesmans K: The surface protein CD72/Lyb-2 is the ligand for CD5. Nature 1991, 351: 662–665
5. Sato Y, Watanabe S, Mukai K, Kodama T, Upton MP, Goto M, Shimosato Y: An immunohistochemical study of thymic epithelial tumors. II. Lymphoid component. Am J Surg Pathol 1986, 10: 862–870
6. De Lellis RA, Tischler AS, Wolfe HJ: Multidirectional differentiation in neuroendocrine neoplasms. J Histochem Cytochem 1984, 32: 899–904

MICROSCOPIC THYMOMA AND MYASTHENIA GRAVIS

A Clinicopathological and Immunohistochemical Study of Two Cases

F. Puglisi,[1] C. Di Loreto,[1] N. Finato,[1] C. Marchini,[2] and C. A. Beltrami[1]

[1]Institute of Anatomic Pathology
[2]Department of Neurology
University of Udine, Italy

1. INTRODUCTION

The term "microscopic thymoma" (MT) was first used by Rosai and Levine[1] to describe an occasionally discovered microscopically sized thymic lesion with the histological features of a thymoma. Since then, to the best of our knowledge, other 5 cases of MT were described in patients suffering from myasthenia gravis (MG).[2–4] Approximately 30–60% of patients with thymomas develop MG but probably this percentage is underestimated because of the possible presence of thymomas with very small dimensions in some myasthenic patients. In a previous paper we suggested the importance of establishing the unequivocal presence of a thymoma in myasthenic patients by obtaining histological samples of the entire gland, especially in those cases without macroscopical evidence of thymoma.[3] In the current paper we describe the histopathological and immunohistochemical features of two cases of MT detected after sampling of the surgically removed thymuses from myasthenic patients.

2. CASE REPORTS

2.1. Case 1

In the first case a diagnosis of MG was performed in a 56 year old man suffering from diabetes mellitus. The patient presented to the hospital with a bilateral palpebral ptosis, diplopia and easy fatigability. The clinical suspicion of MG was confirmed by means of an anticholinesterase test, repetitive nerve stimulation and positive assay of ace-

Epithelial Tumors of the Thymus, edited by Marx and Müller-Hermelink.
Plenum Press, New York, 1997

tylcholine receptor antibodies. In order to investigate the presence of an associated thymic abnormality, a computed tomography of the chest was made. No image consistent with thymic lesions was seen. However, a thymectomy was performed with the aim of obtaining a therapeutic response. The patient is well over a follow up period of two years, his medical treatment consisting of anticholinesterase agents.

2.2. Case 2

A 57 year old man with diabetes mellitus presented to the hospital because of generalized weakness, easily fatigability, mostly of the lower limbs, and diplopia. The presence of a 70% reduction in the amplitude of the evoked muscle action potential and the positivity of the assay for acetylcholine receptors antibodies supported the diagnosis of MG. A computed tomographic scan was unable to detect the presence of a mediastinal mass. Nevertheless, also in this case the patient underwent to thymectomy for therapeutic purposes. After thymectomy, the patient is well over a follow up period of a year, his only treatment consisting of daily prednisone per os (50 mg).

3. MATERIALS AND METHODS

The entire thymuses from both patients were processed for conventional histology. Hematoxylin-eosin stained sections were studied. In addition, sections of the two cases were examined immunohistochemically by the avidin-biotin-peroxidase complex technique (Vectastain ABC Elite Kit, Vector, Burlingame, CA) using commercially available antibodies directed against cytokeratins (AE-1, AE-3), MIB-1, p53, bcl-2 and CD45 RO (table 1). After blockage of the endogenous peroxidase, the slides were heated in a 750 W microwave oven set at maximum power for two minutes and at 100 W for 8 minutes, then were cooled and washed twice in PBS. The slides were incubated overnight in primary antibodies. In the immunohistochemical procedure each step was followed by washes with PBS, and the peroxidase reaction was developed in 3,3′-diaminobenzidine tetrahydrochloride (Sigma, St. Louis, MO) and H_2O_2. The slides were counterstained in Mayer's hematoxylin, dehydrated and mounted with Permount. Opportune negative controls were carried out.

An image analyser (IBAS2000, Kontron) was used to measure the microscopic dimensions of the thymic lesions.

Table 1. Monoclonal antibodies used for the immunohistochemical analysis

Clone	Antigen	Source
DO-7	p53	Dako
124	bcl-2	Dako
UCHL1	CD45-RO	Dako
MIB-1	Ki-67	Immunotech
AE1/AE3	keratins of acidic and basic subfamilies	Oxoid

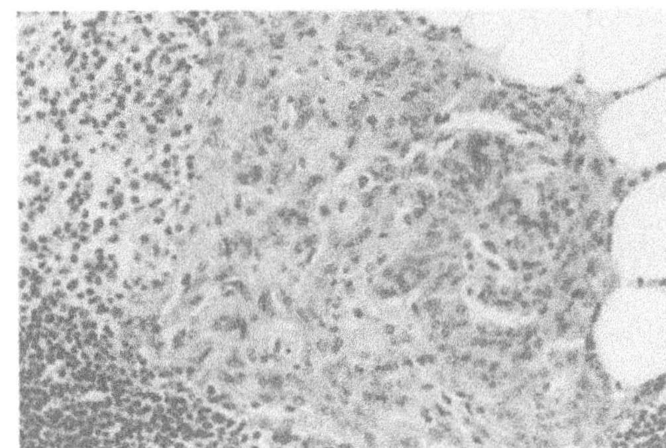

Figure 1. Microscopic thymoma (case 1). Small island of epithelial round-oval cells with dispersed chromatin and inconspicuous nucleoli is evident. (Haematoxylin and eosin, original magnification x 250).

4. RESULTS

The surgical specimen excised in case 1 consisted of a lobulated soft yellow thymic gland weighing 30 g.

On histological examination, several islands of epithelial round-oval cells with dispersed chromatin and inconspicuous nucleoli were detected in a thymus with a variable degree of involution. Mitotic figures were not found. We interpreted these epithelial nests as multiple foci of MT (figure 1). The largest island measured 0.27 x 0.07 mm.

The surgical specimen of the case 2 weighed 35g and showed a cystic surface. On histology, small nests of round to oval epithelial cells were discovered (figure 2); the largest island measured 0.5 x 0.5 mm.

The immunohistochemical pattern was similar in case 1 and case 2. The neoplastic epithelial nests showed a strong immunoreactivity for cytokeratins. In addition, a cytoplasmic positivity for bcl-2 protein was observed in all epithelial islands (figure 3). On the contrary, p53 and MIB-1 were not expressed by the cells in the foci of microscopic thymoma. Bcl-2 and CD45 RO were expressed in intermingling thymocytes (figure 4).

5. DISCUSSION

The evidence that microscopic thymoma represents a true pathological entity suggests that thymuses removed from patients suffering from myasthenia gravis should be examined entirely to look for the presence of microscopic epithelial islands. In order to

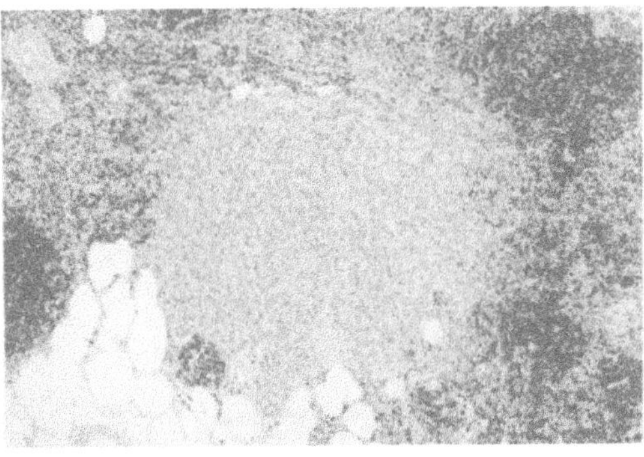

Figure 2. Microscopic thymoma (case 2). A small nest of oval cells with dispersed chromatin and inconspicuous nucleoli is evident. (Haematoxylin and eosin, original magnification x 100).

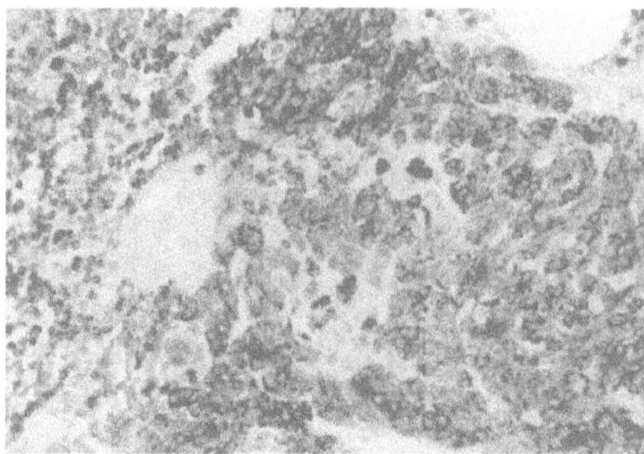

Figure 3. Photomicrograph of immunohistochemical staining showing homogeneous bcl-2 immunoreactivity in tumor cells (original magnification x 250).

highlight the microscopic foci of tumour the sections can be immunostained for cytokeratins.

Since a link between microscopic and larger thymomas has not be demonstrated, MT could be hypothesized to represent an early stage in the progression of thymic epithelial tumors, or otherwise a multifocal lesion without risk of neoplastic evolution. In our study we examined microscopic thymomas for proteins involved in the control of the cell proliferation or cell death.

Alterations in cell cycle can be determined by mutations in genes encoding proteins acting as positive or negative regulators of cell proliferation. Abnormal control of the cell cycle can be in turn associated with the loss of the tissue homeostasis and with the development of neoplastic clones.

The p53 gene is a tumour suppressor gene that encodes a protein involved in the regulation of cell proliferation. After a cell damage, the wild-type p53 protein acts by preventing the passage from G1 to S phase of the cell cycle to allow the repair of the cellular damage. However, if the damage can not be repaired, p53 induces apoptosis. A mutation of the p53 gene determines a loss of these mechanisms and may lead to the selection of abnormal cell clones. Mutations of the p53 gene have been reported in various malignant tumours.[5] Although the immunohistochemical detection of the wild-type p53 protein is not possible because of its short half-life, mutations in the p53 gene produce a protein with longer half-life and detectable by immunohistochemistry.

In a recent paper, Tateyama et al suggested that with progression of epithelial thymic tumours there is an increasing accumulation of mutant p53 protein.[6] Our data would

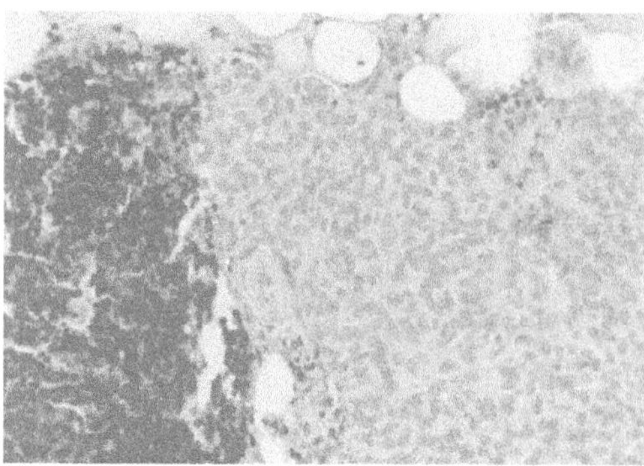

Figure 4. Immunostaining for CD45 R0 was detec ted in thymocytes near a tumoral focus (origina magnification x 250).

appear to indicate that there is not p53 mutant protein when the tumor is smaller than 1 mm in diameter.

Bcl-2 is a proto-oncogene that encodes a protein that protects cells from death by apoptosis. Bcl-2 protein is normally expressed in various organs including the breast, thyroid, skin, nervous systems, pancreas, lymphoid tissue and also in most of epithelial cells of the fetal thymic medulla.[7,8] Recently, Brocheriou et al reported the bcl-2 expression in epithelial cells of spindle-cell thymomas and in the spindle component of mixed thymomas. On the contrary, bcl-2 protein was not detected in cortical thymomas.[9] In both of our cases bcl-2 protein was detected in the epithelial neoplastic foci. This finding suggests that bcl-2 could act early in the tumorigenesis of microscopic thymomas by inhibiting cell death.

In addition, the absence of immunoreactivity for MIB-1 in microscopic epithelial islands may be interpreted as sign of low cell proliferation and even more supports the main role of inhibition of apoptosis in thymomas of smaller dimensions.

In conclusion, our data indicate that microscopic foci of thymoma can be detected more easily by immunostaining for cytokeratins and that p53 expression is not characteristic of the neoplastic epithelial islands. Moreover, the negative immunoreactivity for MIB-1 could be correlated with a less aggressive growth of the MT, whereas the bcl-2 positive expression could be evidence of extension of neoplastic cell survival.

6. REFERENCES

1. Rosai J, Levine GD. Tumors of the thymus. Atlas of tumors pathology, second series. Washington DC: Armed Forced Institute of Pathology, 1976.
2. Pescarmona E, Rosati S, Pisacane A, Rendina EA, Venuta F, Baroni CD. Microscopic thymoma: histopathological evidence of multifocal cortical and medullary origin. Histopathology 1992; 20: 263–6.
3. Puglisi F, Finato N, Mariuzzi L, Marchini C, Floretti G, Beltrami CA. Microscopic thymoma and myasthenia gravis. J Clin Pathol 1995;48:682–683.
4. Poulard G, Mosnier JF, Dumollard JM, Prades JM, Convers P, Boucheron S. Thymome microscopique et myasthenie grave. Ann Pathol 1994; 14: 203–204.
5. Porter PL, Gown AM, Kramp SG, Coltrera MD. Widespread p53 overexpression in human malignant tumours: An immunohistochemical study using methacan-fixed, embedded tissues. Am J Pathol 1992;140:145–53.
6. Tateyama H, Eimoto T, Tada T et al. p53 Protein Expression and p53 Gene Mutation in Thymic Epithelial Tumors. Am J Clin Pathol 1995; 104: 375–381.
7. Hockenbery DM, Zutter M, Hickey W, Nahm M, Korsmeyer SJ. Bcl-2 is topografically restricted in tissues characterized by apoptotic cell death. Proc Natl Acad Sci USA 1991;88:6961–5.
8. LeBrun DP, Warnke RA, Cleary ML. Expression of bcl-2 in fetal tissues suggests a role in morphogenesis. Am J Pathol 1993;142:743–53.
9. Brocheriou I, Carnot F, Briere J. Immunohistochemical detection of bcl-2 protein in thymoma. Histopathology 1995;27:251–5.

13

COMPLEX AND DIFFERENTIAL CYTOKERATIN PROFILES IN THYMOMAS AND CORRELATION WITH NORMAL THYMUS

Kerstin Grommisch,[1] Walter J. Hofmann,[2] Herwart F. Otto,[2]
Kirsten Willgeroth,[3] and Roland Moll[3]

[1]Institute of Pathology
University of Mainz
D-55101 Mainz, Germany
[2]Institute of Pathology
University of Heidelberg
D-69120 Heidelberg, Germany
[3]Institute of Pathology
University of Halle-Wittenberg
D-06097 Halle (Saale), Germany

SUMMARY

Cytokeratins (CKs) are characterized by highly diverse expression patterns and thus serve as potent epithelial differentiation markers. We have studied 31 cases of thymomas (12 cortical, 2 predominantly cortical, 5 mixed, and 9 medullary type thymomas as well as 3 well-differentiated thymic carcinomas) and, for comparison, 15 normal thymi, for the presence of different CK polypeptides. Immunohistochemistry was performed on cryostat sections using the indirect immunoperoxidase method.

In normal medullary epithelial cells, all 16 CKs studied were detected with variable frequencies. Cortical epithelial cells showed less complex patterns, mainly composed of the simple-epithelial CKs 8 and 19 and the stratified-epithelial CK 14. In the subcapsular epithelium, CKs 5, 14 and 19 were predominant.

Analyses of the thymomas revealed a broad spectrum of variably complex CK patterns which, although being fluid, allowed the definition of several quite distinct CK phenotypes. All thymomas co-expressed simple-epithelial (CKs 8, 18, 19) and stratified-epithelial (mainly CKs 5, 14, 15 and 17) CKs. Half of the cortical thymomas revealed a phenotype with predominance of CKs 5 and 15 while 5/9 medullary thymomas showed prevalence of CK 14. Focal expression of CK 6 was more typical of cortical thymomas. CKs 4, 7, 10, 13 and 20 were inconstantly and sparsely expressed, with enhancement of CKs 4, 7 and 13 in cystic structures. "Medullary differentiation" usually was

Epithelial Tumors of the Thymus, edited by Marx and Müller-Hermelink.
Plenum Press, New York, 1997

accompanied by a shift towards enhanced stratified-epithelial CKs. Seven cases contained neurofilaments.

The data demonstrate partial correlations between particular CK patterns and the morphological subtypes of thymomas although there are no simple relations to the normal thymic zones. The possible biological significance of the different CK phenotypes needs to be substantiated with larger series.

INTRODUCTION

Cytokeratins are characterized by highly diverse, differentiation- and cell-type-specific expression patterns and thus may serve as potent epithelial differentiation markers useful for cell lineage tracing in embryology and as histological tumor markers in pathology (Moll et al., 1982, 1992; Moll, 1993; Nagle, 1994; Schaafsma and Ramaekers, 1994).Thymic epithelial cells are known to display a variety of differentiation phenotypes. Early gel electrophoretic studies have suggested an unusually complex cytokeratin expression pattern (Moll et al., 1983). Recently, specific antibodies against most of the 20 human cytokeratins known have become available. This has prompted us to analyze immunohistochemically, on the cellular level, the expression of the individual cytokeratins in normal human thymi as well as in different types of thymomas.

METHODS

Surgical specimens of normal thymi (n = 15) and of thymomas (n = 31) were snap-frozen. For the morphological classification of thymomas (Kirchner and Müller-Hermelink, 1989), H&E-stained cryostat sections cut from the frozen blocks used for immunohistochemistry were assessed in addition to the routine paraffin sections. Since data on associated myasthenia gravis were not available for every case, this feature was not included in the evaluation. Cryostat sections were fixed with cold acetone and immunostained with a large battery of antibodies against different cytokeratins and other intermediate filament proteins using the indirect immunoperoxidase method or, in selected cases, indirect immunofluorescence microscopy (see Moll et al., 1992).

The following *primary antibodies* against cytokeratins were used (for references, see Moll, 1993): (1) Monoclonal mouse antibody (MAb) 34ßB4 against cytokeratin (CK) 1 (from Enzo Diagnostics, Farmingdale, NY, USA); (2) MAb Ks2.342.7.1 against CK 2e (Progen Biotechnik, Heidelberg, Germany); (3) MAb 6B10 against CK 4 (Euro-Diagnostica, Apeldoorn, The Netherlands); (4) MAb AE14 against CK 5 (kindly provided by Dr. T.-T. Sun, New York); (5) MAb Ks6.KA12 against CK 6 (Progen); (6) MAb CK-7 against CK 7 (Boehringer Mannheim, Mannheim, Germany); (7) MAb M20 against CK 8 (Euro-Diagnostica); (8) polyclonal antibodies TY-1 against CK 9 (kindly provided by Dr. L. Langbein, German Cancer Research Center, Heidelberg, Germany); (9) MAb K8.60 against CK 10 (Progen); (10) MAb 2D7 against CK 13 (Euro-Diagnostica); (11) MAb LL001 against CK 14 (Cymbus Bioscience, Southhampton, UK); (12) polyclonal antibodies GP KRIT against CK 15 (kindly provided by Dr. R. Leube, German Cancer Research Center, Heidelberg, Germany); (13) MAb Ks17.E3 against CK 17 (Progen); (14) MAb Ks18.174 against CK 18; (15) MAb Ks19.2 against CK 19 (Progen); (16) MAbs IT-Ks20.3 and IT-Ks20.5 against CK 20 (Progen); as well as (17) the broad-spectrum CK MAb KL-1 (Dianova, Hamburg, Germany).

In addition, the following antibodies against other intermediate filament proteins were applied: (1) MAb VIM-9 against vimentin (Viramed, Martinsried, Germany); (2) MAb D33 against desmin (Dako, Hamburg, Germany); (3) MAb G-A-5 against glial fibrillary acidic protein (GFAP; Boehringer Mannheim); (4) MAb 2F11 against the neurofilament proteins NF-L and NF-H (Biochrom, Berlin, Germany); (5) MAb NR4 against the neurofilament protein NF-L (Boehringer Mannheim); (6) MAb NN18 against the neurofilament protein NF-M (Boehringer Mannheim); (7) MAb N52 against the neurofilament protein NF-H (Sigma, Deisenhofen, Germany).

The slides were evaluated semiquantitatively by assessing the relative proportions of positive (epithelial) cells.The MAb against GFAP consistently produced negative results and thus also served as negative control.

RESULTS

Normal Thymi

The normal thymi studied comprised 5 cases without significant involutory changes (ages 2, 4, 19, 22, 22 years), 5 cases with slight (ages 16 - 26 years) and 5 cases with pronounced involution (ages 19 - 49 years). There were no significant differences in cytokeratin expresssion related to the age or to the degree of involution.

The results of the immunohistochemical staining for the various cytokeratins and intermediate filament proteins are summarized in Table 1; selected staining are illustrated in Fig. 1. Although the expression patterns were generally valid as rules, there were notable interindividual variabilities with respect to certain cytokeratins.

In all thymic zones, the epithelial cells were characterized by a co-expression of cytokeratins of the simple- and the stratified-epithelial type.The broad-spectrum cytokeratin antibody KL1 and the CK 19 antibody exhibited the same, general staining pattern, indicating ubiquitous expression of CK 19 in thymic epithelial cells. CK 14 also was abundantly expressed. In the *subcapsular layer*, certain cytokeratins (predominantly CK 5) were additionally present, with the resulting pattern resembling that of basal cells of mucosal stratified squamous epithelia (Moll, 1993). In the *cortex*, a reduced complexity and a shift towards predominance of simple-epithelial cytokeratins (prominent CK 8 and CK 19) was noted.The *medulla* was characterized by a highly increased complexity of cytokeratin

Table 1. Cytokeratin expression in normal human thymus

Thymic zones	Simple-epithelial cytokeratins					Stratified-epithelial cytokeratins										
CK	7	8	18	19	20	1	2e	4	5	6	9	10	13	14	15	17
Subcapsular layer	–	+	(+)	++	–	–	–	–	++[a]	(+)[b]	–	–	–	++	+	+[c]
Cortex	–	++	+	++	–	–	–	–	(+)[c]	–	–	–	–	++[a]	(+)[c]	(+)[c]
Medulla	(+)[b]	+	+	++	(+)	(+)[b]	(+)	(+)	++[a]	(+)	(+)	(+)	(+)	++	++[a]	+
Hassall corpuscles	(+)	+	+	++	(+)	++	+	+	(+)	+	+	++	(+)	(+)	–	+

++, homogeneously or abundantly positive; +, heterogeneously positive (in subcapsular, cortical, and medullary zones with pronounced interindividual variability of the proportions of positive cells); (+), sparsely positive (up to 20% of cells; variable proportions of negative cases); -, mostly or consistently negative

[a] Some cases with less expression

[b] The majority of cases was negative

[c] Some cases with higher expression

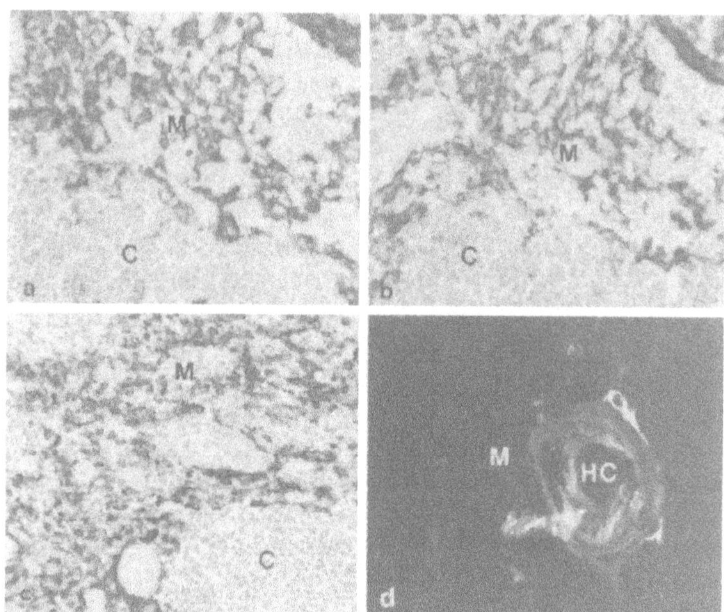

Figure 1. Normal thymus of a two-year-old child, stained with the pan-cytokeratin antibody KL-1 (a) and with antibodies against CK 19 (b), CK 5 (c) and CK 20 (d). Immunoperoxidase (a-c) and immunofluorescence (d) microscopy on cryostat sections. C, cortex; M, medulla; HC, Hassal corpuscle. a, x 280; b, x 280; c, x 220; d, x 280.

expression, resulting in the presence of most of the 16 CK polypeptides studied in variable frequencies, with an overall predominance of stratified-epithelial cytokeratins. Formation of *Hassall corpuscules* was accompanied by the appearance of cytokeratins related to squamous epithelial maturation and keratinization (e.g., CK 1, CK 10), including highly specialized cytokeratins typical of advanced terminal epidermal differentiation (CK 2e) or of palmo-plantar epidermis (CK 9). In addition, some cases exhibited medullary cells expressing desmin (4/15 cases) or neurofilaments, in particular the large neurofilament protein NF-H (5/15 cases). GFAP was negative.

Thymomas

12 cortical, 2 predominantly cortical, 5 mixed, and 9 medullary type thymomas as well as 3 well-differentiated thymic carcinomas were investigated. The results are exemplarily illustrated in Fig. 2 and summarized in Table 2.

In general, a broad spectrum of variably complex cytokeratin patterns was found. All thymomas co-expressed simple-epithelial (CKs 8, 18, 19) and stratified-epithelial (mainly CKs 5, 14, 15 and 17) cytokeratins but the relative proportions of some of these proteins were highly diverse.

Among *simple-epithelial cytokeratins*, CK 19 was - like in normal thymus - consistently and abundantly expressed. Another broadly (but somewhat less consistently) expressed component was CK 8. The level of CK 18 was variable, higher levels being more common in medullary and mixed thymomas as compared to cortical thymomas. CK 7 and CK 20 were irregularly and sparsely expressed, with CK 7 showing some preference of medullary thymomas, and CK 20 being seen in only 6/31 cases.

Among *stratified-epithelial cytokeratins*, the main components expressed were CKs 5, 14, and 15, followed by CKs 17 and 6. CK 15 showed higher levels in cortical thy-

Table 2. Cytokeratin expression in thymomas

Simple-epithelial cytokeratins		Well-differentiated thymic carcinoma	Cortical thymoma	Predominantly cortical thymoma	Mixed thymoma	Medullary thymoma
CK 7	0%[a]	0/2[b]	8/12	2/2	2/5	3/9
	1%-20%	2/2	4/12	0/2	3/5	6/9
	21%-60%	0/2	0/12	0/2	0/5	0/9
	61%-100%	0/2	0/12	0/2	0/5	0/9
CK 8	0%	0/3	0/12	0/2	0/5	0/9
	1%-20%	0/3	0/12	0/2	0/5	0/9
	21%-60%	0/3	3/12	0/2	0/5	0/9
	61%-100%	3/3	9/12	2/2	5/5	9/9
CK 18	0%	0/3	0/12	0/2	0/5	0/9
	1%-20%	0/3	6/12	0/2	0/5	0/9
	21%-60%	0/3	5/12	1/2	1/5	3/9
	61%-100%	3/3	1/12	1/2	4/5	6/9
CK 19	0%	0/3	0/12	0/2	0/5	0/9
	1%-20%	0/3	0/12	0/2	0/5	0/9
	21%-60%	0/3	0/12	0/2	0/5	0/9
	61%-100%	3/3	12/12	2/2	5/5	9/9
CK 20	0%	1/2	11/12	0/2	4/5	8/9
	1%-20%	1/2	1/12	2/2	1/5	1/9
	21%-60%	0/2	0/12	0/2	0/5	0/9
	61%-100%	0/2	0/12	0/2	0/5	0/9
Stratified-epithelial cytokeratins						
CK 1	0%	3/3	12/12	1/2	4/5	9/9
	1%-20%	0/3	0/12	1/2	1/5	0/9
	21%-60%	0/3	0/12	0/2	0/5	0/9
	61%-100%	0/3	0/12	0/2	0/5	0/9
CK 4	0%	1/3	8/12	1/2	3/5	5/9
	1%-20%	1/3	4/12	1/2	2/5	4/9
	21%-60%	1/3	0/12	0/2	0/5	0/9
	61%-100%	0/3	0/12	0/2	0/5	0/9
CK 5	0%	0/3	1/12	0/2	0/5	0/9
	1%-20%	0/3	0/12	0/2	1/5	2/9
	21%-60%	1/3	5/12	1/2	2/5	5/9
	61%-100%	2/3	6/12	1/2	2/5	2/9
CK 6	0%	0/3	2/11	0/1	2/5	5/9
	1%-20%	2/3	6/11	0/1	3/5	4/9
	21%-60%	1/3	3/11	1/1	0/5	0/9
	61%-100%	0/3	0/11	0/1	0/5	0/9
CK 10	0%	0/3	8/11	2/2	3/5	9/9
	1%-20%	3/3	3/11	0/2	2/5	0/9
	21%-60%	0/3	0/11	0/2	0/5	0/9
	61%-100%	0/3	0/11	0/2	0/5	0/9
CK 13	0%	1/3	9/12	2/2	4/5	5/9
	1%-20%	2/3	3/12	0/2	1/5	4/9
	21%-60%	0/3	0/12	0/2	0/5	0/9
	61%-100%	0/3	0/12	0/2	0/5	0/9
CK 14	0%	0/3	1/12	0/2	0/5	0/9
	1%-20%	2/3	8/12	1/2	2/5	1/9
	21%-60%	1/3	1/12	0/2	0/5	3/9
	61%-100%	0/3	2/12	1/2	3/5	5/9
CK 15	0%	0/3	2/12	0/2	0/5	3/9
	1%-20%	2/3	0/12	0/2	3/5	3/9
	21%-60%	0/3	6/12	1/2	1/5	2/9
	61%-100%	1/3	4/12	1/2	1/5	1/9
CK 17	0%	0/3	2/12	0/2	1/5	0/9
	1%-20%	1/3	6/12	2/2	3/5	3/9
	21%-60%	1/3	4/12	0/2	1/5	4/9
	61%-100%	1/3	0/12	0/2	0/5	2/9

[a] Estimated percentage of positively immunostained epithelial tumor cells

[b] Number of cases with indicated expression level / total number of cases analyzed

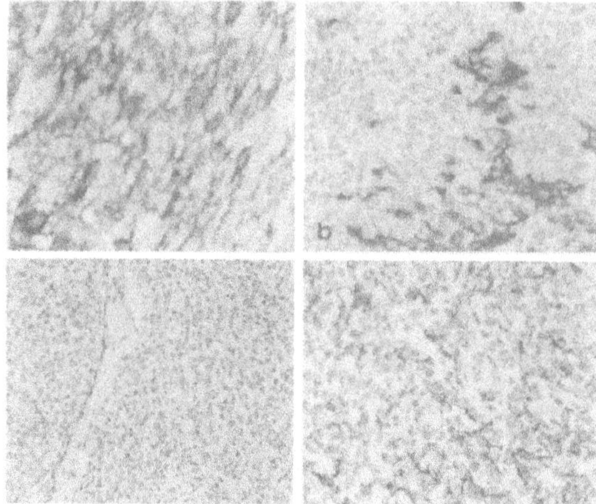

Figure 2. Cytokeratin expression in thymomas. (a, b) Cortical type (CK 5/CK 15 phenotype): Abundant immunostaining for CK 5 (a). In contrast, CK 14 is only focally present (b). (c, d) Medullary thymoma (CK 14 phenotype), showing very little staining for CK 5 that is restricted to some peripherally located cells (c) but staining of most epithelial tumor cells for CK 14 (d). Immunoperoxidase microscopy on cryostat sections. a, x 360; b, x 280; c, x 180; d, x 360.

momas, CK 14 higher expression in medullary thymomas. CK 5 was broadly variable, with slight preference of the cortical type, and CK 17 showed variable, usually minor expression (with occasional major expression in medullary thymomas). CK 6 was moderately expressed, with preference of cortical thymomas. CK 4, CK 10, CK 13 and CK 17 showed low levels of expression in the minority of cases. CK 1 was mostly negative. (CK 16, another possible thymic cytokeratin, was not determined in this study.)

Thus, these differential expression profiles revealed partial correlations with the morphological classification of thymomas. Although the patterns were fluid, and a sharp distinction of the histological types was not possible, several quite distinct cytokeratin phenotypes could be defined. Of the *cortical thymomas*, half (6/12 cases) exhibited a phenotype characterized by *predominance*, among the stratified-epithelial cytokeratins, *of CK 5 and CK 15* (simple-epithelial cytokeratins being also present as stated above). A further third of cortical thymomas (4/12 cases) belonged to another phenotype defined by sparseness of stratified-epithelial cytokeratins in general and, correspondingly, *main* expression of *simple-epithelial cytokeratins*. Interestingly, of the 3 well-differentiated thymic carcinomas studied, one case exhibited CK 5/CK 15 predominance, and one case simple-epithelial cytokeratin predominance, suggesting relationship to cortical thymomas. (Among other thymoma types, these two cytokeratin phenotypes were found only rarely.) More than half of the *medullary thymomas* (5/9 cases) revealed a phenotype with *prevalence*, among the stratified-epithelial cytokeratins, *of CK 14*. (This pattern was observed in only 2 other thymomas.) Two further medullary thymomas, but no other type, was conspicuous by particularly *prominent stratified-epithelial cytokeratins*.

Few neurofilament-positive cells (NF-L, NF-H) were detected in 4/12 cortical, 1/5 mixed, and 1/8 medullary thymomas and in 1/3 well-differentiated thymic carcinomas (cf. Marx et al., 1992). Vimentin appeared to be negative in epithelial thymoma cells but in some cases was difficult to judge due to closely neighbouring lymphocytes. Desmin and GFAP were always negative.

Cells lining *perivascular spaces* did not differ significantly from the other epithelial thymoma cells of the respective case. Cortical thymoma cells bordering at thick *fibrous septa* often showed pronounced staining for CK 14 and CK 17. "*Medullary differentiation*" (observed in cortical and in predominantly cortical thymomas) often showed increased staining for stratified-epithelial cytokeratins (CK 5, CK 14; partly CK 6, CK 17). *Cyst-lining cells* were conspicuous by prominent staining for CK 4, CK 7 and CK 13, which otherwise were sparsely expressed in thymomas, and partly for CK 6.

DISCUSSION

Normal Thymus

We have demonstrated an enormous complexity of cytokeratin expression in normal thymic epithelial cells, including very specialized and body-site-specific cytokeratin subtypes. The present data point to the close relationship between Hassall corpuscule formation and terminal differentiation of stratified squamous epithelia, including epidermis. In a previous report, even hair-type cytokeratins have been detected in medullary epithelial cells and Hassall corpuscules (Heid et al., 1988). Thus, the thymic epithelial reticulum can be regarded as a modified stratified squamous epithelium. In line with this view, the cytokeratin patterns of subcapsular cells and, with certain restrictions, also of cortical cells are compatible with cytokeratin phenotypes of basal cells of stratified squamous epithelia (Moll, 1993; Schaafsma and Ramaekers, 1994). In contrast, maturation-typical cytokeratins appear in subpopulations of medullary cells and, most prominently, in Hassall corpuscules. Using a basal cell-specific cytokeratin as a marker (antibody KB-37; polypeptide no. not defined), Shezen et al. (1995) have proposed a maturation flow from subcapsular epithelium to Hassall corpuscules which is in line with the present, more detailed findings.

On the other hand, also simple-epithelial and glandular features are obvious, including expression of CK 20 which otherwise is restricted to gastrointestinal epithelia, urothelium and Merkel cells (Moll et al., 1992). In view of the high level of stratified-epithelial cytokeratins present in thymic medullary epithelial cells, it is well possible - but remains to be proven by double staining experiments - that these cells co-express CK 20 together with one or several stratified-type cytokeratin(s), which in fact would be an unusual expression pattern (Moll et al., 1992). Simple-epithelial cytokeratins predominated in cortical epithelial cells, which also exhibited the least complex cytokeratin composition.

The abundance and heterogeneity of cytokeratin polypeptides in thymic medullary epithelial cells reflects the broad range of differentiation phenotypes that is realized in the small compartment of the thymic medulla. This may be important for maturation and education processes of T cells, including the induction of self-tolerance. In fact, in terms of cytokeratin expression, the thymus appears to be the most complex epithelial unit of the body.

The present results on the cytokeratin expression in normal human thymus confirm and extend previous studies (Viac et al., 1980; Moll et al., 1983; Laster et al., 1986; Ochs et al., 1986; Savino and Dardenne, 1988; Colic et al., 1990; Fukai et al., 1993; Meireles de Souza and Savino, 1993; Shezen et al., 1995). In contrast to other studies, we found less expression of CK 13. Some authors (Savino and Dardenne, 1988; Colic et al., 1990; Meireles de Souza and Savino, 1993) reported CK 8 and/or CK 18 to be restricted to (human) medulla while we detected both cytokeratins also in the cortex, cytokeratin 8 even at a higher level as compared to the medulla. Such discrepancies may be due to different antibodies and techniques used.

THYMOMAS

Only few previous studies are available reporting on cytokeratin polypeptide profiles of thymomas, and limited antibody panels have been used in those studies (Savino and Dardenne, 1988; Kirchner and Müller-Hermelink, 1989; Fukai et al., 1993). As far as comparisons are possible, our data are generally in agreement with the previous data; however, Fukai et al. (1993) found higher levels of CK 13 expression in most polygonal cell (cortical) thymomas while we noted lower degrees.

In the present extensive cytokeratin analysis of thymomas, we have found partial (but not sharp) correlations between the cytokeratin patterns and the morphologically defined thymoma types. When normal thymic epithelial cells (cortical, medullary) are compared to the corresponding thymoma types (cortical, medullary), the *overall patterns* rarely show correspondence but rather contrary features (e.g., predominance of CK 5 and CK 15 in some cortical thymomas while in normal cortex CK 14 is the major stratified-epithelial cytokeratin). This seeming discrepancy might be explained by the idea of expansion of minor subpopulations of cells expressing the appropriate patterns, which in fact are present in each thymic zone. Alternatively, many studies dealing with different cell types of the body have established a considerable plasticity of cytokeratin phenotypes, even within a given lineage, e.g. upon changes in the microenvironment, upon cell damage, and upon malignant transformation (for review, see Moll, 1993). Therefore, formal cytokeratin differences between normal and tumor cells do not necessarily contradict histogenetic classification schemes. Overlap in antigenic profiles, including cytokeratin expression, between the different thymoma types has also been noted in several previous studies (Kirchner and Müller-Hermelink, 1989; Fukai et al., 1993).

One of the major results of the present study is the identification of subgroups of thymomas on the basis of distinct cytokeratin phenotypes. Their possible biological significance needs to be substantiated with larger series of tumors. Such studies are meanwhile facilitated by the fact that most of the cytokeratins dealt with in this study can now, using special enhancement methods, be visualized on paraffin sections of routinely processed tissue (e.g., Demirkesen et al., 1995).

ACKNOWLEDGMENTS

The authors thank Dipl. Med. A. Behringer and Mrs. F. Thaler for their assistance in the preparation of the poster and the manuscript.

REFERENCES

Colic M, Dragojevic-Simic V, Gaslic S, Duljic A: Interspecies differences in expression of cytokeratin polypeptides within thymic epithelium: A comparative immunohistochemical study. Developm Compar Immunol 14: 347–354 (1990)

Demirkesen C, Hoede N, Moll R: Epithelial markers and differentiation in adnexal neoplasms of the skin: an immunohistochemical study including individual cytokeratins. J Cutan Pathol 22:518–535 (1995)

Fukai I, Masaoka A, Hashimoto T, Yamakawa Y, Mizuno T, Tanamura O: Cytokeratins in normal thymus and thymic epithelial tumors. Cancer 71:99–105 (1993)

Heid HW, Moll I, Franke WW: Patterns of expression of trichocytic and epithelial cytokera- tins in mammalian tissues: II. Concomitant and exclusive synthesis of trichocytic and epithe- lial cytokeratins in diverse human and bovine tissues (hair follicle, nail bed and matrix, lingual papilla, thymic reticulum). Differentiation 37:215–230 (1988)

Kirchner T, Müller-Hermelink HK: New approaches to the diagnosis of thymic epithelial tumors. In: Progress in Surgical Pathology, Vol. 10. Field and Wood, Philadelphia, pp.167–189 (1989)

Laster AJ, Itoh T, Palker TJ, Haynes BF: The human thymic microenvironment: Thymic epithelium contains specific keratins associated with early and late stages of epidermal kerati- nocyte maturation. Differentiation 31:67–77 (1986)

Marx A, Kirchner T, Greiner A, Schalke B, Müller-Hermelink HK: Neurofilament epitope expression in thymic epithelial tumors and anti-axonal autoantibodies in myasthenia gravis: A model for autoimmunity by abnormal T cell selection. Verh Dtsch Ges Path 76:256–261 (1992)

Meireles de Souza LR, Savino W: Modulation of cytokeratin expression in the hamster thymus: Evidence for a plasticity of the thymic epithelium. Developm Immunol 3:137–146 (1993)

Moll R, Franke WW, Schiller DL, Geiger B, Krepler R: The catalog of human cytokeratins: Patterns of expression in normal epithelia, tumors and cultured cells. Cell 31:11–24 (1982)

Moll R, Krepler R, Franke WW: Complex cytokeratin polypeptide patterns observed in certain human carcinomas. Differentiation 23:256–269 (1983)

Moll R, Löwe A, Laufer J, Franke WW: Cytokeratin 20 in human carcinomas: A new histo- diagnostic marker detected by monoclonal antibodies. Am J Pathol 140:427–447 (1992)

Moll R: Cytokeratins as markers of differentiation : Expression profiles in epithelia and epithelial tumors. Progress in Pathology, vol. 142. Gustav Fischer Verlag, Stuttgart, Jena, New York. pp 1–197 (1993)

Nagle RB: A review of intermediate filament biology and their use in pathologic diagnosis. Mol Biol Reports 19:3–21 (1994)

Ochs BA, Hofmann W, Franke WW, Otto HF: Immunhistochemische und biochemische Unter- suchung der Cytokeratine im normalen menschlichen Thymusepithel und in Thymomen. Verh. Dtsch. Ges. Path 70:591 (1986)

Savino W, Dardenne M: Immunohistochemical studies on a human thymic epithelial cell subset defined by the anti-cytokeratin 18 monoclonal antibody. Cell Tissue Res 254:225–231 (1988)

Schaafsma HE, Ramaekers FCS: Cytokeratin subtyping in normal and neoplastic epithelium: Basic principles and diagnostic applications. In: Rosen PP, Fechner RE, eds. Pathology Annual, part 1, vol. 29. Appleton & Lange, Norwalk. pp 21–62 (1994)

Shezen E, Okon E, Ben-Hur H, Abramsky O: Cytokeratin expression in human thymus: immunohistochemical mapping. Cell Tissue Res 279:221–231 (1995)

Viac J, Schmitt D, Staquet MJ, Thivolet J: Epidermis-thymus antigenic relations with special reference to Hassall's corpuscles. Thymus 1:319–328 (1980)

14

UNUSUAL RECURRENCE OF MIXED THYMOMA IN BREAST

I. C. Kiricuta[1] and Th. Kirchner[2]

[1]Department of Radiation Oncology
University of Würzburg, Würzburg, Germany
[2]Department of Pathology
University of Erlangen, Germany

1. INTRODUCTION

Malignant thymomas are by definition locally invasive with extrathoracic spread being unusual. Metastasis to the breast has been documented in only 2 patients (1, 5). The breast is, in general an uncommon site for metastases, comprising only 1.2% of all breast tumors in one large series (4). However, carefull post-mortem examination of the breast in cases of malignant neoplasm would probably reveal more cases (7). The commonest primary tumors that metastasize to the breast are contralateral breast cancer, melanoma, lymphoma and leukaemia (2, 7).

Solitary manifestation in the breast from mixed thymoma has not been documented. In the case reported here, the patient presented a subcutaneous nodule in the left breast 9 1/2 years after surgery of a mediastinal mixed thymoma.

1.1. Case Report

A 54-year-old white woman was refered to our radiation oncology department with a 9 1/2 years old history of a mediastinal mixed thymoma. In 1980 she was operated for an anterior mediastinal tumor (160 gr). In May 1990 she showed a subcutaneous nodule in the left breast (upper/inner quadrant) (Figure 1), which was resected and classified as recurrence of the previous thymoma. Four month later, a 7 x 4 x 3.8 cm well encapsulated lobulated recurrence of the thymoma in the anterior mediastinum was resected (Figure 2). A postoperative adjuvant radiotherapy up to a total dose of 57.2 Gy was delivered. The treatment volume included the anterior mediastinum and the quadrant of the breast where the subcutaneous nodule was excised. Myasthenia gravis is present. Until June 1995, the patient was with no evidence of disease.

Epithelial Tumors of the Thymus, edited by Marx and Müller-Hermelink.
Plenum Press, New York, 1997

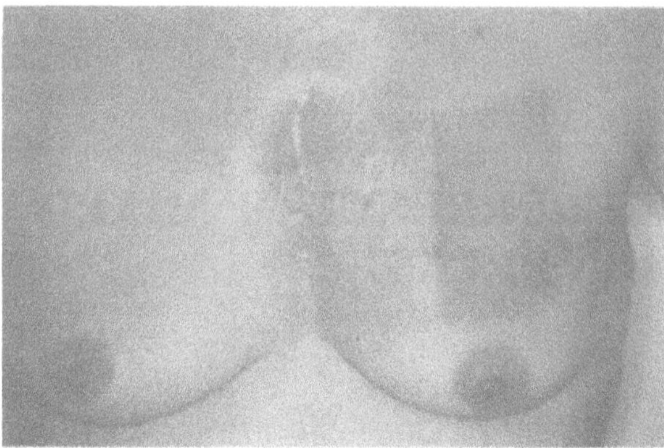

Figure 1. General view of the chest wall after radiotherapy (February 1991). Note the midline scar after the primary thymectomy (December 1980) and the scar after local excision of the subcutaneous nodule in the left breast (May 1990).

1.2. Pathology

The primary tumor and the recurrences (Figure 3, 4) were histologically reevaluated and classified as mixed thymoma according to criteria described by Kirchner and Müller-Hermelink (3). A resection in sano could not be confirmed for the primary tumor mass, and that could explain the late local recurrence. Histologically, the subcutaneous nodule in the left breast was not different from the primary and the recurrence.

2. DISCUSSION

Although most thymomas appear benign, some may invade tissue locally, and rarely, thymomas may metastasize. Operative trauma may contribute to tumor dissemination.

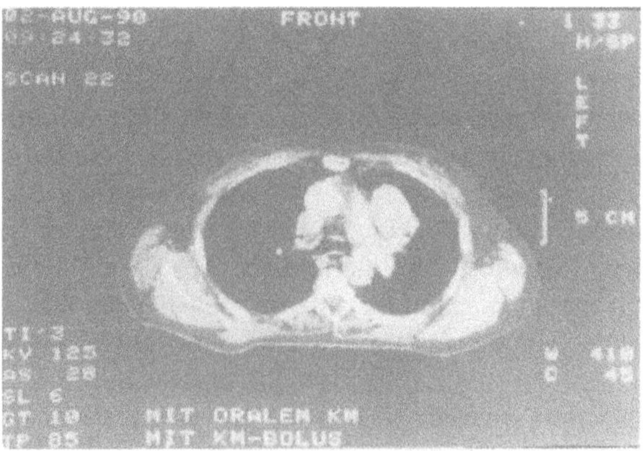

Figure 2. Computer tomographic findings before surgery of the intrathoracic recurrence (August 1990).

Figure 3. Overview of the intrathoracic recurrence of the mixed thymoma showing an encapsulated tumor without invasion.

Two cases of distant spread of thymoma in the breast have been previously reported (1, 5). Both reports do not specify the subtype of thymoma. According to previous studies the mixed type of thymoma of our case is considered to be a benign tumor without risk of metastasis. Incomplete resection of the primary tumor could explain the late local mediastinal recurrence. Most probably the distant spread into the breast is not due to vascular dissemination, since other metastases were missing. It might rather be explained by mechanical spreading and implantation of the tumor tissue either by surgical procedure or by postoperative drainage (Figure 5). Another way of spread could be through the disturbed lymphatics of the mediastinum and chest wall after the first operation. Most probably, mixed thymomas might recur in rare cases also due to incomplete resection and implantation of tumor tissue at the reoperation, as it has been described for other benign neoplasms e. g. pleomorphic adenoma of the salivary glands.

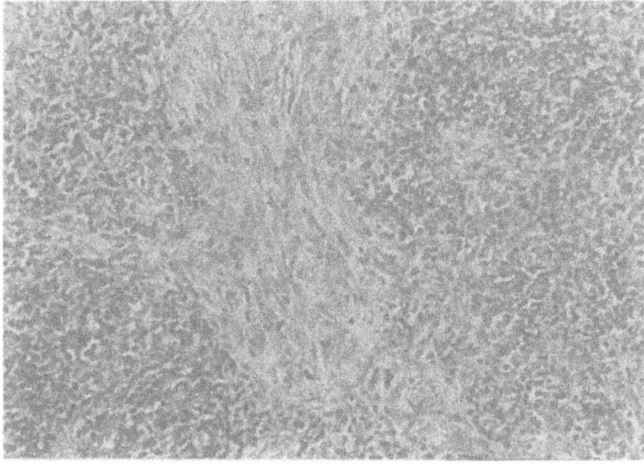

Figure 4. Detail of the recurrence of mixed thymoma with spindle cells of medullary type between lymphocyte-rich areas of cortical differentiation.

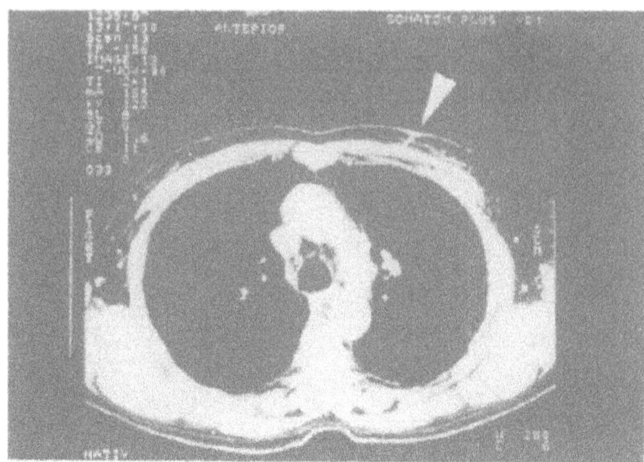

Figure 5. Computer tomographic findings after surgery of the subcutaneous nodule in the left breast and the intrathoracic recurrence (November 1990). Note the subcutaneous scar in the left breast after removal of the subcutaneous nodule (white arrow).

The involvement of the subcutaneous space in the left breast—as it was seen in our patient—was not described until now. In all cases reported in the literature, the extrathoracic spread was associated with local invasiveness of the primary tumor. This locally invasive character was not present at the initial or subsequent surgery.

REFERENCES

1. Guillan R. A., Zelman S., Smalley R. L., Iglesias P. A. Malignant thymoma associated with myastenia gravis, and evidence of extrathoracic metastases. An analysis of published cases and report of a case. Cancer 27: 823–830, 1971.
2. Hajdu S. L., Urban J. A. Cancers metastatic to the breast.Cancer 29: 1691–1696, 1972.
3. Kirchner Th., Müller-Hermelink H. K. New Approaches to the Diagnoses of Thymic Epithelial Tumors. Progr. Surg. Pathol. 10: 167–189, 1989.
4. Landon G., Sneige N., Ordonez N. G., Mackay B., Carcinoid metastatic to breast diagnosed by fine-needle aspiration biopsy. Diagn Cytopathol 3: 230–233, 1987.
5. Maggi G., Giaccone G., Donadio M., Ciufreda L., Dalesio O., Leria G., Trifletti G., Casadio C., Palestro G., Mancuso M., Calciati A. Thymomas - A review of 169 cases, with particular reference to results of sugical treatment. Cancer 58: 765–776, 1986.
6. Moir G. C., Carpenter R., Bass P., Royle T. G. Metastatic carcinoid of the breast: An unusual screen-detected breast cancer. Eur. J. Surg. Oncol. 19: 92–94, 1993.
7. Sandison A. T. Metastatic tumors in the breast. Br. J. Surg. 47:54–58, 1959.

15

HISTIOCYTOSIS -X OF THE THYMUS

Development of Myelomonocytic Leukemia 5 Years after Thymectomy

Wiesław T. Dura and Małgorzata J. Dura

Department of Pathology
Children's Memorial Health Institute (CMHI)
Warsaw, Poland

1. INTRODUCTION

Histiocytosis - X [H-X, "Langerhans' cell histiocytosis"] is a nonneoplastic but often biologically aggressive proliferation of Langerhans' cells [LC] which primary function is an uptake, processing and presentation of an antigen in squamous epithelia.[5,7,8,27] Despite observations of impaired immunity in H-X, the cause of H-X remain largely unknown and its neoplastic potential is practically indeterminable upon histopathology alone.[8] The following main non-histopathologic criteria for predicting a poor prognosis have been found: [i] organ involvement which has to be assessed on the basis of a score system; [ii] dysfunction of organs that are involved in the diseases; [iii] rapid progression and poor response to therapy and finally [iv] very young age, especially when related to pediatric patients.[3,12,15,21,25,27] Thymic primary presentation of H-X is rare. No LC are found in normal thymus, instead corresponding function is ascribed to interdigitating cells (IDC) which constitute a cellular substrate for intrathymic negative selection process.[26,29,30,31] Both LC and IDC are believed to develop from common ancestral cells based within the bone marrow monocytic precursor compartment.

We report three cases of histiocytosis X in thymic region for four reasons. First, for its rarity as the only anatomical presentation of disease, second for the development of myelomonocytic (M4 of FAB) type of leukemia 5 years after thymectomy and chemotherapy, third, because of concomitant "dysplastic" thymic pathology, and finally, to reconsider prognostic value of Masaoka's [17] criteria of "thymoma" staging (invasiveness) if applied to thymic H-X.

2. MATERIAL AND METHODS

All three patients have been admitted to Children's Memorial Health Institute in Warsaw during the period of one year. Surgical material have been personally received,

Epithelial Tumors of the Thymus, edited by Marx and Müller-Hermelink.
Plenum Press, New York, 1997

viewed and diagnosed by authors. One of the cases (case 3) have already been presented to the workshop of European Association for Hematopathology in 1989 in Wurzburg. Fresh tumor tissue have been snap frozen, sectioned and stored in -60 °C for further immunomorphologic study. Small fragments were fixed in glutaraldehyde and routinely embedded in Epon for electron microscopic evaluation. Number of paraffin blocks submitted for histology varied from 15 to 23. About 25–30 imprints from fresh cut surfaces have also been taken, subsequently air dried, fixed in acetone and stored in -60 °C for further immunocytochemical study. In two cases (case 1 and 3) adjacent to tumor thymic tissue have been grossly identified and separately submitted for frozen and for paraffin blocks. Since leukemic M4/M5 transformation have been diagnosed elsewhere, bone marrow preparation as well clinical charts, including laboratory and radiological studies have been obtained and reviewed. Immumomorphologic study was based on APAAP technique with the use of following monoclonal antibodies: CD1a, CD2, CD3, CD4, CD8, CD11a, CD13, CD33, CD54, CD14, CD20, CD23, DRC-1, CD45RO, CD68, HLA-DR and anticytokeratine MNF-116 (from Dakopatts, Danmark), CD16 and CD57 as markers for natural killer cells, (from Novocastra, U.K.), β-integrin, pan αβTCR, pan γδTCR (from Genzyme. USA) and finally specific markers for thymic epithelium Mas-251, Mas-252, Mas-253 (from Seralab, U.K.).

3. RESULTS

The three reported cases of histiocytosis- X in the thymic region together with similar cases found in the literature are summarized in the Table I.

3.1. Case Reports

Case 1. The 2 years and 6 month old boy has been presented to family doctor with symptoms of dyspnoe, upper trunk vein distention and cyanosis. Suspected to have congenital heart disease referred to CMHI. Upper anterior mediastinal tumor have been identified on chest X-ray. Fine needle aspiration biopsy was diagnostically inconclusive. He underwent thoracotomy but infiltration/adherence of "thymic tumor" to the major vessels and pericardium, had prevented from radical resection. The diagnosis of "Langerhans cell granulomatosis" (H-X) was done upon resected specimen. All 7 lymph nodes identified in the surgical material showed extensive H-X infiltrate. Thymus has been identified both, within H-X infiltrate as well at the periphery of resected lesion and its histology was consistent with dysplasia of "severe thymic atrophy" type. His bone marrow was screened tree times for H-X cells, buy apart from nonspecific changes no Langerhans cells have been found. Liver biopsy was histologally normal as well X-rays of skeleton. Bearing in mind partial resection of the lesion, lymph node invasion, and inability (dysplastic thymus) of organ function assessment, the boy received four drug chemotherapy (as for disseminated H-X) and subsequently mediastinal irradiation. After 9 month of treatment he was asymptomatic without evidence of recurrence. 4 years and 7 month later he was admitted to hospital with hepatosplenomegaly and severe trombocytopenia. Myelomonocytic (M4 of FAB) leukemia have been diagnosed and appropriately treated. First M4 relapse was identified 19 month and the second 13 month later. He is now well and alive 7 month after the end of third round of treatment.

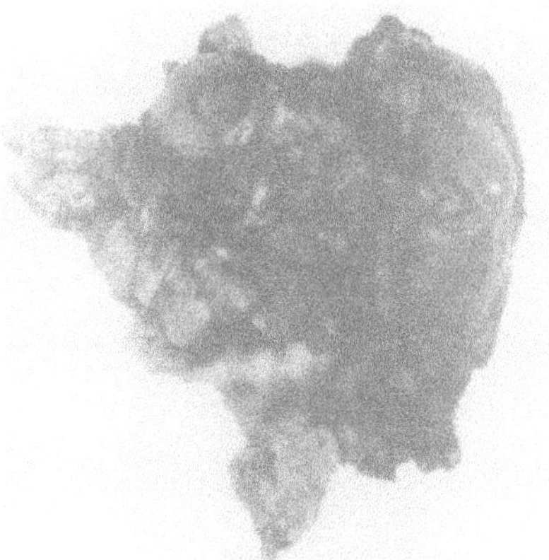

Figure 1. Histiocytosis-X of the thymus-gross appearance of the resected specimen (case 3) measuring 9 cm x 13 cm.

Case 2. This 4 years old boy was admitted to CMHI because of "temporary appearing, cough induced", 2 cm x 2 cm lump in suprasternal notch with grossly visible superior vena cava stasis. X-ray, NMR and venograms showed retrosternal mass (Fig. 1). Fine needle aspiration biopsy strongly suggested Langerhans cell histiocytosis. Biopsy of suprasternal mass was unsuccessful hence thoracotomy was done and the lesion with adjacent fragment of pericardium was completely resected. Diagnosis of H-X was confirmed. Yamshidi liver biopsy showed no evidence of H-X. Eight lymph nodes found in the vicinity of the mediastinal mass disclosed heavy infiltrate by H-X Langerhans cells. This, along with dimension of the lesion, its adherence to pericardium, were reasons why boy underwent heavy, four drug chemotherapy, followed by radiotherapy, both concluded 9 month after surgery. There was no evidence of H-X in two aspirate of bone marrow. The boy was fine 3 years and 11 month when readmitted with pancytopenia, weight loss and malaise. M4 leukemia was diagnosed and he was placed on adequate treatment protocols. After the second relapse he underwent unsuccessful bone marrow transplant (from his brother). Now he is well and alive 15 month after last chemotherapy.

Case 3. A 1,5 years old boy spend in the different hospital his last 6 month. When admitted to CMHI he presented upper mediastinal widening, progressive dyspnoe and circulation insufficiency. Thoracotomy was than performed and a huge, flat, hard mass was partially resected. Laterally tumor infiltrated phrenic nerves and was closely adherent to inner sternum. There was no hepatosplenomegaly, lympadenopathy or skin lesions. Bone marrow was normal. H-X diagnosis was followed by skeleton X-ray which showed no lytic lesions. Finding of five H-X invaded lymph node in resected specimen, partial resection of the tumor and bilateral hydrothorax had motivated oncologist to introduce three and subsequently four drug chemotherapy. That was concluded 11 month thereafter. Boy was fine until at the age of 5 and 8 month when noticed a lump above left eye. Fine needle aspiration cytology suggested "malignancy possibly rhabdomyosarcoma or PNET". When he developed huge hematoma in the place of aspiration biopsy, elaborate hematological investigation disclosed 90% bone marrow replacement by myelomonocytic (M4/M5 according to FAB) cells. Retrospective review of retrobulbar aspiration cytology revealed specific ASD esterase positive cytology consistent with "histiocytic/granulocytic sarcoma". He was placed on treatment and currently, 19 month after first relapse, he is alive and well.

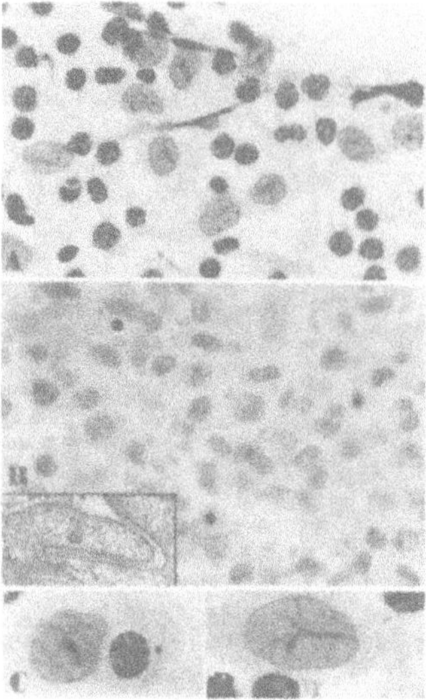

Figure 2. Cytological (A, C & D) and histological (B) appearance of Langerhans' cells in thymic H-X. Note characteristic nuclear envelope grooving, Birbeck granules formation on outer membrane and rarely observed phagocytosis. HE, A&B-650x, C&D-1200x, window on B-35000x.

3.2. Pathology

All three resected mediastinal lesions were irregular, solid, hardly encapsulated, rather circumscribed (Fig.2), soft (in case 1) or hard and "fibroid" as in case 2 and 3. Adjacent thymic tissue and lymph nodes were easily identifiable in two children (case 1 and 2). In the third one, thymus and lymph nodes were found only after careful microscopic search as being embedded in histiofibrotic tissue. There were no apparent yellowish necrotic zones. Resected specimens measured from 5 cm x 11cm (case 3) to 9 cm x 13 cm (the biggest in case 2).

The histopathology of infiltrate was similar in all cases and otherwise typical of Langerhans' cell histiocytosis. Main constituent was that of a bland looking, histiocytic

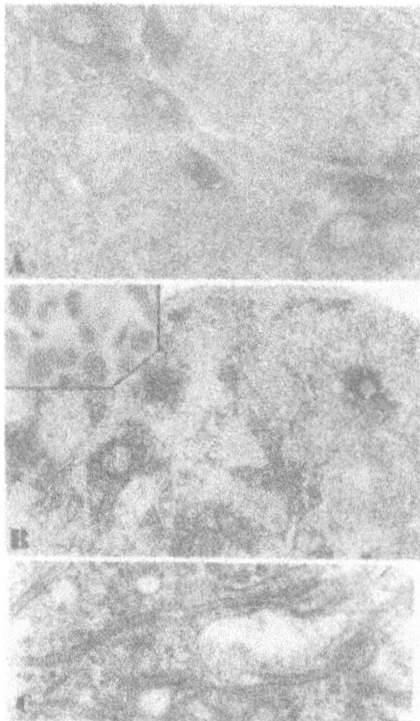

Figure 3. H-X of the thymus infiltrating regional lymph nodes. Note characteristic location of LC in T-cell areas (A & B), living intact B-cell follicles. In some instances (A) nodule forming infiltrate closely resembles features observed in dermatopathic lymphadenopathy. Intracytoplasmic Birbeck granules (C) were always observed. H&E, A & B - 75x, window on B - 650x, C - 36 000x

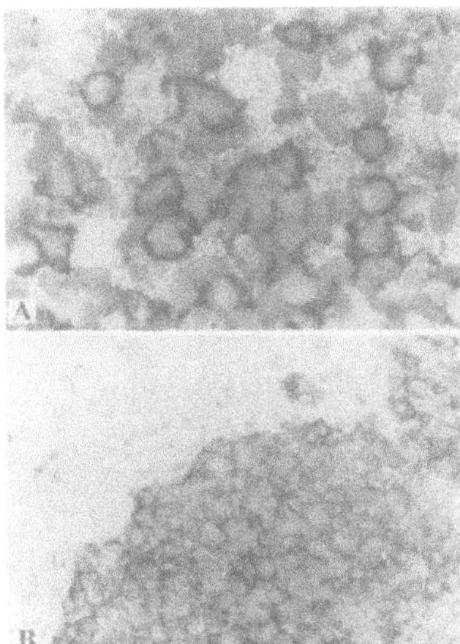

Figure 4. CD1a molecule expression on needle aspiration biopsy specimen (A) shown on fig.2a and on frozen section (B). A- 690x, B- 250x ; Mab CD1a, unstained.

cells (Fig. 3 and 4) with characteristic excentrically positioned, folded or intended, clear, "open face" nuclei. Small, nonbasophilic, one or two nucleoli, seen near the center of nuclei were usually attached to one of the nuclear clefts. H-X cells were non adhesive in growth pattern with well delineated borders of eosinophilic, abundant cytoplasm. Multinucleated cells were very rare. H-X infiltrate in the lymph nodes almost always left intact B-cell follicles, infiltrating clearly T cell dependent areas. Spectrum of eosinophilic component varied from case to case, even from field to field. In most instances, number of eosinophils was small or even absent. Mitotic figure were exceedingly rare as well no

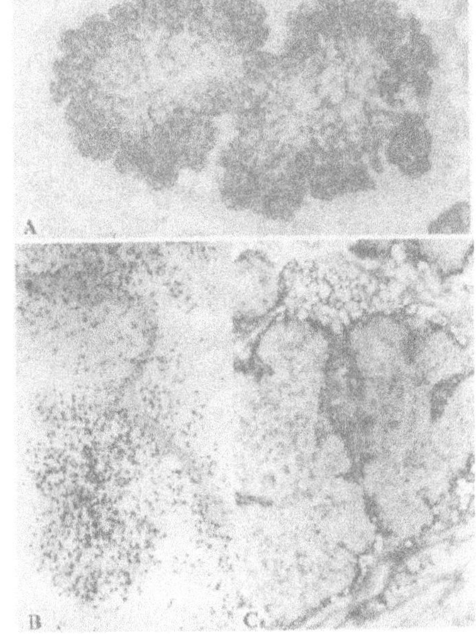

Figure 5. Immunoprofile of dysplastic (A & C) and severely atrophied thymuses (B) observed in thymic histiocytosis X. Note characteristic, rounded shape of the lobules in dysplasia, epithelial network positivity (A) with anti-HLA-DR. Cortical epithelium is present only on outer limits of the dysplastic lobules. CD8a positive lymphoid cells were found (B) located mostly outside of rudimentary epithelium. A - HLA-DR, 250x, B - CD8a - 100x, C - Mas-252, x 150,unstained.

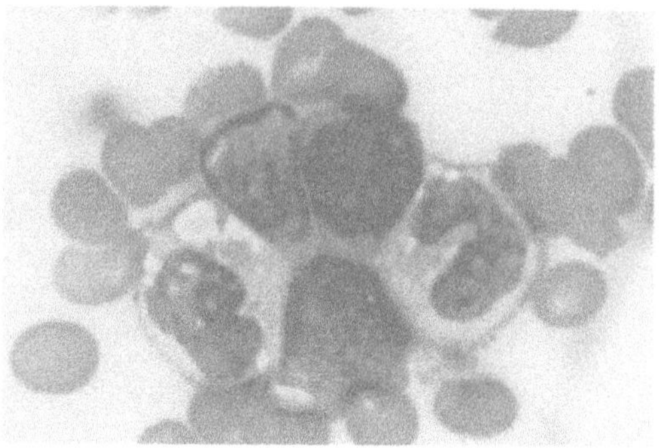

Figure 6. Representative cluster of M4/M5 leukemic cells observed in case 3. Wright, 1200x.

overtly atypical cells was present. Electron microscopic pictures of H-X cells was characterized by the presence of multiple, easy to find and very polymorphic Birbeck granules, ranging from small intendation of cellular membrane to long, intracytoplasmic structures connected or not to cytoplasmic organelles.

Almost all H-X cells disclosed strong expression of CD1a molecules in addition to HLA-DR and β-integrin (Fig.5). CD54 and CD11a molecules were also constantly strongly expressed on H-X cells as well on the fibrohistiocytic cells (as in case 3), making specificity of staining difficult to judge. Fine needle aspiration cytology was adequate and diagnostic in only one case (case 1). Combined with immunomorphologically evidenced CD1a molecule, it served as excellent adjunct to the preoperative diagnosis.

Residual thymic tissue was found in all cases : part of them as peripherally located, collapsed network of thymic epithelium without lymphoid component and in part, within tumor H-X infiltrate. In a few instances, Langerhans' histiocytic infiltration of thymic epithelium resembled "histioepithelial lesion" of the skin. That was particularly well expressed, when thymic epithelium have been delineated by immunocytochemical visualization of cytokeratin. All thymic tissues presented features consistent with so-called "dysplasia": one classified as simple, two as "dysplasia of severe atrophy type" (Fig. 5). Both showed immunoprofile of medullary type of thymic epithelium, as delineated by Mas-252 antibody. Most of lymphocytes in dysplastic thymuses, showed mature lymphoid profile, namely that of αβTCR, CD3 and CD4/C8 as well CD45RO. Number of CD14 or CD68 positive cells varied from abundant to few and they were not identifiable as belonging to H-X population. Myeloid markers, namely CD13 and CD33, were negative.

Bone marrow smears (Fig.6), obtained when leukemic transformation occurred, were almost identical in all studied cases and showed over 75% replacement of marrow by myelomonocytoid cells, corresponding to M4 leukemia (in FAB classification). In the case 3, shift to the monoblasts was much more conspicuous. Morphology of leukemic proliferation did not changed considerably after first or second relapse observed in all cases.

4. DISCUSSION

Review of literature, however certainly not complete, disclosed 2054 reported cases[1,2,4,6,7,9–11,14,16,19,21,23,35,28] of H-X, among which, only 7 had primary anatomical presentation in the thymic region[13,19,28] and 16 were described as having minor H-X of the thymus at the time of autopsy. None of these showed transformation into leukemia or hematologic malignancy (Table 1). Siegal et al.[28] had reported 4 own cases and found 3 others in the literature.

Authors concluded, that H-X, which first appears in the region of thymus, does not act clinically the same as when it is a part of systemic disease. Five out of seven thymic H-X they considered as uniorgan disease, despite the fact of incomplete resection of thymic tumor. That support Komp [12] assessment, that if less than two organs are involved in H-X, no mortality is seen. If this applies for thymic tumors in the setting of H-X as disease, it cannot be true when applying Masaoka's criteria [17] for anatomic invasiveness of thymic tumors. According to this classifications, any sign of local invasiveness and in consequence, only partial resection of thymic tumor, results in categorizing it as stage III, prognosticaly poorer group. Indeed, surgeon usually is not aware of histological matter of "thymoma" being resected and status of art inquire him to apply Masaoka'a criteria for thymic tumors. This disconcordance clearly shows, that final histological diagnosis of Langerhans cell histiocytosis shall incline us to abandon usual criteria of "thymoma" invasiveness. Important to note is the fact, that outcome of all 10 reported cases of thymic region H-X, was fairly and equally good among all cases and no H-X recurrence was observed.

Perithymic lymph nodes involvement was observed in all our cases as well in 3 cases reported in literature. Behavior of H-X in the lymph node alone is, according to study of Lennert's [20] group, similar to eosinophilic granuloma of bone and benign, even when a group of regional lymph node is involved in the process. Those authors did not found differences in clinical behavior between patients with localized lympadenopathy and those with a widespread lymph node involvement. The most remarkable observation made by Motoi and al.[20] was, that lymph node based H-X, may even be a selfhealing process, without therapy. It would be difficult to accept from both clinical and immunobiologic standpoint, that thymus and regional lymph nodes shall be considered as one functional region, nevertheless Table 1 clearly shows, that thymic H-X should be considered as biologically a benign disease.

Involvement of bone marrow, even in prognosticaly unfavorable (disseminated plus multiorgan dysfunction) group of H-X is rare. In contrast to whole spectrum of immune system proliferation's in children, it seems, that in general, biology of H-X cells is not oriented to bone marrow spread. McClain et al.[11] found cytological evidence of bone marrow involvement in 5 of the 28 patients (18%) with disseminated H-X. Such high number however, has not been confirmed by any other recently reported series [7,8,15,22] Certainly, thymic location was not an anatomic site favoring bone marrow spread, quite contrary, none of reported thymic H-X cases, including ours, had Langerhans cells identified in marrow aspirates.

Leukemic transformation of H-X into histiomonocytic leukemia is exceedingly rare. We found only one case report describing direct transformation of disseminated H-X into monocytic leukemia in 12 month old baby [24]. We do not relate M4/M5 leukemia, which developed in our cases, directly to the H-X. The most plausible speculation is, that it resulted from constellation of spectrum of factors, from severe (four drugs) cytotoxic treatment, to severe depression of immune system in those children, as reflected by "dysplastic" histology of the thymuses. Two of Siegal's et al reported thymic H-X cases, despite incomplete resections of the lesions, had not been treated at all and remain well. This, as well several clinically oriented staging systems anlysis[8,12], underline far too often complication resulting from overtreatment of H-X and drug cytotoxicity .

Coexistence of considerable thymic pathology and H-X, however in autopsy material, have been noted previously by Nezelof group [21] and Hamoudi et al. [10]. We would like to confirm this by adding above observation on surgical material. In our experience, based on 18 autopsies of children died form H-X, 11 presented thymic pathology consistent with dysplasia of different types and 7 presented borderline changes, between severe thymic at-

Table 1. Reported cases of histiocytosis -X of the thymic region */

Patient	Sex	Age	Presenting symptoms	Extrathymic involvement	Surgical treatment	Postoperative treatment	Follow up
1.	M	2,5y	Mediastinal mass; sup. vena cava syndrome	Mediastinal (perithymic) lymph nodes)	Partial excision	Chemotherapy (4 drugs) plus radiation	M4 leukemia after 4 years. Two relapses A&W 4.5 y
2.	M	1,5	Mediastinal mass	Perithymic lymph nodes	Complete excision	Chemotherapy (4 drugs)	M4 leukemia after 5 years, one relapse A&W 5 y
3.	M	4	Huge mediastinal mass, sup. vena cava syndrome.	Perithymic lymph node, great vessels, pleura	Partial excision	Chemotherapy (4 drugs) and radio therapy	M4/M5 leukemia after 4 years. Two relapses, unsuccessful B M transplant A&W
4.	M	5	Lump in suprasternal notch. Mediastinal widening	None	Partial excision	Radiation	A&W 5 y
5.	F	8	Incidental X-ray finding, anterior mediastinal mass	Mediastinal lymph node	Complete excision	Unknown	A&W;14 y
6.	F	5	Antero-superior mediastinal mass	Bone - multiple lytic lesions	Complete excision	Chemotherapy	A&W; 4 y
7.	M	0.2	Respiratory difficulty; ant. mediastinal mass	None	Partial excision	Radiation	A&W; 3,3 y
8.	M	12	Mediastinal widening	None	Total excision	None	A&W 2 y
9.	M	3	Suprasternal notch swelling overlying thyroid gland	None	Biopsy only	None	A&W 2 y
10.	M	1	Mediastinal mass, cough	Bone & skin	Total excision	Chemotherapy	A&W

*/ Cases 1-3: this report; cases 4-10: Siegal et al. [28]. A&W - alive and well

rophy and dysplasia. Significance of this coincidence in not known. Enough to say, that most, if not all children with disseminated H-X presents severe, but sometimes transient, immune deficiency. In contrast, in Siegal's three cases, where histology of the thymus was recorded, it did not show any comparable dysmorphic thymic pathology.

Last three years brought important progress and discoveries regarding H-X. One, and the most important, was the demonstration in HX of LC clonality [29,30,31]. It seems from this works, that H-X is a clonal proliferation and its clonality is independent from clinical (anatomic) presentation. This does not necessary confirm biologic malignancy - it implicates, that proliferating Langerhans' cells disclose palpable genomic mutation (locus Humara on chromosome X) . If clonality detection in aggressive forms would not be so surprising, occurrence of the same genomic abnormality confirmed in "simple and unifocal" eosinophilic granuloma, is intellectually somewhat astonishing. It is however still possible, that prognostically different clinical forms differ, because genomic mutations do not necessary concern the same locus. The second major discovery is understanding of signaling pathway in LCs. Since the principal proliferating stimuli for activation of LC lays in GM-CSF [5], we may expect in H-X mutation to be found in close proximity of this cytokine signaling pathway. On the other hand GM-CSF plays a principal growth factor role in myeloid/histiocytic compartment of the bone marrow. Involvement of this cytokine in the development of M4 leukemia in our patients, seems to be an attractive speculation. It remains also to be elucidated if CD1a molecule, which is to date the best diagnostic marker of LC in H-X, is involved in GM-CSF receptor/signaling pathway.

5. REFERENCES

1. Avery ME, McAfee J.G., Guild H G. The course and prognosis of reticuloendotheliosis (eosinophilic granuloma, Schuller Christian Disease and Letterer Siwe disease) Am.J. Med. 23:636-652,1957.
2. Bokkering JP., De Vaan G.A.M. Histiocytosis X Eur. J,. Pediatr. 135: 129-146, 1980.
3. Broadbent V, Gadner H., Komp D.M., Ladisch S. (The Clinical Writing Group of the Histiocyte Society) Histiocytosis syndromes in Children: II Approach to the clinical and labolatory evaluation of children with Langerhans cell histiocytosis. Med.Ped.Oncol. 17:492-495, 1989.
4. Daneshbod K., Kissane J. Idiopathic differentiated histiocytosis.Am.J.Clin.Pathol. 76:381-389,1978,
5. Emile JF, Peuchmaur M, Fraitag S., Bodemer C, Brousse N. Immunochistochemical detection of granulocyte/macrophage Colony stimulating Factor in Langerhans cell histiocytosis. Histopathology 23: 327-332, 1993
6. Enriquez P., Dahlin D. ,Hayles A. ,Henderson E.D. HistiocytosisnX : a clinical study. Mayo Clin. Proc 42: 88-99,1967.
7. Favara B., McCarty R.C., Mierau G.W. Histiocytosis -X. Hum.Pathol. 14:663-676,1983,
8. Favara BE, Jaffe R The histopathology of Langerhanse cell histiocytosis. Br. J. Cancer 70: S17-S23, 1994.
9. Hartman K. Histiocytois-X: a review of 114 cases with oral involvement . Oral Surg.49:38-54.1980.
10. Hamoudi AB, Newton WA Jr, Mancer K. Thymic changes in Histiocytoses. Am.J.Clin Pathol. 77: 169-174, 1982.
11. McClain K., Ramsay NKC., Robison L., Sundberg RD, Nesbit M. Jr. Bone marrow involvement in Histiocytosis X. Med. Ped. Oncol. 11:167-171.1983.
12. Komp D. Concepts in staging and clinical studies for treatment of Langerhan's cell histiocytosis. Sem. Oncol. 18: 18-23, 1991.
13. Lemos L, Hamoudi AB. Malignant thymic tumor in an infant (malignant histiocytoma) Arch. Pathol Lab.Med. 102: 84-89.1978.
14. Lieberman P, Jones C., Dargeon H., Begg C. A reappraisal of eosinophilic granuloma of bone, Hand Schuler Christian syndrome and Letterer Siwe syndrome. Medicine 48: 375-400, 1969.,
15. Leiken SL. Immunobiology of Histiocytosis-X. Hematol/Oncol North Am. 1:49-61, 1989
16. Lichtenstein L. Histiocytoisis-X . J.Bone Joint Dis. 46:76-90,1964,
17. Masaoka A, Monden Y, Nakahara K et al. Follow up study of thymoma with special reference to their clinical stages. Cancer 48:2485-2492, 1981
18. McLand et al. A flow cytometric study of Langerhans cell histiocytosis. Br.J. Dermat. 120: 485-91, 1989.,
19. McKeown F. Letterer-Siwe disease a report of two cases J.Path.Bact. 68:147-154.1955
20. Motoi M., Helbron D., Keiserling E., Lennert K. Eosinophilic granuloma of lymph node - a variant of histiocytosis X. Histopathology 4:585-606, 1980.
21. NezelofC., Frileux-Herbert F., Cronier-Sachot J. Disseminated histiocytosis X Analysis of prognostic factors based on a retrospective study of 50 cases. Cancer 44:1824-1838.1979,
22. Ornvold K. et al. Immunochistochemical study of the abnormal cells in Langerhans cell histiocytosis. Virchows Arch A 416: 403-10, 1990,
23. Oberman HA. Idiopatic histiocytosis A clinico-pathologic study of 40 cases and review of the literature. Pediatrics 28:307-319, 1961
24. Pollak A., Radaszkiewicz R., Wesenbacher G. Untersuchung zur Frage der Verwandtschaft zwischen Histiocyten und monocyten an Hand einer Letterer-Siweschen Erkrankung mit Ubergang in Monozytenleukemie. Wien.Klin.Wochenschrift.85:841-44,1973.,
25. Raney R.B., D'Angio G.J. Langerhans' cell histiocytosis (histiocytosis X) - experience at the Childrens' Hospital of Philadelphia 1970-1984. Med.Ped.Oncol. 17:20-28,1989
26. Rausch E. Kaiserlink E., Goos M. Langerhans Cells and Interdigitating reticulum cells in the thymus dependent region in human dermatopathic lymphadenitis. Virchowa Arch. B. Cell Pathol. 25: 327-343,1977,
27. Starling AK, Fernbach DJ. Histiocytosis. In: Clinical Pediatric oncology; Sutow WW , Vietti TJ, Fernbach DJ (Eds), C.V. Mosby, St Luis 19973, p.337-358.,

28. Siegal G. et al. Histiocytosis X (Langerhans'cell granulomatosis) of the thymus. Am. J.Surg. Path. 9:117-124, 1985.
29. Willman CL, Busque L., Griffith BB. Langerhans cell histiocytosis: a clonal proliferative disease. N.Engl. J.Med. 331:154-60, 1994.
30. Yu RC , Chu C, Buluwela L, Chu AC. Clonal proloferation of Langerhans cells in Langerhans' cell histiocytosis. Lancet 1: 767-7, 1994.
31. Yu RC, Chu AC. Lack of T-cell receptor gene rearrangement in cell involved in Langehans' cell histiocytosis. Cancer 75:1162-6

16

T CELL DEVELOPMENT IN THE HUMAN THYMUS

Bart Vandekerckhove, Dominique Vanhecke, and Jean Plum

Department of Clinical Chemistry, Microbiology and Immunology
University Hospital
Blok A 4 de verdieping
Depintelaan 185, 9000 Gent, Belgium

T cell differentiation occurs in the thymus. In the thymus $CD4^+$ helper cells and $CD8\alpha\beta^+$ cytotoxic cells are generated under tight MHC control. Besides intrathymic T cell generation, T cells are generated outside the thymus. Peripheral expansion of mature T cells, which may or may not be antigen driven, is a major source of peripheral T cells, as well as de novo formation of T cells. Extrathymic T cell development mainly gives rise to CD4-CD8 double negative or $CD8\alpha\alpha^+TCR\alpha\beta^+$and $TCR\gamma\delta^+$ cells which reside mainly in bone marrow and epithelia.

MODELS FOR THE STUDY OF HUMAN T CELL DEVELOPMENT

For a long time the study of human T cell development was restricted to phenotypic analysis of hematopoietic organs and thymus. In 1988, the SCID-hu mouse was described[1]. In this model, a source of hematopoietic stem cells are co-implanted with a fragment of human fetal tissue in a severe combined immunodeficiency (SCID) mouse. After implantation, human stem cell differentiate to mature T cells and continue to do so for more than one year, allowing for the first time manipulation of human T cell development. Besides this *in vivo* animal model, an *in vitro* model was described based on the murine fetal thymic organ culture (FTOC) as first described by Dr. Owen. Either mouse or human fetal thymus lobes are isolated and cultured[2–4]. Endogenous cells are killed either by deoxyguanosine or irradiation and human precursors are introduced. During the following 5–6 weeks these human cells differentiate to mature $CD4^+$ and $CD8\alpha\beta^+$ T cells. The characteristics of these systems are compared in table 1.

Epithelial Tumors of the Thymus, edited by Marx and Müller-Hermelink.
Plenum Press, New York, 1997

Table 1. Experimental systems for the study of human T cell differentiation

Model	SCID-hu	Human FTOC	Hybrid FTOC
Publication:	McCune et al 1988	Galy et al 1993	Fischer et al 1991
Description:	Precursor cells and human fetal thymus is implanted in a SCID mouse	Precursor cells are injected in irradiated human fetal thymus and cultured.	Precursor cells are introduced in fetal SCID or deoxyguanosin depleted fetal mouse lobes.
Major advantages:	1. cell recovery is high 2. steady state differentiation	easily manipulated	1. easily manipulated 2. genetically engineered mice can be used
Major disadvantages:	1. requires human fetal tissue 2. in vivo model 3. HLA marker required to discriminate endogenous from injected cells	1. requires human fetal tissue 2. limited cell recovery 3. HLA marker required to discriminate endogenous from injected cells	1. artificial human-mouse cell interactions 2. limited cell recovery

PRECURSOR CELLS SEEDING TO THE THYMUS

Multipotent $CD34^{+}CD38^{-}$ hematopoietic stem cells give rise to T cells when artificially introduced in human thymus. This observation clearly shows that no pre-commitment of the hematopoietic precursor outside the thymus is required. $CD34^{+}CD38^{-}$ hematopoietic cells were observed in the human thymus at low frequency, suggesting that indeed uncommitted multipotent precursors seed the thymus and that these cells differentiate to T cells probably under the influence of the environment[5,6]. On the other hand, Galy et al [7] reported that in the bone marrow, $CD10^{+}CD45RA^{+}CD34^{+}CD38^{+}$ cells were detectable with limited lineage differentiation potential: T cells, B cells, NK cells and dendritic cells. In the mouse model, finally, cells were found in cord blood which are already committed to the T cell lineage and some of these had D to J rearrangements in the TCRβ locus[8]. In conclusion, differentiation from multipotent to T committed stem cell may occur outside as well as inside the thymus but which pathway is the most important under physiologic conditions is still unclear.

EARLY T CELL DEVELOPMENT IN WILD TYPE AND GENETICALLY ENGINEERED MICE

Our understanding of the mechanics of early T cell differentiation has grown tremendously due to the study of "knock-out" mice(KO)[9]. Early T cell differentiation turns out to be very similar to B cell development. Precursor cell start rearranging TCRβ VDJ genes, at the double negative stage. RAG-1 and RAG-2 KO mice cannot complete these rearrangements and fail to make double positive (DP) thymocytes. The TCRβ may be rearranged in frame or out of frame. This is tested in the thymus. When the receptor is in frame, a TCRβ protein is generated, which associates with a pseudo-α chain, the CD3 complex and $p56^{lck}$. This complex interacts with an unknown ligand, possibly CD81, on thymus epithelium and signals inside the cell to stop β rearrangement, begin α rearrange-

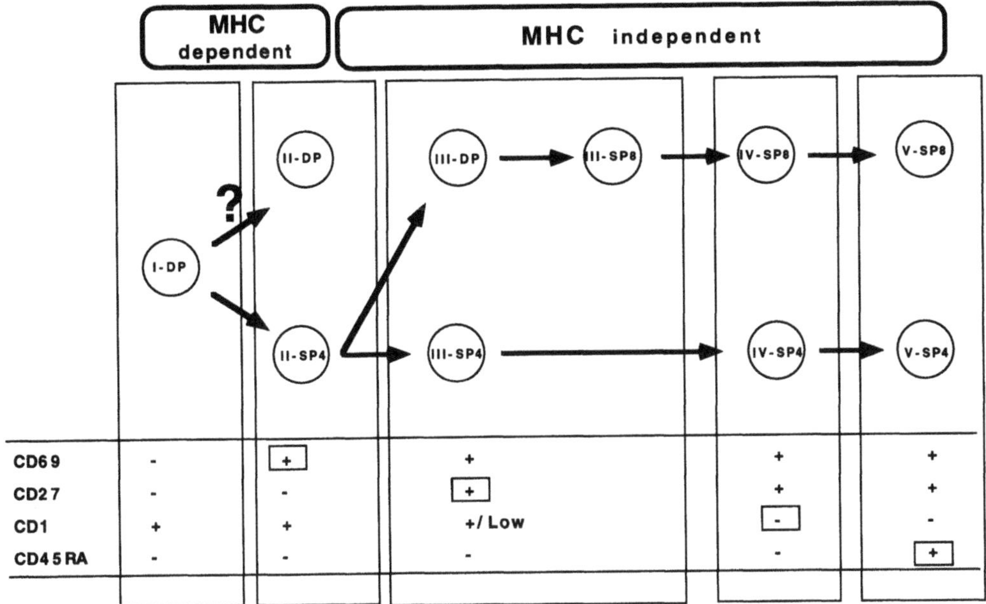

Figure 1. Positive selection and terminal differentiation in the human.

ment and become CD4⁺CD8⁺ DP thymocytes. Pseudo-α KO, CD3ε KO, $p56^{lck}$ KO have no DP thymocytes. TCRα rearrangement can be in frame or out of frame. In frame rearrangements give rise to TCRα protein which associates with the TCRβ protein to form the TCRαβ dimer. These dimers are tested on MHC. Fitting complexes signal via ZAP-70 to stop TCRα rearrangement and to become single positive T cells. This process is called positive selection and is accompanied by the expression of an activation marker CD69. TCRα KO, ZAP-70 KO and MHC KO have no CD69 expression in the thymus and no single positive mature T cells in the thymus.

POSITIVE SELECTION AND TERMINAL DIFFERENTIATION IN THE HUMAN

As in the mouse, CD69 expression is the hallmark of positive selection since $CD69^-$ cells contain mRNA for RAG and $CD69^+$ cells are negative for RAG mRNA. $CD69^+$ cells have therefore lost the ability to rearrange TCR genes.

As shown in figure 1, a number of discrete phenotypes were defined in the $CD69^+$ population. The sequential changes in expression of CD69, CD27, CD1 and CD45RA in combination with CD4 and CD8β defined 3 discrete DP stage, 3 $CD8^+$ SP stages and 4 $CD4^+$ SP stages[10]. The asymmetry between $CD4^+$ SP and $CD8^+$ SP cells was due to the existence of a $CD27^-$ $CD4^+$ SP stage absent in the $CD8^+$SP population. SCID-hu mice as well as hybrid FTOC were used for testing the precursor activity of the various cell population. After 1 to 3 weeks the progeny was analyzed phenotypically. Large DP $CD3^-$ cells, as expected[11], gave rise to mature $CD4^+$ and $CD8^+$SP cells. Of the $CD69^+$ DP populations, only the $CD27^+$ cells gave rise to mature $CD1^-$ cells: $CD8^+$ SP only. Surprisingly, $CD27^-$ $CD4^+$SP cells gave rise to $CD4^+$ as well as $CD8^+$ SP cells (Vanhecke et al , unpublished).

All cells, $CD4^+$ or $CD8^+$ SP, matured and became CD1-, CD27+ CD45RA+ T cells. Finally, we could show that mainly $CD1^-$ $CD45RA^+$ cells and some $CD1^-$ $CD45RA^-$ cells leave the thymus[10].

Functional maturity was not acquired together with positive selection, but much later[12]. All DP stages as well as $CD27^-$ SP were completely unable to produce IL-2 upon proper stimulation, nor were they clonable. $CD1^-$ thymocytes, on the other hand, were comparable in proliferation on IL-2, production of cytokines and cloning efficiency to naive peripheral cells.

These data suggest that at least two stimuli are necessary for full maturation:

- Positive selection and the acquisition of CD69. We could show in FTOC using MHC KO mice, that this step is MHC dependent.
- A continuous stimulus which drives differentiation from non-functional intermediates to $CD27^+$, $CD1^-$ $CD45RA^+$ functionally competent cells. This step is thymus dependent but MHC independent (Vanhecke et al, unpublished).

NEGATIVE SELECTION IN THE HUMAN

Staphylococcal enterotoxin B (SEB) is a superantigen, which in combination with MHC stimulates T cells using a particular Vβ. $V\beta3^+$ cells react with SEB, whereas $V\beta2^+$ T cells do not. Injection of SEB in SCID-hu mice results in a strong reduction in $V\beta3^+$ thymocytes, whereas the percentages of $V\beta2^+$ cell increased. This is the case in the DP as well as in the SP thymocyte population, indicating that negative selection can occur at any $CD3^+$ differentiation stage[13].

It is unlikely that clonal elimination of SEB reactive cells reflects the physiologic situation. Analysis of the repertoire of SP thymocytes from unmanipulated child thymus showed that the percentage of $V\beta2^+$ cells is 2 to 3 times higher within the $CD4^+$ than in the $CD8^+$ SP cells (Vandekerckhove et al, unpublished). The difference in percentages in the $CD4^+$ and $CD8^+$ lineage could be due to differential negative selection. Measurements of $V\beta2^+$ cells within the various subsets are compatible with the selective elimination of $V\beta2^+$ in the $CD8^+$ lineage. Percentages of $V\beta2^+$ cells were identical in $CD69^-$ DP cells, mature CD4+SP cells and all intermediate stages . The percentage of $V\beta2^+$ cells dropped slightly from $CD69^-$DP to $CD69^-CD27^+$DP, the immediate precursor of the $CD8^+$ SP cells, and dropped to a larger degree from $CD69^-CD27^+$DP to mature $CD8^+$ SP cells. Since positive selection occurs at the acquisition of CD69 and the fall in the percentage of $V\beta2^+$ cells is dissociated from the acquisition of CD69, we think this phenomenon reflects negative selection of these cells. These data suggest therefore that although negative selection can occur at any stage in differentiation, under physiologic conditions negative selection may occur after positive selection and before the cells are functionally mature.

REFERENCES

1. McCune, J. M., R. Namikawa, H. Kaneshima, L. D. Schultz, M. Lieberman, and I. L. Weissman. 1988. The SCID-hu mouse: murine model for the analysis of human hematolymphoid differentiation and function. *Science* 241:1632.
2. Galy, A., A. Barcena, S. Verma, and H. Spits. 1993. Precursors of CD3+CD4+CD8+ in the human thymus are defined by expression of CD34. Delineation of early events in human thymic development. *J. Exp. Med.* 178:391.

3. Fischer, A.G., L. Larson, L. K. Goff, D.E. Restall, L. Happerfield, and M. Merckenschlager. 1991. Human thymocyte development in organ cultures. *Int. Immunol* 3:1.
4. Plum, J., M. De Smedt, M-P. Defresne, G. Leclercq, and B. Vandekerckhove. 1994. Human CD34+ fetal stem liver cells differentiate into T cells in a mouse thymic microenvironment. *Blood* 84:1587
5. Spits, H., L. L. Lanier, and J. H. Phillips 1995 Development of human T and NK cells. *Blood*. 85:2654
6. Barcena, A., A. H. M. Galy, J. Punnonen, M.O. Muench, D. Schols, M. Roncarolo, J. E. de Vries, and H. Spits . 1994. Lymphoid and myeloid differentiation of fetal liver CD34+ lineage- cells in human thymic organ cultures. *J Exp Med* 180:123.
7. Galy, A., M. Travis, D. Cen, and B. Chen. 1995. Human T, B, natural killer, and dendritic cells arise from a common bone marrow progenitor cell subset. *Immunity* 3:459.
8. Rodewald, H-R. 1995 Pathways from hematopoietic stem cells to thymocytes. *Current Opinion in Immunology* 7:176.
9. Kisielow, P., and H. Von Boehmer. 1995. Development and selection of T cells: facts and puzzles. *Adv in Immunol.* 58:87.
10. Vanhecke, D., G. Leclercq, J. Plum and B. Vandekerckhove. 1995. Characterization of distinct stages during differentiation of human CD69+CD3+ thymocytes and identification of thymic emigrants. *J. Immunol* 155: 1862.
11. Kraft, D. L., I. L. Weissman, and E. K. Waller. 1993. Differentiation of CD3-CD4-CD8- human fetal thymocytes in vivo: characterization of a CD3-CD4+CD8- intermediate. *J. Exp. Med.* 178:965.
12. Vanhecke, D., B. Verhasselt, V. Debacker, G. Leclercq, J. Plum and B. Vandekerckhove. 1995. Differentiation to T Helper cells in the thymus: gradual acquisition of T helper cell function by CD3+ CD4+ cells. *J. Immunol* 155: 1862.
13. Baccala, R., B. A. E. Vandekerckhove, D. Jones, D. H. Kono, M.-G. Roncarolo, A. N. Theofilopoulos. 1993. Bacterial superantigens mediate T cell deletions in the mouse severe combined immunodeficiency-human liver/thymus model *J. Exp. Med* 177: 1481.

17

INTRATHYMIC AUTOANTIGENS AND THEIR ROLE IN THE SHAPING OF THE AUTOIMMUNE T LYMPHOCYTE REPERTOIRE

Hartmut Wekerle, Monika Bradl, Georg Kääb, Kimikazu Kojima, Christopher Linington, Alexander Marx, Scott Peterson, and Markus Reindl

Max-Planck-Institute of Psychiatry
D-82152 Martinsried, Germany

The physical deletion of self-reactive lymphocytes from the immune repertoire is the only way to provide an absolute guarantee for continued maintenance of self tolerance. In fact, deletion of self-reactive T cell clones does occur in the development of the immune repertoire. However, this deletional, self-tolerogenic mechanism is restricted to a limited set of autoantigens, especially those available in the thymus at high concentration. This is not the case for the majority of tissue specific autoantigens, and expression of the autoantigen does not lead to the complete elimination of specific self-reactive T cells. As a consequence all healthy organisms harbor unexpectedly high numbers of self reactive T cells, some of which possess the potential to attack the body's own tissue and to cause disease.

The function of such autoimmune and potentially autoaggressive T cells in the healthy immune system is uncertain. Many immunologists doubt that these clones simply persist by neglect and thus represent a permanent hazard to the body's integrity, but the mechanisms that prevent their accidental activation are also poorly understood. It appears unlikely that a mere lack of activation of the T cell clones would be sufficient to prevent autoimmune disease throughout life, but so far no regulatory pathway acting in the resting immune system has been identified with certainty.

Here, we summarize recent work from this laboratory, which was undertaken to analyze autoantigen expression within the thymus, and to identify potentially autoreactive T cells within the immune system. We will then speculate about the role of intrathymic autoantigen expression for the formation of the autoimmune T cell repertoire.

EXPRESSION OF MYELIN BASIC PROTEIN (MBP) WITHIN THE THYMUS

MBP is an integral membrane component of the myelin sheath in the nervous system and is widely used as an autoimmunogen. In fact, immunization of experimental animals

Epithelial Tumors of the Thymus, edited by Marx and Müller-Hermelink.
Plenum Press, New York, 1997

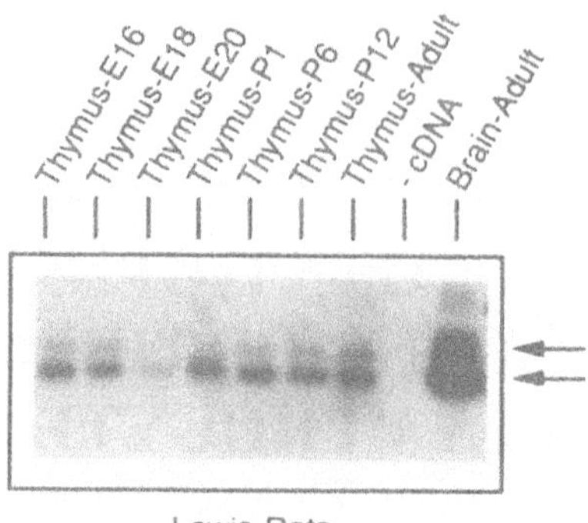

Figure 1. Expression of MBP in the thymus of the Lewis rat. Total RNA isolated from thymi and brains of developmentally staged Lewis rats was analyzed by PCR (embryonic day 16, 18 and 20, postnatal day 1, 6, 12 and adult animals) using primers specific for MBP and ß-actin (internal standard). The amplified products were transferred to nylon membranes and probed with digoxigenin-labelled oligonucleotide probes specific for the amplified gene transcripts. MBP specific transcripts were present in all samples analyzed.

with MBP results in an autoimmune disease termed experimental autoimmune encephalomyelitis (EAE), which serves as a valid model for initial inflammatory events in multiple sclerosis. Some isoforms of MBP are expressed widely - even in thymus and spleen of mice[5,17], man[19], and rats (own, unpublished observation, Fig. 1). In spite of this rather ubiquitous expression, MBP specific, autoaggressive T cells can be easily detected, both in MBP-primed and naive animals.

MBP SPECIFIC, ENCEPHALITOGENIC T CELL LINES FROM ANTIGEN PRIMED LEWIS RATS

MBP specific, $CD4^+$ T cells can be readily isolated from lymph nodes of immunized Lewis rats, and have a number of unusual properties in that they are almost exclusively specific for the MBP epitope 68–88, recognized in context of MHC class II gene elements and use the Vß8.2 gene element in their αß T cell receptor. Furthermore, the diversity of their CDR3 sequences is remarkably simple, with a relative deficit in N region additions[9,25]. This property is typically seen in T cells during early stages of ontogeny, e.g. in the pre- or neonatal immune system[8,2].

This bias in TCR selection may have been generated at several levels. Most trivially, it could have occurred during in vitro establishment of the lines which are derived from donor animals immunized with MBP in complete Freund's adjuvant, an experimental manipulation which may itself introduce a bias in TCR selection. Alternatively, utilization of Vß8.2 for MBP specific TCRs could be a natural property of the immune repertoire of the Lewis rat.

To distinguish between these possibilities, and, in particular, to probe the natural immune repertoire, we used a primary limiting dilution method which allows the isolation of MBP specific TCLs directly from the thymuses of *naive*, unprimed Lewis rats.

MBP SPECIFIC, ENCEPHALITOGENIC T CELL LINES FROM THE THYMUS OF NAIVE, UNPRIMED LEWIS RATS

We isolated MBP reactive TCLs from naive thymuses, which were, with respect to antigen recognition and TCR usage, indistinguishable from "classical" MBP reactive T cells derived from *in vivo* primed rats[1]. They recognized the immunodominant epitope p68–88 from MBP in context of MHC class II products (RT1.B[l]), were encephalitogenic, and expressed the αβ TCR at high levels. Moreover, FACS analyses using Vß specific monoclonal antibodies (MAbs)[22], as well as cloning and sequencing analyses of genes encoding the ß chain demonstrated that, with one exception, all MBP specific TCLs from naive thymuses used the Vß8.2 gene for their TCR, as did virtually all anti-MBP TCLs derived from MBP primed animals[6,4].

Furthermore, two TCL obtained from naive thymus contained the amino acid sequence AspSer, one of the CDR3 motifs most commonly used in conventional MBP specific Lewis rat TCLs[6,9,25]. Unexpectedly, MBP specific TCLs from naive thymus differed from their standard counterparts in their abnormally low levels of membrane CD4.

Our examination of MBP specific, encephalitogenic T cells in the natural thymic T cell repertoire of Lewis rats demonstrated that the biased utilization of the Vß8.2 gene by MBP specific T cells does not depend on *in vivo* priming with MBP in Freund's adjuvant, but seems to be a property of the natural T cell repertoire. We could thus extend our previous studies[20] demonstrating, that autoaggressive T cells are normal components of the healthy immune system, and could show the presence of these T cells in the thymus, a tissue where their complementary autoantigen, MBP, has been recently found to be present at considerable concentrations[11,17,19].

EXPRESSION OF S100ß WITHIN THE THYMUS

Recent observations indicated, that intrathymic co-existence of tissue specific autoantigens with complementary autoreactive T cells is not limited to MBP. In fact, this seems to apply to many other autoantigenic structures.

S100ß, a cytosolic calcium binding protein, is expressed in the central nervous system (CNS) by astrocytes, in peripheral nerves by Schwann cells, and in the eye by Müller glia cells[26]. Interestingly, S100ß was also found in immune organs of some species[16,23]. PCR analyses of brain or thymus cDNA using S100ß-specific primers revealed the presence of S100ß mRNA in these organs. Moreover, immunocytochemical staining located S-100ß protein in two distinct sets of thymic medullary cells, both implicated in intrathymic negative selection events[3]: In cells located near medullary microvessels, resse-bling interdigitating cells, and in medullary epithelial cells.

But would the thymus of an untreated Lewis rat harbor both S100ß protein and at the same time S100ß specific, autoaggressive T cells?

S100ß SPECIFIC, AUTOAGGRESSIVE T CELL LINES FROM THE NAIVE THYMUS

We examined the naive thymic T cell repertoire for the presence of S100ß-specific T cell clones. To this end, the primary limiting dilution approach that had allowed to identify MBP specific T cells in naive thymuses[15], was used. Four S100ß-specific TCLs could be isolated. These TCLs all expressed the rat αß TCR and were pathogenic. They induced a severe inflammatory response throughout the CNS, in spite of an inappropriately mild clinical course, and were thus indistinguishable from conventional S100ß specific T cells[14]. Again, S100ß reactive TCLs from naive thymuses displayed a reduced expression of CD4.

We could thus unequivocally demonstrate coexistence of autoantigen and autoimmune T cells. Interestingly, these reaction partners were both present in the thymic medulla, where negative T cell selection is thought to take place.

Our experiments investigating the development of autoimmune T cells in the naive thymus provided strong though indirect evidence that interactions between thymus stroma and differentiating T lymphocytes influence the shaping of the natural autoreactive T cell repertoire. In an attempt to elucidate cellular/molecular mechanisms possibly involved in these process, we recapitulated the development of the Lewis rat immune system by transplanting lymphohemopoietic progenitor cells into immunodeficient SCID mice.

RECONSTITUTION OF SCID MICE WITH LEWIS RAT FETAL LIVER

SCID mice were reconstituted with liver cells from 16 d old fetal Lewis rats (SCID.FL chimeras). These chimeras were immunologically reconstituted by rat T cell precursors seeding into the SCID thymus and developing there to immunocompetent T lymphocytes[21,10]. The thymuses of these chimeras contained all stromal components required for the correct differentiation of rat T cells: A thymus epithelium from the mouse, and bone-marrow-derived stroma cells, including interdigitating cells and macrophages from rat fetal liver stem cells.

In untreated SCID mice, thymuses are usually atrophic and disorganized[21]. In SCID.FL animals, however, the thymuses grew to considerable size and contained large numbers of lymphocytes expressing the rat αß TCR, some of which bound Vß8.2 specific MAbs. The chimeric thymuses also developed a marked cortico-medullary architecture. To investigate the encephalitogenic T cell response of SCID.FL chimeras, we isolated MBP specific TCLs from *in vivo* primed donor mice. In our chimeras, immunization never resulted in clinical EAE, as described by others[12,13]. All the TCLs obtained recognized the immunodominant epitope of MBP (p68–88) in context of Lewis rat MHC class II products ($RT1.B^l$), were $CD4^+CD8^-$, encephalitogenic in Lewis rats, and thus corresponding to TCLs isolated from primed intact Lewis rats[24] . However, in marked contrast to their Lewis rat derived MBP specific counterparts, these cells used a very broad TCR repertoire. Only one out of 12 SCID.FL derived, epitope p68–88 specific TCLs used Vß8.2.

RECONSTITUTION OF SCID MICE WITH LEWIS RAT FETAL LIVER AND THYMUS

We next compared SCID.FL derived T cells with a selection of MBP specific TCLs isolated the same way from SCID mice reconstituted by Lewis fetal liver *plus* E16 embryonic thymuses grafted beneath the recipients' kidney capsules, SCID.FL/FT chimeras. In these animals, rat T cell precursors seed both into the orthotopic mouse thymus as well as

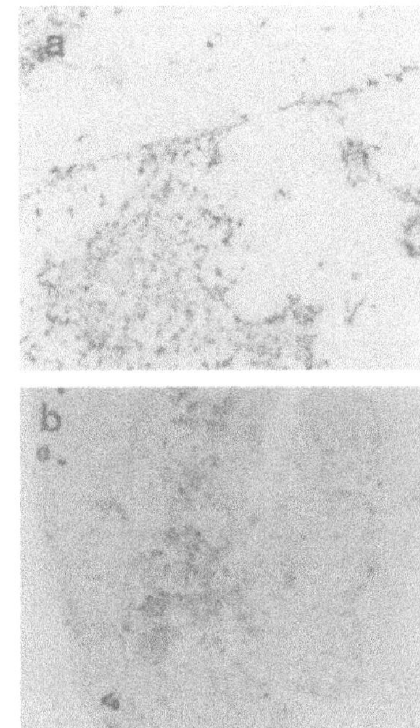

Figure 2. Immunocytochemical analysis of the chimeric thymus of SCID.FL(a) and the grafted thymus of SCID.FL/FT(b). In SCID.FL, the rat MHC class II specific antibody OX-6 specifically stains rat derived macrophages and dendritic cells, which are localized within the thymic medulla. Thymic epithelial cells are only stained in the transplanted SCID.FL/FT thymus.

into the rat thymus transplant, providing an intact rat thymic milieu (including epithelium, IDC and macrophages) which would allow correct differentiation as in an unmanipulated Lewis rat.

The chimeras were immunized, and MBP specific $CD4^+CD8^-$ rat T cells were isolated. All SCID.FL/FT TCLs were restricted exclusively by MHC class II products of the Lewis rat, recognized epitope p68–88 and were encephalitogenic in Lewis rats. In marked

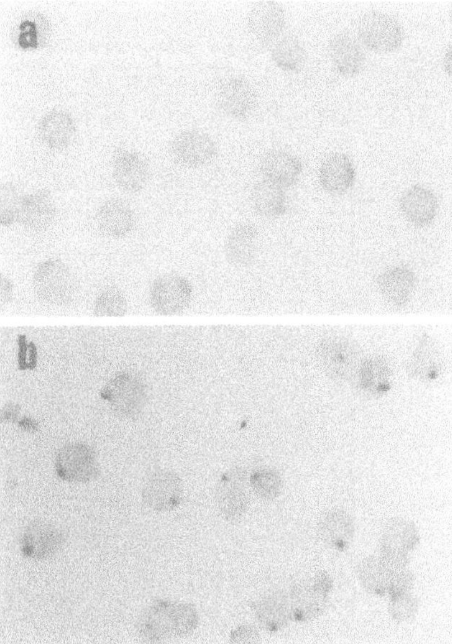

Figure 3. *In situ* hybridization of wild type (a) and TK-tsA transgenic (b) T lymphocytes. Transgenic T cells carry a genetic marker which can be visualized as a nuclear dot.

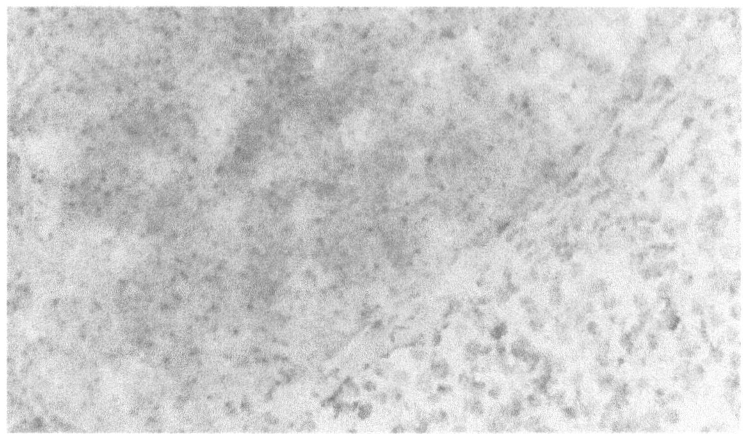

Figure 4. *In situ* hybridization of a wild type thymus graft of a SCID.FL/FT chimera reconstituted with TK-tsA transgenic fetal liver cells. Numerous TK-tsA DNA^{+}, fetal liver derived cells are seen in the graft.

contrast to their SCID.FL counterparts, however, SCID.FL/FT derived MBP specific TCLs used, without exception, Vß8.2 in their TCR.

But did these MBP-specific, Vß8.2+ T cells mature in the transplanted thymus? To answer this question, we constructed SCID.FL/FT chimeras by combining genetically marked transgenic fetal liver cells with wildtype thymus grafts. The marked liver cells were from transgenic Lewis rat embryos carrying a non-expressed transgenic marker with high copy number.

Transgenic T cells were identified by *in situ* hybridization using a transgene specific DNA probe, both in the grafted wild type thymus lobes and in MBP specific TCLs. They did not differ with respect to antigen recognition, MHC restriction, surface markers and TCR usage from wildtype TCLs derived from SCID.FL/FT chimera or intact Lewis rats. They all used Vß8.2.

Table 1. Characterization of TCLs derived from thymuses of unprimed and MBP-primed animals. All TCLs were specific for the priming/selecting antigen, which is recognized in the context of MHC class II (RT1.B^{l}), and express the αß TCR. MBP specific encephalitogenic T cells exclusively use the Vß8.2 TCR gene[15]

	Antigen specificity			TCR expression		
	No Ag	MBP	PPD	ConA	αß	Vß8.2
Unprimed TCL						
D10G2	51^{+}/-7	2767^{+}/-361	47^{+}/-3	4821^{+}/-291	100	NT
F6	3^{+}/-1	1775^{+}/-257	6^{+}/-2	2667^{+}/-428	100	97
B3	67^{+}/-4	9740^{+}/-318	54^{+}/-15	8948^{+}/-585	100	99
D10	15^{+}/-3	3980^{+}/-478	6^{+}/-1	6785^{+}/-814	100	98
E10	69^{+}/-1	12224^{+}/-87	24^{+}/-4	15330^{+}/-214	100	98
D3	182^{+}/-37	14295^{+}/-912	204^{+}/-75	20409^{+}/-2753	100	96
D2.1	15^{+}/-4	2086^{+}/-278	10^{+}/-4	5876^{+}/-798	100	2
MBP-primed TCL						
P25	200^{+}/-1	7475^{+}/-420	180^{+}/-20	10907^{+}/-2050	100	99
P26	66^{+}/-7	2265^{+}/-276	11^{+}/-4	8840^{+}/-1382	100	97

CONCLUSION AND SUMMARY

We have shown that the immune system of intact Lewis rats contains autoimmune T cells which have differentiated within the thymus, in the presence of autoantigens. Thus, negative selection of autoreactive T cell clones by local intrathymic autoantigens seems to be a rather leaky process. Alternatively, the unusual diversity of thymic autoantigens could also have a positive role in shaping the immune system's TCR diversity, possible in the sense of an "immunological homunculus", as postulated by Cohen[7].

REFERENCES

1. Ben-Nun, A., Wekerle, H., and Cohen, I.R. (1981). The rapid isolation of clonable antigen-specific T lymphocyte lines capable of mediating autoimmune encephalomyelitis. Eur. J. Immunol. *11*, 195–199.
2. Bogue, M., Candéias, S., Benoist, C., and Mathis, D. (1991). A special repertoire of a:b T cells in neonatal mice.. EMBO J. *10*, 3647–3654.
3. Burkly, L.C., Degermann, S., Longley, J., Hagman, J., Brinster, R.L., Lo, D., and Flavell, R.A. (1993). Clonal deletion of Vb5$^+$ T cells by transgenic I-E restricted to thymic medullary epithelium.. J. Immunol. *151*, 3954–3960.
4. Burns, F.R., Li, X., Shen, N., Offner, H., Chou, Y.K., Vandenbark, A.A., and Heber-Katz, E. (1989). Both rat and mouse T cell receptors specific for the encephalitogenic determinant of myelin basic protein use similar Va and Vb chain genes even though the major histocompatibility complex and encephalitogenic determinants being recognized are different. J. Exp. Med. *169*, 27–39.
5. Campagnoni, A.T., Pribyl, T.M., Campagnoni, C.W., Kampf, K., Amur-Umarjee, S., Landry, C.F., Handley, V.W., Newman, S.L., Garbay, B., and Kitamura, K. (1993). Structure and developmental regulation of *Golli-mbp*, a 105 kilobase gene that encompasses the myelin basic protein gene and is expressed in cells in the oligodendrocyte lineage in the brain.. J. Biol. Chem. *268*, 4930–4938.
6. Chluba, J., Steeg, C., Becker, A., Wekerle, H., and Epplen, J.T. (1989). T cell receptor b chain usage in myelin basic protein-specific rat T lymphocytes. Eur. J. Immunol. *19*, 279–284.
7. Cohen, I.R. (1992). The cognitive paradigm and the immunological homunculus.. Immunol. Today *13*, 490–494.
8. Feeney, A.J. (1991). Junctional sequences of fetal T cell receptor b chains have few N regions. J. Exp. Med. *174*, 115–124.
9. Gold, D.P., Offner, H., Sun, D., Wiley, S., Vandenbark, A.A., and Wilson, D.B. (1991). Analysis of T cell receptor b chains in Lewis rats with experimental allergic encephalomyelitis: Conserved complementary determining region 3.. J. Exp. Med. *174*, 1467–1476.
10. Greiner, D.L., Shultz, L.D., Rossini, A.A., Mordes, J.P., Handler, E.S., and Rajan, T.V. (1991). Recapitulation of normal and abnormal BB rat immune system development in SCID mouse/rat lymphohemopoietic chimeras.. J. Clin. Invest. *88*, 717–719.
11. Grima, B., Zelenika, D., and Pessac, B. (1992). A novel transcript overlapping the myelin basic protein gene.. J. Neurochem. *59*, 2318–2323.
12. Jones, R.E., Bourdette, D.N., Whitham, R.H., Offner, H., and Vandenbark, A.A. (1993). Induction of experimental autoimmune encephalomyelitis in severe combined immunodeficient mice reconstituted with allogeneic and xenogeneic hematopoietic cells.. J. Immunol. *150*, 4620–4629.
13. Jones, R.E., Whitham, R.H., Sullivan, T., Mass, M., and Bourdette, D.N. (1995). Encephalitogenic T lymphocytes develop from SJL/J hematopoietic cells transplanted into severe combined immunodeficient (SCID) mice.. J. Neuroimmunol. *57*, 155–164.
14. Kojima, K., Berger, T., Lassmann, H., Hinze-Selch, D., Zhang, Y., Gehrmann, J., Wekerle, H., and Linington, C. (1994). Experimental autoimmune panencephalitis and uveoretinitis in the Lewis rat transferred by T lymphocytes specific for the S100b molecule, a calcium binding protein of astroglia.. J. Exp. Med. *180*, 817–829.
15. Lannes-Vieira, J., Goudable, B., Drexler, K., Gehrmann, J., Torres-Nagel, N.E., Hünig, T., and Wekerle, H. (1995). Encephalitogenic, myelin basic protein specific T cells from naive rat thymus: Preferential use of the T cell receptor gene Vb8.2 and expression of the CD4$^-$CD8$^-$ phenotype.. Eur. J. Immunol. *25*, 611–616.
16. Lauriola, L., Michetti, F., Stolfi, V.M., Tallini, G., and Cocchia, D. (1984). Detection by S-100 immunolabelling of interdigitating reticulum cells in human thymuses. Virchows Arch. *45*, 187–195.

17. Mathisen, P.M., Pease, S., Garvey, J., Hood, L., and Readhead, C. (1993). Identification of an embryonic isoform of myelin basic protein that is expressed widely in the mouse embryo.. Proc. Natl. Acad. Sci. USA *90*, 10125–10129.
18. Max, H., Halder, T., Kalbus, M., Gnau, V., Jung, G., and Kalbacher, H. (1994). A 16mer peptide of the human autoantigen calreticulin is a most prominent HLA-DR4Dw4 associated self-peptide.. Hum. Immunol. *41*, 39–45.
19. Pribyl, T.M., Campagnoni, C.W., Kampf, K., Kashima, T., Handley, V.W., McMahon, J., and Campagnoni, A.T. (1993). The human myelin basic protein gene is included within a 179-kilobase transcription unit: Expression in the immune and central nervous system.. Proc. Natl. Acad. Sci. USA *90*, 10695–10699.
20. Schluesener, H.J. and Wekerle, H. (1985). Autoaggressive T lymphocyte lines recognizing the encephalitogenic region of myelin basic protein: In vitro selection from unprimed rat T lymphocyte populations. J. Immunol. *135*, 3128–3133.
21. Surh, C.D. and Sprent, J. (1991). Long-term xenogeneic chimeras. Full differentiation of rat T and B cells in SCID mice. J. Immunol. *147*, 2148–2154.
22. Torres-Nagel, N.E., Gold, D.P., and Hünig, T. (1993). Identification of rat Tcrb-V 8.2, 8.5, and 10 gene products by monoclonal antibodies.. Immunogenetics *37*, 305–308.
23. Ushiki, T., Iwanaga, T., Masuda, T., Takahashi, Y., and Fujita, T. (1984). Distribution and ultrastructure of S-100-immunoreactive cells in the human thymus. Cell Tiss. Res. *235*, 509–514.
24. Wekerle, H., Kojima, K., Lannes-Vieira, J., Lassmann, H., and Linington, C. (1994). Animal models.. Ann. Neurol. *36*, S47-S53.
25. Zhang, X.-M. and Heber-Katz, E. (1992). T cell receptor sequences from encephalitogenic T cells in adult Lewis rats suggest an early ontogenic origin.. J. Immunol. *148*, 746–752.
26. Zimmer, D.B., Cornwall, E.H., Landar, A., and Song, W. (1995). The S100 protein family: History, function and expression.. Brain Res. Bull. *37*, 417–429.

18

T CELL EPITOPES OF THE ACETYLCHOLINE RECEPTOR AND THE PATHOGENESIS OF MYASTHENIA GRAVIS

Arthur Melms,[1] Robert Weissert,[1] Alexej Schmidt,[1] Claudia Müller,[2] Günther Jung,[3] and Georg Malcherek[1]

[1]Department of Neurology
[2]Department of Medicine
Tübingen University Medical Center
[3]Institute of Organic Chemistry
University of Tübingen
D 72076 Tübingen, Germany

INTRODUCTION

CD4-positive T cells are required for sustained antibody production. T and B lymphocytes recognize cognate determinants of an antigen and communicate by direct cell to cell interactions including the CD40/CD40-ligand and B7-CTLA4 pairs of accessory molecules (reviewed in Clark and Ledbetter, 1994). In addition, T cell derived cytokines promote growth and differentiation signals for antibody-producing B cells (Coffman et al., 1988). In the animal model of myasthenia gravis (MG), experimental autoimmune myasthenia gravis (EAMG), the depletion of T lymphocytes prevents the production of autoantibodies after immunization with acetylcholine receptor (AChR; Lennon et al., 1976). T helper cells recognize antigen in the context of MHC class II molecules. Inhibition of antigen recognition by monoclonal antibodies to MHC class II molecules has been reported to suppress the immune response to AChR and prevent EAMG in vivo (Waldor et al., 1983). MHC class II molecules bind peptides in a preformed binding groove and allelic products differ in their binding requirements which have been described as allele-specific ligand or binding motifs (Rammensee et al., 1995). For example, the bm-12 mutation of murine MHC class II molecules I-A alters the peptide binding site of MHC class II molecules, hence, animals with the bm-12 mutation respond to a different set of AChR peptides compared to the wild type and are resistant to the induction of EAMG (Bellone et al., 1991). This underscores the strong influnence of MHC class II molecules on the determinant selection and the immune response regarding the susceptibility to develop an autoimmune disease.

Epithelial Tumors of the Thymus, edited by Marx and Müller-Hermelink.
Plenum Press, New York, 1997

In humans, there is also circumstantial evidence for T cells playing a significant role in the pathogenesis of MG. First, the thymus and thymoma in MG are enriched with AChR-specific T cells (Melms et al., 1988; Sommer et al., 1990). Since AChR is expressed on myoid epithlial cells as normal constituents of the thymus medulla, a chain of events has been proposed which argues for an intrathymic pathogenesis of MG (Wekerle et al., 1981). Thymoma cells i.e. neoplastic thymic epithlial cells do not express AChR polypeptides, however, they express determinants shared by the AChR (Kirchner et al., 1988; Marx et al., 1990) suggesting mechanisms linking the paraneoplatic immune response to AChR by immunological mimicry (Fujinami and Oldstone 1985). Functionally, neoplastic thymic epithlial are capable to process and present antigens (Marx et al., 1994) including the AChR and stimulate autoreactive T cells (Gilhus et al., 1995). In the non-neoplastic thymus, there is an accumulation of B lymphocytes producing considerable amounts of AChR-autoantibodies forming germinal centers and after thymectomy there is a significant drop in AChR autoantibody titer (Vincent et al., this volume) often associated with amelioration of myasthenic symptoms. This scenario briefly illustrates the pivotal role of the thymus and the thymus-dependent immune responses in the autoimmune escalation eventually leading to MG (Wekerle 1993).

During the past decade, much effort was spent in several laboratories to study T cell responses in myasthenia gravis. It was expected from experimental conditions that the identification of T cell determinants should foster the development of a T cell directed selective immunotherapy to control the autoimmune deviation by tuning down autoreactive AChR-specific T helper cells. This might give insight not only into the pathophysiology of autoimmune T cells but also about the mechanisms initiating the autoimmune response focused on AChR.

THE AChR AS A MODEL MULTIDETERMINANT AUTOANTIGEN

The AChR is a multideterminant antigen-complex containing numerous antigenic determinants for B- and T-lymphocytes. The majority of autoantibodies in MG patients are directed against a conformation-dependent epitope including the sequence α67–76 on the extra-cellular part of the AChR α-subunit termed the main immunogenic region (MIR; Tzartos et al., 1988). By contrast, T cells recognize antigen fragments generated by intracellular degradation in antigen-presenting cells, hence, they may respond to determinants from all over the molecule including epitopes on intra-/extra- and transmembrane segments of the AChR. Progress in technology has greatly facilitated the study of T cell determinants on the peptide level. In an ambitious approach, a battery of overlapping peptides spanning all subunits of the human AChR was synthesized by Conti-Tronconi and associates and examined for peptides that evoked T cell responses in MG patients (reviewed in Protti et al., 1993). They found a striking heterogeneity of candidate epitopes which clearly showed that the AChR is a highly immunogenic protein antigen inducing a rather heterogeneous T cell response. This is in some contrast with a more restricted pattern in strains of experimental animals. Moreover, given our current understanding of the physiology of antigen processing , it is not known whether all AChR candidate epitopes survive the intracellular degradation and how they succeed in the competition for binding to MHC molecules eventually being presented on the cell surface hence whether they equivalents of naturally processed antigen fragments. Traditionally, we prefer raising T cell lines and clones with intact antigens thereby avoiding a bias in processing by predetermined peptides and then using peptides to map T cell determinants in a second step (Hawke et al. 1996).

AChR-PEPTIDES BINDING TO HLA-DR3(17)

The association in young adult caucasians of MG and HLA-DR3 (Compston et al.1980) prompted us to examine the role of HLA-DR3 (the new nomenclature is DR17 or DRB1*0301) as a restriction molecule for autoreactive, AChR-specific T helper cells. We expected that the analysis of peptides bound to and presented by HLA-DR3(17) would give new insight about autoantigenic T cell determinants of the AChR and why the DR3(17)haplotype confers an increased risk for MG.

First, we have determined the binding requirements of peptides naturally bound to HLA-DR3(17) and extracted a motif for DR3(17)-binding ligands which is a pattern of 4 conserved residues of a nine-mer core segment fitting the DR17 binding groove (Malcherek et al., 1993 and Table 1). The contribution of specific contact sites as anchors in peptide-MHC-interaction was systematically evaluated by alanine-substituted analogues of prominent natural ligands (Malcherek et al., 1994). This information provided the basis to select.candidate protein sequences biased for binding to HLA-DR3(17). Here we describe the features of preselected DR17-motif peptides of the AChR and their features as T cell epitopes. During the past few years, ligand motifs have been determined for many MHC-alleles which refined our view about the peptide-MHC interaction. The rapidly expanding base of information should be a useful guide to study antigen-recognition in various allelels predicting novel T cell determinants in the future (Rammensee et al. 1995).

Table 1. Binding capacity of DR17-motif -peptides from human acetylcholine receptor α-subunit

DR3(17)-bindung motif	1 * * 4 * 6 * * 9	
(peptide core)	L D K Y	
	I R F	**$C_{50\%}$ inhibition**
	F E R	**DR17-agonist**
	M Q hydrophobic	**binding**
	V aliphatic/ aromatic	**μM**
natural DR17-ligand (agonist)		
ApoB(2877-92)	I S N Q L T L **D** S **N** I K **Y** F H K	**1.0**
acetylcholine receptor peptides (motif peptides)		
α7-24	L V A K **L** F K **D** Y S S V **V** R P V E D	**38**
α37-54	L I Q L **I** N V **D** E V N Q **I** V T T N V	>200
α63-80	Y N L K **W** N P **D** D Y G G **V** K K I H I	>200
α82-99	S E K I **W** R P **D** L V L Y **N** N A D G D	**46**
α131-148	I V T H **F** P F **D** E **Q** N C S M K L G T	>200
α145-162	K L G T **W** T Y **D** G S V V **A** I N P E S	**40**
α231-248	L V F Y **L** P T **D** S G E K **M** T L S I S	>200
α310-327 human	N W V R K **V** F I **D** T I P N **I** M F F S	**2**
α310-327 torpedo	Q W V R K **I** F I **D** T I P N **V** M F F S	**2**
α338-355	D K K **I** F T **D** I D I S D I S G K P	**70**
α382-399	I A E T **M** K S **D** Q **E** S N **A** A A E W K	**127**
α400-417	K Y V A **M** V M **D** H I L L G V F M L V	**4**

The α-subunit of the AChR is the most immunogenic in humans and experimental animals (Hohlfeld et al., 1987; Fujii and Lindstrom, 1988). It contains eleven DR17-motif peptides which have in the nine-mer core segment fitting the DR17-binding groove hydrophobic aliphatic or aromatic residues at relative position 1 and the DR17-specific anchor site aspartate at relative position 4 (Table 1). In addition, some peptides had compatible residues at positions 6 and 9. These peptides were synthesized according to the size of natural ligands previously isolated from purified DR3(17)-molecules (Malcherek et al., 1993 and 1994). Table 1 shows the binding performance of α-subunit motif peptides in competition with a high affinity natural ligand. The range of this assay is about 200 μM to measure half-maximal inhibition of agonist binding but there is evidence that peptides exceeding this value still retain some activity for DR3(17)-binding. Although several peptides share identical anchor residues like α310–327 and α37–54 they differ considerably in their binding capacity (in this example by a factor of more than 200). This is in accordance with our earlier observation that the primary peptide sequence especially charged non-anchor neighbour residues (aspartate, D and glutamate, E) have adverse influences on the binding performance. Nevertheless, among this set of eleven AChR motif peptides, two were active like natural high affinity ligands, five bound reasonalbly well and only four peptides were rather less competitive antagonoists of naturally bound peptides. T cells ignore the majority of natural DR3(17)-ligands like the peptides from apolipoprotein B, transferrin receptor and others membrane-associated proteins and their ligands. Therefore, MHC-binding capacity is certainly a major prerequisite for a given peptide to be immunogenic, however, it is the T cell repertoire and the presence of specific T cells which makes a processed peptide a T cell epitope.

Following this issue, we examined the ability of AChR-motif peptides to evoke proliferation of peripheral blood lymphocytes from a panel of DR3-positive donors, both MG patients and normal healthy volunteers. We noted in primary peptide-stimulated cultures that virtually all motif-peptides although with individual preferrences evoked significant responses that exceeded the controls. However, there was no difference in the pattern between DR3-positive healthy individuals and DR3-positive MG patients. Unexpectedly, AChR-peptide responses were more frequent and stronger in normal DR3-positive individuals than in MG patients who were not on immunosupression. Motif-peptides located on the extra-cellular part of the α-subunit (α1–216) were not strikingly immunogenic, however, the peptides α231–248, α310–327 and α338–355 were the prominent T cell determinants recognized in the DR17-positive population. A minority of non-DR3(17) controls also responded to some peptides which can be explained by the presence of additional motifs in the primary peptide sequences. For example, there is a cluster of motifs in α310–327 compatible with binding to DR1, DR3 and DR4.

Several T cell clones were raised from limiting dilution cultures stimulated with AChRα338–355, which was the most prominent determinant recognized by more than 2/3 of all DR17-positive individuals and by all DR17-positive normal donors. These monospecific T cells allowed a series of experiments to study motif-peptide recognition in more detail. Figure 1 shows that T cells responded vigorously to AChR peptide α338–355 but obviously ignore all the longer antigen stimuli containing this particular sequence. Moreover, another T cell clone from a DR17-positive MG patient recognized AChR α310–327 (Figure 2). This peptide has previously been reported as a T cell epitope from several different laboraories (Brocke et al., 1988; Protti et al., 1993, Matsuo et al., 1995) and happens to be one of the best DR17-binding peptides that we found (Table 1 and Malcherek et al., 1994). We have used DR3-transfected L-cells to confirm that AChRα310–327 is recognized in the context of DR3(17) (data not shown). Comparing the core-sequences from

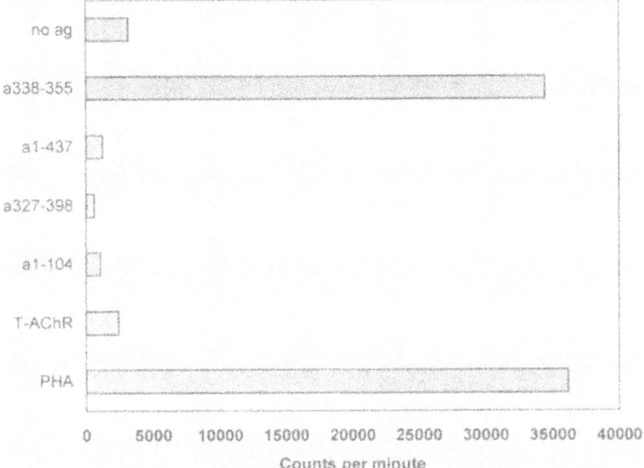

Figure 1. T cells raised from limiting dilution cultures of a DR3(17)-positive donor were challenged with autologous antigen presenting cells and the selecting AChR motif-peptide α338–355, or recombinant AChR polypeptides, or torpedo AChR. Bars indicate T cell proliferation measured as counts per minute of ^{3}H-thymidine incorporation.

human and torpedo-AChR, there are just two conservative exchanges at compatible anchor residues of AChRα310–327 making both peptide cores indistinguishable for the T cell receptor. However, if such α310–327 peptide-specific T cells were challenged with the α-subunit polypeptide or torpedo-AChR both antigens failed to stimulate these T cells (Figure 2). When we tested truncated variants of α310–327 we noted a significant reduction of the T cell stimulation after removing residue 311W, tryptophane (Figure 3). The DR17-motif resides between residues valine (V) 315 and isoleucin (I) 322 and truncation outside this core-segment did not affect the binding performance (α312–325 bound even slightly better than α310–327, data not shown). A systematic alanine-scan of α310–327 showed that, as expected, exchanges at certain sites inside the binding core did also affect immunogenicity, however, the exhange of 311W for alanine (A) severly impaired the an-

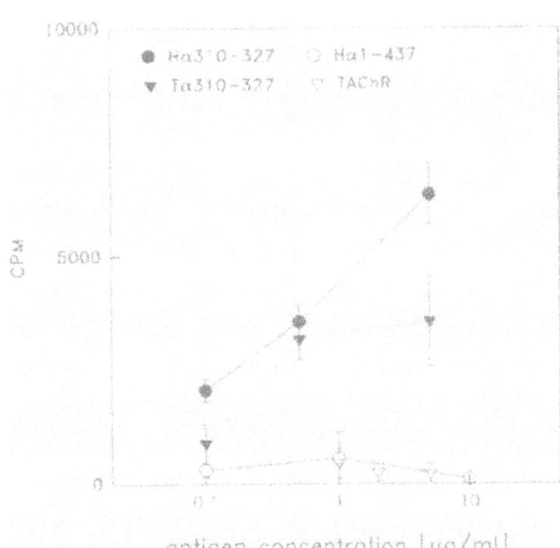

Figure 2. T cells specific for AChR motif peptide α310–327 stimulated with autologous antigen presenting cells and antigens as indicated in the legend.

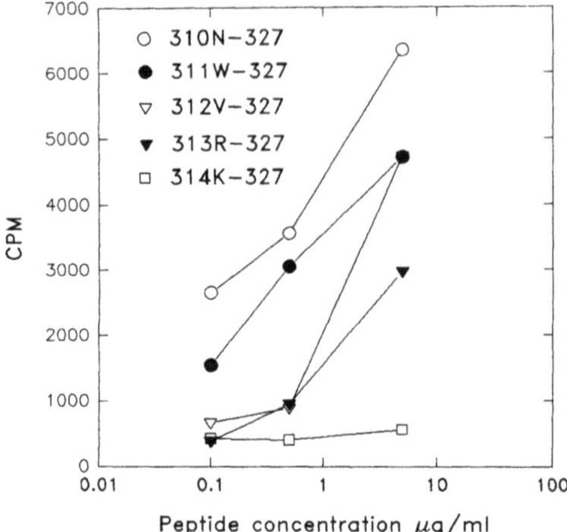

Figure 3. Dose-response analysis and effect of N-terminal peptide truncation in T cells specific for AChR motif peptide α310–327.

tigenicity of non-truncated ala-substitited peptide variant. Together this argues that at least one specific extra-core contact at 311W is required for the full activation of this particular T cell clone. With regard to the failure of the long-sized antigens to activate α310–327-specific T cells, one possible explanation is that antigen-processing fragments are generated lacking residue 311W or more at the N-terminus. Therefore, peptide-specific T cells, apparently, do not reflect the true repertoire of autoreactive AChR-specific T helper cells. Supporting this view of non-physiological processing of preselected AChR-peptides, Willcox and collegues analysed similar T cells and noted that prolonged antigen storage or digestion by trypsin which is not involved in the proteolytic antigen degradation in lysosomes created products that were active and stimulated α310–327-specific T cells in vitro (Matsuo et al., 1995).

This situation is in marked contrast with our results with DR17-motif peptides from a foreign antigen, tetanus toxin (TT). Chosing a set of eleven DR17-motif-peptides from tetanus toxin, there was a perfect correlation between the binding performance of TT-motif peptides and their nature as T cell determinants. In particular, on the clonal level motif-peptides could be shown as equivalents of naturally-processed fragments of tetanus toxin (Malcherek et al., manuscript submitted).

Currently, the physiological role of AChR-peptide-specific T cell as described here remains unclear. They certainly reflect some of the ability of the encyclopedic T cell repertoire to respond in principle to high affinity ligands. As they do not recognize the antigen proper, they are unlikely, at first sight, to be involved in the pathogenesis of MG. Sercarz and collegues have launched the concept of antigenic spreading to cryptic epitopes and their role in autommunity requires further investigation (Lehmann et al., 1992). Motif-peptides like the ones described here tend to have good MHC binding capacities. Recent observations, however, suggest that autoreactive T cell may have escaped the thymic selection process by recognizing low affinity ligands (Gammon end Sercarz, 1990; Liu et al., 1995). In addition, it is apparent that not all possible peptides from a self antigen are presented, hence, T cell tolerance is restricted to epitopes that were physiologically presented (Schild et al., 1990). We are now much better prepared to address these issues in human autoimmune diseases in our future experiments.

SUMMARY

We have applied the DR17-ligand motif to select from the sequence of the AChR α-subunit a set of peptides which in majority had good binding capacities. Hence, the DR17-motif in peptide sequences correlated with DR17-binding. All AChR-motif peptides evoked significant proliferation in peripheral blood lymphocytes from a panel of DR17-positive donors. Whereas high affinity motif peptides from tetanus toxin were found equivalent of naturally processed antigen fragments, T cells selected with AChR peptides did not recognize AChR polypeptides containing the respective sequences. There is evidence that some DR17-motif peptides of AChR are simply not generated after processing of AChR polypeptides in antigen-presenting cells. Therefore, peptide-specific T cells do not reflect the true repertoire of autoreactive AChR-specific T helper cells in myasthenia gravis. Regarding peptides forming T cell determinants, it appears that high affinity peptides of AChR do not follow the rules of foreign antigenic peptides. This is in accordance with observations arguing that autoreactive T cells may have escaped thymic tolerance induction by recognizing low affinity determinants. These issues are now being addressed with regard to the pathogenesis of myasthenia gravis.

ACKNOWLEDGMENTS

We thank U. Gern for expert technical assistance. Work in the laboratory of A.M. was supported by the DFG, Sonderforschungsbereich 120 and a grant from the Sandoz Stiftung für Therapeutische Forschung. G.M. was supported by a fellowship from the fortüne-Programm of the University of Tübingen.

REFERENCES

Bellone M, Ostile N, Lei S, Wu XD, Conti-Tronconi B. 1991. The I-A^{bm12}mutation, which confers resistence to experimental autoimmune myasthenia gravis, drastically affects the epitope repertoire of murine CD4+ cells sensitized to nicotinic acetylcholine receptor. J Immunol. 147:1484–1491

Brocke S, Brautbar C, Steinman L, Abramsky O, Rothbard J, Neumann D, Fuchs S, Mozes E. 1988. In vitro proliferative responses and antibody titers specific to human acetylcholine receptor synthetic peptides in patients with myasthenia gravis and relation to HLA class II genes. J. Clin. Invest. 82:1894–1900

Clark EA, Ledbetter JA. 1994. How T and B cells talk to each other. Nature 367:425–428

Coffman RL, Seymour BW, Lebman DA, Hiraki DD, Christiansen JA, Shrader B, Cherwinski HM, Savelkoul HF, Finkelman FD, Bond MW, Mossmann TR. 1988. The role of helper T cell products in mouse B cell differentiation and isotype regulation. Immunol. Rev. 102: 5–28

Compston DAS, Vincent A, Newsom Davis J, Batchelor JR. 1980. Clinical, pathological, HLA antigen and immunological evidence for disease heterogeneity in myasthenia gravis. Brain 103, 579–601

Fujinami RS, Oldstone MBA. 1985. Amino acid homology between the encephalithogenic site of myelin basic protein and virus: mechanism for autoimmunity. Science 230:1043–1045

Fuji Y, Lindstrom J. 1988. Specificity of the T cell response to acetylcholine receptor in experimental autoimmune myasthenia gravis . Response to subunits and synthetic peptides. J. Immunol. 140: 1830–1837

Gammon G, Sercarz E. 1989. How some T cells escape tolerance induction. Nature 342:183–185

Gilhus NE, Willcox N, Harcourt G, Nagvekar N, Beeson D, Vincent A, Newsom-Davis J. 1995. Antigen-presentation by thymoma epithelial cells from myasthenia gravis patients to potentially pathogenic T cells. J. Neuroimmunol. 56: 65–76

Hawke S, Nagvekar, Nicolle M, Malcherek G, Melms A, Willcox N. 1996. Autoimmune T cells in myasthenia gravis: Heterogeneity and potential as target for therapy. Immunol today in press

Hohlfeld R, Toyka KV, Tzartos SJ, Carson W, Conti-Tronconi B. 1987. Human T helper lymphocytes in myasthenia gravis recognize the nicotinic receptor alpha subunit. Proc. Natl. Acad. Sci. USA 84:5379–5383

Kirchner T, Tzartos S, Hoppe F, Schalke B, Wekerle H, Müller-Hermelink HK. 1988. Pathogenesis of myasthenia gravis: Acetylcholine receptor-related determinants in tumor-free thymuses and thymic epithelial tumors. Am. J. Pathol. 130:268–280

Lehmann PV, Forsthuber T, Miller A, Sercarz EE. 1992. Spreading of T cell autoimmunity to cryptic determinants of an autoantigen. Nature 358: 155–157

Lennon VA, Lindstrom JM, Seybold ME. 1976. Experimental autoimmune myasthenia gravis: Cellular and humoral immune responses. Ann. N.Y. Acad. Sci. 274, 283–299

Liu GY, Fairchild PJ, Smith RM, Prowle JR, Kioussis D, Wraith DC. 1995. Low avidity recognition of self-antigen by T cells permits escape from central tolerance. Immunity 3:407–415

Malcherek G, Falk K, Rötzschke O, Rammensee H-G, Stevanovic S, Gnau V, Jung G, Melms A. 1993. Peptide motif of two HLA molecules associated with myasthenia gravis. Intl. Immunol. 5:1229–1237

Malcherek G, Gnau V, Stevanovic S, Rammensee HG, Jung G, Melms A. 1994. Characterization of allele-specific contact sites of DR17 ligands. J. Immunol. 154: 1141–1149

Marx A, O'Connor R, Geuder KI, Hoppe F, Schalke B, Tzartos S, Kalies I, Kirchner T, Müller-Hermelink HK. 1990. Characterization of a protein with an acetylcholine receptor epitope from myasthenia gravis associated thymomas. Lab. Invest. 62: 279–286

Marx A, Schömig D, Schultz A, Gattenlöhner S, Jung S, Kirchner T, Melms A, Müller-Hermelink HK. 1994. Distribution of molecules mediating thymocyte-stroma interactions in human thymus, thymitis and thymic epithelial tumours. Thymus 23: 83–93

Matsuo H, Batocchi A-P, Hawke S, Nicolle M, Jacobson L, Vincent A, Newsom-Davis J, Willcox, N. 1995. Peptide-selected T cell lines from myasthenia gravis patients and controls recognize epitopes that are not processed from whole acetylcholine receptor. J. Immunol. 155: 3683–3692

Melms A, Schalke B, Kirchner T, Albert E, Müller-Hermelink HK, Wekerle H. 1988. Thymus in myasthenia gravis: Isolation of T lymphocyte lines specific for the nicotinic acetylcholine receptor from myasthenic patients. J. Clin. Invest. 81:902–908

Protti MP, Manfredi A, Horton RM, Bellone M, Conti-Tronconi BM. 1993. Myasthenia gravis: recognition of a human autoantigen at the molecular level. Immunol. Today 14:363–368

Rammensee HG, Friede T, Stevanovic S. 1995. MHC ligands and peptide motifs: first listing. Immunogenetics 41:178–228

Schild HJ, Rötzschke O, Kalbacher H, Rammensee HG. 1990. Limit of T cell tolerance to self proteins by peptide presentation. Science 247: 1587–1589

Sommer N, Willcox N, Harcourt GC, Newsom-Davis J. 1990. Myasthenic thymus and thymoma are selectively enriched in acetylcholine receptor-reactive T cells. Ann. Neurol. 28:312–319

Tzartos SJ, Kokla A, Walgrave SL, Conti-Tronconi BM. 1988. Localization of the main immunogenic region of human muscle acetylcholine receptor to residues 67–76 of the α-subunit. Proc. Natl. Acad. Sci. USA 85: 2899–2903

Waldor MK, Sriram S, McDevitt HO, Steinman LS. 1983. In-vivo therapy with monoclonal anti-I-A antibody suppresses immune response to acetylcholine receptor. Proc. Natl. Acad. Sci. USA 80: 2713–2717

Wekerle H. 1993. The thymus in myasthenia gravis. Ann. N.Y. Acad. Sci. 681: 47–55

19

THYMUS IN THYMOMA-ASSOCIATED MYASTHENIA GRAVIS

Transplantation of Thymoma and Extrathymomal Thymic Tissue into SCID Mice

A. Sarropoulos,[1] A. Marx,[2] R. Hohlfeld,[1,3] H. Wekerle,[1] and S. Spuler[1,3*]

[1]Department of Neuroimmunology
Max-Planck-Institute, Martinsried
[2]Department of Neurology
University of Munich
[3]Department of Pathology
University of Würzburg

1. INTRODUCTION

The SCID mouse model of myasthenia gravis (MG) has given some insight into the pathogenesis of autoimmune MG associated with lymphofollicular hyperplasia of the thymus[1,2]. In this model, small pieces of thymic tissue were transplanted under the kidney capsule of SCID mice. The transplant induced a longlasting production of anti-acetylcholine receptor antibodies (anti-AchR-abs) in these mice. In contrast, the injection of single cell suspensions containing 100fold more cells than thymus transplant resulted only in an initial, transient rise of anti-AchR-abs. When investigated immunohistochemically, the transplants had retained the characteristic features of thymus tissue. Some myoid cells had differentiated further into myotubes. This study demonstrated that the hyperplastic thymus in autoimmune MG contains all elements necessary to induce and maintain an immune response against the AchR.

The pathogenesis of paraneoplastic MG is different from autoimmune MG. Here, the thymic abnormalities consist not of lymphofollicular hyperplasia but of epithelial neoplasias. Using the classification of thymic tumors introduced by Kirchner and Müller-Hermelink[3] the cortical thymoma and the well differentiated thymic carcinoma are strongly associated with the development of paraneoplastic MG. The AchR is not expressed in these thymomas[4]. Pa-

* Correspondence to: Dr. Simone Spuler, Dept. of Neurology, Mayo Clinic, Rochester, MN 55905, USA. Fax: 507-284-5831.

Epithelial Tumors of the Thymus, edited by Marx and Müller-Hermelink.
Plenum Press, New York, 1997

Table 1. Characteristics of patients with thymoma-associated MG

Patient and sex	Age (a)	Type	Anti-AchRAb titer(nmol/l)	Anti-striated muscle abs	Histology
W.D., m	32	generalized	>20	n.t.	cortical thymoma
W.S., m	74	generalized	34	pos.	well differentiated thymic carcinoma
A.M., f	54	generalized	56	pos.	cortical thymoma
P.T., m	44	generalized	96	neg.	cortical thymoma and lymphofollicular hyperplasia in the restthymus

n.t.: not tested

tients with paraneoplastic MG commonly have very high anti-AchR ab titers, are often also positive for anti-striational ab and usually do not respond well to thymectomy.

To investigate the role of the thymus in paraneoplastic MG we transplanted small pieces of thymoma tissue and of extrathymomal thymic remnant under the kidney capsule of SCID mice. The serum of the mice was assayed for the presence of human IgG, anti-striational abs and antiAchR abs at regular intervalls and all transplants were investigated by immunohistochemistry.

2. MATERIALS AND METHODS

2.1. Patients

The clinical data of the patients are summarized in Table 1.

2.2. Methods

Figure 1 shows an overview of the experiment.

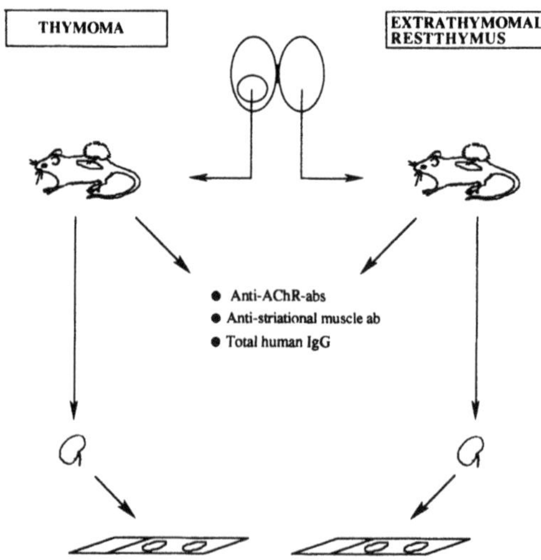

Figure 1. Method.

Table 2. Monoclonal antibodies used for immunocytochemistry

Antibody	Concentration or dilution	Epitope	Reference or company
OKT 4	1:100	CD 4 molecule	ATCC, USA
T 8	1:2	CD 8 molecule	Coulter Electronics, FRG
Leu 14	1:25	CD 22 molecule	Becton-Dickinson, FRG
L 234	1:2	HLA-DR molecule	ATCC, USA
MAS 114p	1:250	HLA-ABC molecule	Seralab
KS 1A3	1:100	Cytokeratin pepitide 13	Sigma, FRG
mab 155	1.0 mm/ml	AChR-a371-378, cross-reactive with troponin I	7,8

2.3. Immunocytochemistry

For immunoperoxidase stains, the tissue was fixed in acetone for 5 min at -20 °C. After fixation, the free binding sites were blocked. Monoclonal abs against different surface markers were added at the optimal concentration in the same solution for 30 min. The abs used in this study are listed in Table 2.

Afterwards the reaction was further enhanced with a three step peroxidase staining, developed with diaminobenzidine (Sigma, Munich, FRG) and counterstained with hematoxylin.

2.4. Detection of Human IgG, Specific Anti-AChR Abs and Anti-Striational Muscle Abs

The concentration of whole human IgG was measured by a two-site ELISA. The plates were read at O.D. 405 nm using a Titertek Multiskan® (Flow Laboratories, Meckenheim, FRG). Ig standards were obtained from Dianova (ChromePure ™). The assay was sensitive to an Ig concentration of 10 ng/ml.

The concentration of human anti-AchR abs was measured with a radioimmunoprecipitation assay as described by Lindstrom et al [5].

Abs against striated muscle components were determined by immunofluorescence staining. Briefly, the sera were incubated with rat muscle and binding of anti-striational muscle ab detected by staining with FITC-labeled goat anti human IgG.

3. RESULTS

3.1. Examination of the MG-Thymus Grafts after Transplantation into SCID Mice

3.1.1. Thymoma Transplants. Fig.2a shows the H&E overview of the thymoma transplant not infiltrating the mouse kidney, but remaining separated by a connective tissue capsule. Stainings against HLA-ABC and -DR confirm the non-invasive growth of the thymoma transplants. The mainly epithelial character of the thymoma is demonstrated by a stain against cytokeratine p13 (Fig. 2b). All thymomas had CD 4 (Fig. 2c) and CD 8 positive T-cells whereas CD 22+ B-cells never occurred. Fig. 2d shows a stain with mab 155 which was positive in all thymoma transplants, but typical myoid cells were never present.

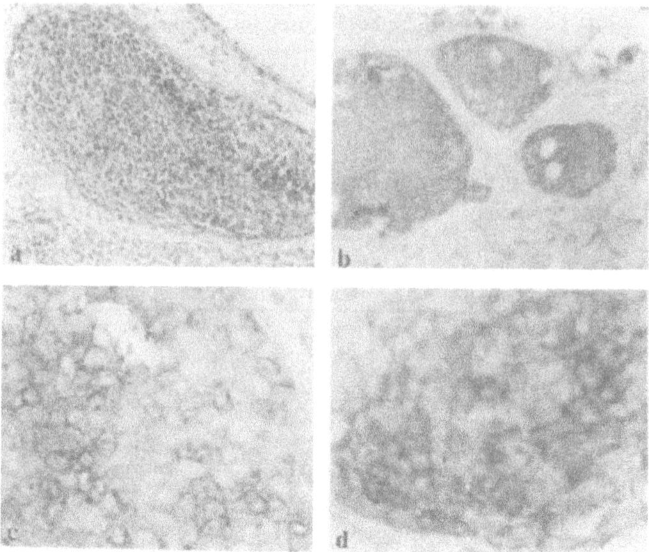

Figure 2. Histology of the thymoma-transplants, consecutive sections of the same kidney. (a) H&E overview (40x), (b) anti-cytoceratine p13 (30x), anti-CD4 (60x), mab 155 (60x).

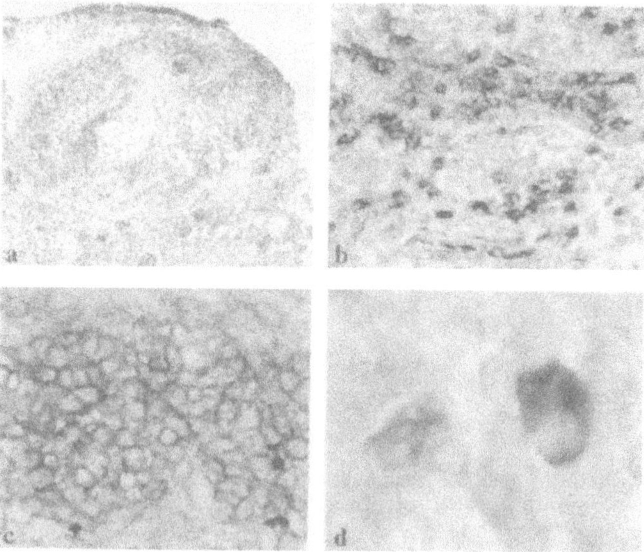

Figure 3. Histology of the hyperplastic restthymus, consecutive sections of the same kidney. (a) H&E stain (20x), (b) anti CD4 (40x), (c) anti CD22 (60x), mab 155 (1200x).

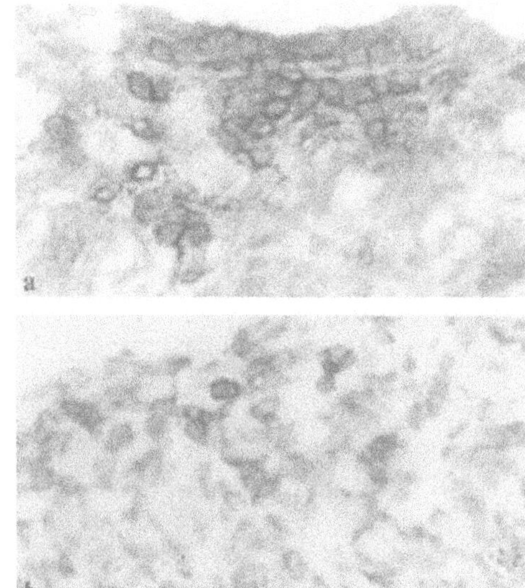

Figure 4. Histology of the involuted restthymus, consecutive sections of the same kidney. (a) anti HLA-ABC (600x), (b) anti CD22 (600x).

3.1.2. Transplants with Extrathymomal Thymic Tissue. The histology of the extrathymomal thymic tissue shows a different degree of involution and in one case, the extrathymomal restthymus was hyperplastic (Patient P.T.)

Fig. 3a shows the H&E overview of this hyperplastic thymus tissue. In all hyperplastic thymus transplants HLA-ABC, HLA-DR, cytokeratine p13, CD 4+(Fig. 3b), CD 8+ and CD 22+ (Fig. 3c) cells were detectable. Staining with mab 155 shows typical myoid cells (Fig. 3d).

The total amount of human cells found in the involuted thymic transplants was smaller, but they also contained CD 22+ B-cells (Fig. 4b) in areas positive for anti-HLA-ABC (Fig. 4a) and HLA-DR.

3.2. Human Anti-AChR Abs Measurement, Whole Human IgG and Anti-Striational Muscle Abs in the Serum of Transplanted SCID Mice

No anti-AchR abs could be detected in SCID mice transplanted with thymoma tissue (n=24). Anti-AchR abs were also absent in sera of mice that had received involuted thymic tissue (n=11) (not shown). Fig. 5 shows the graph of the aAchR ab titers of the trans-

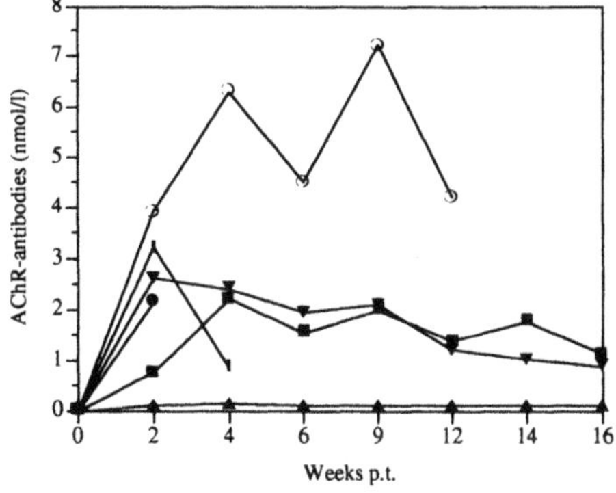

Figure 5. Anti-AChR abs titers after transplantation of hyperplastic restthymus.

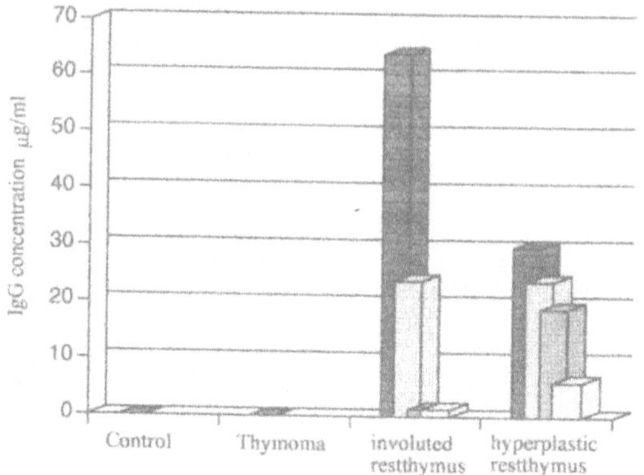

Figure 6. Whole human IgG in the SCID-mice sera.

plants with hyperplastic thymus tissue (n=6), where one can see in agreement with previous results a high production of anti AchR abs for periods of three to four months[1].

The ELISA for the whole human IgG titers shows no human antibodies in SCID sera tested from thymoma-transplanted mice. In contrast, human IgG was detected in all sera from SCID mice that had been transplanted with extrathymomal thymic tissue, regardless of whether these transplants were hyperplastic or involuted (Fig. 6).

Anti-striational muscle abs were negative in all transplanted mice.

4. DISCUSSION

In regard to their myasthenic symptoms, patients with thymoma associated MG usually do not benefit from thymectomy in contrast to MG-patients with lymphofollicular hyperplasia of the thymus [6]. This may be explained by removal of a major source of anti-AchR ab producing B-cells in hyperplastic thymi. B-cells were completly absent from thymoma tissue, no specific anti-AchR-abs and no human IgG was produced by thymoma fragments transplanted into SCID mice.

However, B-cells are present in the extrathymomal thymic tissue. Those B-cells secrete human IgG in SCID mice. Although the patients had very high anti-AchR ab titers, these autoabs were not detected in the SCID sera, except in one case, where the extrathymomal thymic remnant showed lymphofollicular hyperplasia.

Although the thymus in thymoma associated MG is not a source of autoab-production the thymus still seems to be involved in the pathogenesis of the disease.

Cortical thymomas and the well differentiated thymus carcinoma, which have the strongest association to MG [3] express a protein (p153) which was found on thymic epithelial cells and is recognized by mab 155[7,9]. In our study p153 could also be detected in the thymoma transplants. Although the function of p153 is unknown, it is possible that T-cells are sensitized in thymomas against p153, which cross-react with epitopes on the AchR. Those T-lymphocytes could activate B-lymphocytes in the peripherial immune system to produce autoabs against native AchR [10]. This could explain the persistence of MG symtoms and the poor reduction of autoantibody-producing B-cells after thymectomy.

Here it has been shown, that neither thymoma tissue nor involuted restthymus is able to induce an anti-AchR-ab production after transplantation into SCID mice.

5. REFERENCES

1. Schönbeck S, Padberg F, Hohlfeld R, Wekerle H. Transplantation of thymic autoimmune microenvironment to severe combined immunodeficient mice. A new model of myasthenia gravis. J Clin Invest 1992; 90: 245–250
2. Spuler S, Marx A, Kirchner T, Hohlfeld R, Wekerle H. Myogenesis in thymic transplants in the SCID mouse model of myasthenia gravis: differentiation of myoid cells into striated muscle cells. Am J Pathol 1994; 145: 766–770
3. Kirchner T, Müller-Hermelink HK. New approaches to the diagnosis of thymic epithelial tumors. In: Progress in Surgical Pathology, 10. CM Fenoglio-Preiser, M Wolff & F Rilke, Eds Field and Wood Inc. Philadelphia, 1989; 167–186
4. Geuder KI, Marx A, Witzemann V, Schalke B, Kichner T, Müller-Hermelink HK. Genomic organization and lack of transcription of the nicotinic acetylcholine receptor subunit genes in myasthenia gravis-associated thymoma. Lab Invest 1992; 66: 452–458
5. Lindstrom J, Seybold ME, Lennon VA, Whittingham S, Duane DD. Antibody to acetylcholine receptor in myasthenia gravis. Prevalence, clinical correlates, and diagnostic value. Neurology 1976; 26: 1054–1059
6. Oosterhuis HJGH. Observations of the natural history of myasthenia gravis and the effect of thymectomy. Ann NY Acad Sci 1981; 377: 678–690
7. Marx A, Osborn M, Tzartos S, Geuder KI, Schalke B, Nix W, Kirchner T, Müller-Hermelink HK. A striational muscle antigen and myasthenia gravis-associated thymomas share an acetylcholine-receptor epitope. Develop Immunol 1992; 2: 77–84
8. Tzartos S, Langeberg L, Hochschwender S, Swanson LW, Lindstrom J. Characteristics of monoclonal antibodies to denatured Torpedo and to calf acetylcholine receptors: species, subunit and region specificity. J Neuroimmunol 1986; 10: 235–253
9. Marx A, O'Connor R, Geuder KI, Kirchner T, Müller-Hermelink HK. Characterization of a protein with an acetylcholine receptor-epitope from myasthenia gravis-associated thymomas. Lab Invest 1990; 62: 279–286
10. Hohlfeld R. Myasthenia gravis and thymoma: paraneoplastic failure of neuromuscular transmission. Lab Invest 1990; 62:241–243

20

THYMIC TUMOR PROGRESSION IN SV40T TRANSGENIC MICE MODEL

Suggestion of Thymoma–Thymic Carcinoma Sequence

Seung-Sook Lee,[1,2] Ja-June Jang,[2] Jeong Wook Seo,[2] Chul Woo Kim,[2] Sung Hoe Park,[2] Jeong-Sun Seo,[3] and Je Geun Chi[2]

[1]Department of Pathology
Korea Cancer Center Hospital
[2]Department of Pathology
Seoul National University College of Medicine
[3]Transgenic Mice Center
Cancer Research Institute and Department of Biochemistry
Seoul National University College of Medicine
Seoul, Korea

INTRODUCTION

Large T antigen of simian virus 40 (SV40 Tag) is a nuclear protein necessary to synthesize DNA and is a potent oncogene, determining both immortalization and transformation of multiple cell types not only in culture system but also in vivo.[1,2] Transgenic mice offer the potential for studying the biological effects of gene expression under physiological conditions that cannot be reproduced in culture, thus providing a system that may accurately emulate in differentiated tissues the behavior of pathological processes, such as neoplastic transformation.[3] Transgenic mouse harboring SV40 Tag gene has been used as an animal model of spontaneous carcinogenesis by regulating its expression with a variety of trans-criptional elements. Choroid plexus tumor and pancreatic islet cell tumors were developed in most studies for SV40 T transgenic mice.[4–10] In addition, SV40 large Tag induced a variety of neoplasm i.e., lymphoma, rhabdomyosarcoma, osteosarcoma, stomach carcinoma, hepatoma, melanoma, retinoblastoma, or hibernoma,[11–21] depending on the transcriptional signals used for its expression. Although thymic hyperplasia has been reported as incidental findings in transgenic mice, there were no reports on thymic carcinoma in transgenic mice. Thymic hyperplasia was observed incidentally in some cases of transgenic mice producing choroid plexus tumors[4,6,7,10] and also as a main event in transgenic mice harboring a growth hormone-releasing factor(GRF) promoter fused with simian virus 40 large T antigen [22,23]. Recently Teitz et al[24] reported a mixed type thymoma in

Epithelial Tumors of the Thymus, edited by Marx and Müller-Hermelink.
Plenum Press, New York, 1997

transgenic mice expressing SV40 Tag under the control of an erythroid specific enhancer. This is the first report on frank thymic epithelial tumor in transgenic mice expressing SV40 Tag. Besides SV40 Tag, there was a report on Thy1-myc transgenic mice developed complex lymphoid and epithelial thymic tumors.[25]

We have established a stable line of transgenic mice which consistently produce thymic tumor within a predictable time span in all cases. A 248 line of transgenic mice, harboring SV40 Tag gene under the transcriptional control of viral promoter and enhancer regions, reproducibly developed thymic carcinoma at the age of 5 to 7 months. They lost weight and manifested breathing difficulties and anterior chest wall bulging by 20 weeks of age. In our preliminary study, all SV40T transgenic mice (248 line) presenting with the above signs developed thymic tumors and kidney abnormalities with no evidence of choroid plexus tumor. The thymic tumors developed in symptomatic mice were all thymic carcinomas and kidney abnormalities included dysplastic tubules, adenomas, and carcinomas.

There have been only a few human case reports for thymic carcinoma associated with mixed type thymoma, indicating a gradual transition of epithelial cells of thymoma progressed to become malignant cells.[26,27,28] There has been no full-scale study for thymoma-carcinoma sequence or thymic hyperplasia-carcinoma sequence neither in human nor animal models. In laboratory animals, spontaneously occuring thymomas are uncommon.[29,30] Therefore a transgenic mouse model of thymus tumorigenesis should exhibit a heritable and reproducible pattern of lesion development, perhaps with separate steps in the sequence of events culminating in neoplasia. We attempted to elucidate the pathogenesis of thymic carcinoma using this animal model with 100% penetration for thymic carcinoma.

We studied sequential change of thymus in SV40 T transgenic mice by means of a morphological and immunohistochemical approach at different time points in animals from 3 to 32 weeks of age. In this study, we tried to provide an evidence for transition between benign thymoma and thymic carcinoma, indicating thymic epithelial cell changes during malignant transformation with time sequence. We focused on the morphologic change and tried to immunohistochemical study and electron microscopy to characterize origin and nature of the thymic tumor.

MATERIALS AND METHODS

Animals and Tumor Induction

Construction of SV40 Large T Antigen Transgene. A 3.0kb BamHI-KpnI fragment carrying the SV40 early region gene was cloned into the multicloning site of pUC19 DNA vector (pSVT). This plasmid contains a SV40 large T and small t antigen under the control of its own enhancer-promoter region. For the microinjection into the fertilized egg, pSVT DNA was linearlized with Sal I digestion and 5.7kb DNA fragments including vector sequence were isolated using glass bead(Qiagen, USA). Production and screening of transgenic mice. SV40 Tag transgene in pSVT DNA was microinjected into the male pronucleus of the fertilized zygotes obtained from F1 hybrid mice (C57BL x CBA) and then eggs were implanted into the pseudopregnant ICR foster mother as described.[31] The offsprings were screened for the presence of the transgene by southern blot analysis or PCR for SV40 Tag gene in DNA isolated from the tails as described.[4] Positive founders were maintained by crossing them with normal C57BL/6J mice or positive littermates.

Table 1. Summary of thymic mass shown in SV40T transgenic mice

		No. of	Mass size (cm)			Diagnosis			
Mouse group	Age(wks)	cases	<1	1–1.5	>1.5	NT	BT	FCa	MCa
Nontransgenic	4–30	7	5						
Transgenic I	3–5	5	5	0	0	4	1		
II	6–7	4	4	0	0	1	3		
III	9–10	5	1	2	2		5		
IV	12–14	10	0	4	6		6	4	
V	15–16	10	0	3	7		4	2	4
VI	17–19	8	0	2	6		1	0	7
VII	20–21	20	0	4	16		3	1	16
VIII	23–32	8	0	0	8				8

NT; No definite tumor, BT; Benign thymoma, FCa: Focal or multifocal carcinoma in the background of benign thymoma, MCa; Definite mass-forming large carcinoma

Tissue Collection and Preparation

Selection of Animal. To study the progressive development of lesions in the thymus of the 248 transgenic line, mice were sacrificed between 3 and 32 weeks after birth (Table 1), after confirming the integration of SV40 Tag to mouse DNA. A total of 70 transgenic mice were examined and 7 transgene-negative littermates of mice from the 248 line were analyzed in parallel as controls for the different stages of tumorigenesis.

Tissue Preparation. After whole thymus was removed the samples were snap-frozen for immunohistochemistry and fixed in 10% buffered formalin, and glutaraldehyde for light micro-scopy and electronmicroscopy, respectively. Other solid organs such as liver, spleen, lung, kidney, testis, salivary gland and brain were also sampled for light microscopic examination. After snap freezing of fresh thymic tissue in cooled isopentene in liquid nitrogen, it was kept in liquid nitrogen until used. The frozen tissue was embedded on OCT compound for sectioning. Six-micron sections were fixed for 5 minutes in ice-cold acetone.

Gross Examination and Histologic Study

Each thymus was measured and weighed. Paraffin sections were stained with H&E. Three pathologists examined the thymus lesions independently and divided into four groups based on the histological features; Group A with no tumor(NT), group B with benign thymoma(BT), group C with focal or multifocal thymic carcinoma in the background of benign thymoma (FCa), and group D with definite mass-forming thymic carcinoma(MCa). The thymic carcinoma was classified into well-differentiated thymic carcinoma(WDTC) and high-grade thymic carcinoma. The diagnosis of high-grade thymic carcinoma was based on the morpho-logical criteria of Troung et al[32]; frequent mitoses(more than 10/10 high power fields), tumor cell necrosis, virtual absence of lymphoepithelial mixture, and nuclear atypia including large cell size, high nuclear/cytoplasmic ratio and prominent nucleoli. WDTC has a clear pre-dominence of epithelial cells, which exhibit a solid growth pattern and containing organotypical features such as epithelial palisading or perivascular space. The round-to-oval epithelial cells have mild to moderate cytologic atypia and occasional mitotic figures, and the tumor contains fewer lymphocytes than cortical thymoma.[33–37]

Immunohistochemical Study for Characterization of Tumor and Localization of SV40T Antigen

Proliferating cell nuclear antigen (PCNA) was performed on paraffin sections by the avidin-biotin-peroxidase complex (ABC) method (Vectastain ABC mouse kit, Vector Laboratories, Burlingame, CA, USA) in the three representative cases in each group, using the monoclonal anti-PCNA antibody (Dako). For negative control, anti-PCNA antibody was replaced by phosphate-buffered saline. The percentage of PCNA-positive cells was determined by counting at least 500 cells. The positive cells for PCNA showed nuclear staining with granular or diffuse pattern and varied in intensity of staining, but all identifiable staining was regarded as positive.

Polyclonal cytokeratin(Zymed) was used in paraffin sections of all cases to elucidate the epithelial nature of the tumor.

Th-3, monoclonal antibody for stromal cells of thymic cortex and Th-4, monoclonal antibody for stromal cells of thymic medulla, provided by Dr. K. Hirokawa (Tokyo Metropolitan Institute of Gerontology, Tokyo, Japan) were applied to the frozen tissue section of the thymic lesions.[38] Rat monoclonal antibody for anti-mouse thymic epithelial cells (Biosource, MS-017-SN) was applied to frozen tissue to elucidate thymic medullary, perivascular and subcapsular epithelia. Thy1.1, Thy1.2(Becton Dickinson), J11d[39], and anti-mouse CD4 (GK1.5) were also used to frozen section. Thy1.2 and thymic epithelial cells were reacted with anti-rat IgG as secondary antibody using ABC method (Vectastain, Burlingame, CA) and others were reacted with anti-mouse immunoglobulin (LSAB Dako kit). These were performed in the three representative cases from both thymic carcinoma and thymoma of pre-malignant stage.

Monoclonal antibody against mouse anti-SV40T antigen (C-terminal) (Chemicon, MAB990) was applied to both frozen and paraffin embedded thymic tissue using ABC method and immunoflorescence. SV40 Tag was demonstrated by nuclear staining using immunohisto-chemical method.

Electron Microscopy

Fifteen cases of thymic tumors were examined by transmission electron microscope (TEM). Thymic tissue for TEM were obtained from the grossly recognizable thymic tumor portion from 13 weeks to 30 weeks of age. The samples consist of 10 malignant tumors and 5 benign tumors. Epithelial cells in the tumor masses were selectively sampled and examined (Table 2). The tissue samples were fixed in 2.5% glutaraldehyde and 1% formaldehyde in 0.1 M cacodylate buffer, for 2 hours and processed routinely. Sections stained with 5% uranyl acetate and Reynold's lead citrate and examined.

Flow Cytometry

Flow cytometry (FCM) analysis were carried out for fresh thymic tumor tissue and cultured cell lines on a Becton Dickinson FACScan as described previously[39]. Antibodies used included Th-3 and Th-4[38], monoclonal anti-mouse thymic epithelial cells (Biosource, MS-017-SN), anti-Thy1.2 (Becton Dickinson), anti-Thy1.1, anti-mouse CD4 (GK1.5), J11D39, cytokeratin and epithelial membrane antigen. Biotinylated antibodies were used

Table 2. Summary of thymic mass shown in SV40T transgenic mice

Increased lymphocyte proliferation with architectural irregularity
(Thymic hyperplasia or not)
↓
Epithelial proliferation with imbalanced epithelial zone expansion
(Cortical thymoma or Organoid thymoma)
↓
Emergence of malignant epithelial cell foci
(Transformation of activated cortical epithelial cells)
↓
Well-differentiated thymic carcinoma(WDTC)
↓
Rapid tumor growth with necrosis
(WDTC or High-grade thymic carcinoma)

with luorescein isothio-cyanate (FITC) conjugated streptavidin, 1:50. Immunolabelling was done by standard indirect immunofluorescence. The data were analyzed on a FACScan flow cytometer (Becton Dickinson) using FACScan software. Dead cells were excluded by forward and side scatter.

RESULTS

I. Morphological Findings

Gross Findings. Thymus change of SV40 T transgenic mice are summarized in Table 1. Before 5 weeks of age (group I), the thymus did not form any tumor-like mass. However, the size and weight increased slightly compared to those of transgene-negative littermate. It was a diffuse enlargement with preservation of its lobular architecture. At the age of 6–7 weeks (Group II), the size and weight of thymus doubled those of group I (Fig. 1A). At 9 weeks of age (Group III), the thymus enlarged markedly up to twenty-five times of control thymus, measuring more than 1 cm in maximal diameter, and formed a gross tumor mass and lost its lobular architecture. As shown in Table 1, there was a progressive

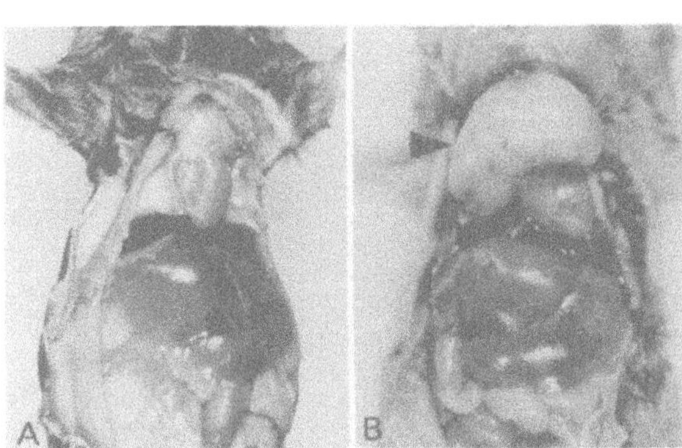

Figure 1. Gross photograph in situ. A: Enlarged thymus (arrowhead) of a 6-week-old TG mouse harbouring SV40T. Thymus enlarged to about 5 folds of age-matched control mice. B: The thymic mass (arrowhead) at 20 weeks of age. A large ovoid mediastinal mass pushes heart and lungs posteriorly.

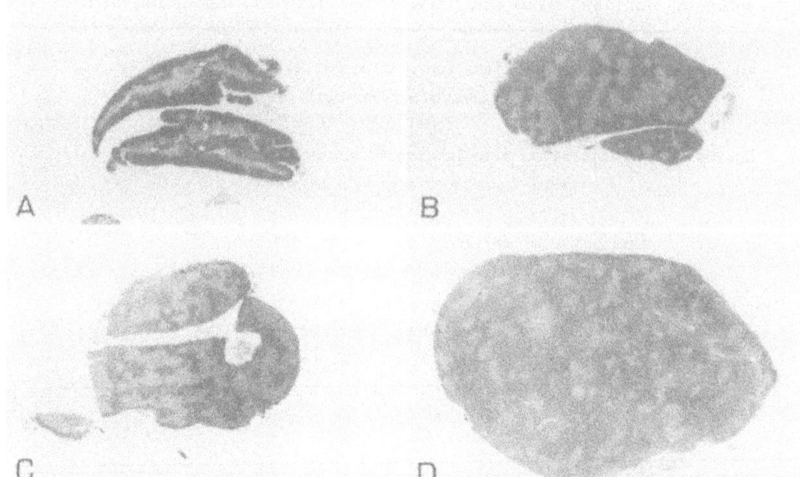

Figure 2. Low power view of thymus of TG mice and non-transgenic control mice in different age group (H & E, x2.5). A: Thymus of non-transgenic control mouse; it shows normal thymic architecture with preserved outer-cortical/inner-medullary pattern B: Group I TG mice (3–5 weeks); slightly enlarged thymus shows an irregular arrangement of cortical zone and medullary epithelial zone with clear distinction between the cortical and medullary zone. Cortical lymphocyte zone is relatively expanded. C: Group II (6–7 weeks) shows irregular and farther expanded medullary zone. D: Group III (9–10 weeks); The cortico-medullary junctions are indistinct and blurred because of irregularly increased epithelial cells.

enlargement of thymus by age. By 20 weeks of age, most thymi reached up to 2cm in size (Fig. 1B). On cut sections of the thymi, the thymic masses showed two different features; one was whitish gray smooth and glistening appearance, and the other was yellowish gray, granular appearance with necrosis. These two distinctive features were microscopically confirmed to be benign thymoma and high-grade thymic carcinoma, respectively. Thymic carcinoma often showed grossly visible necrosis. In some animals, these two features were noted in a same thymic mass. Metastases to lung were detected in some of the animals.

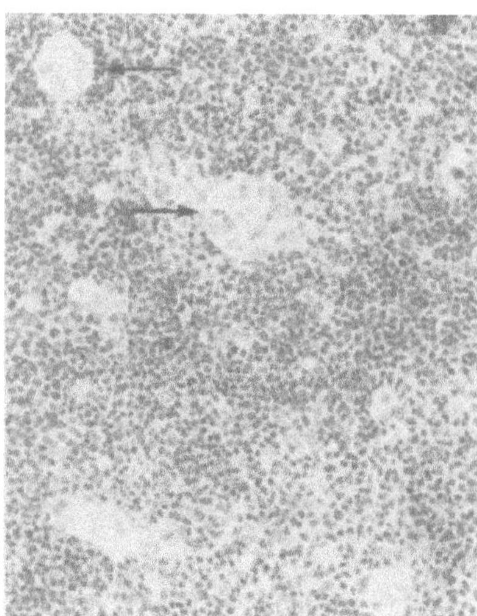

Figure 3. A few foci of small epithelial cell clusters that are composed of 5 to 30 bland-looking epithelial cels (arrows) (H&E, x66).

Microscopic Findings. Microscopic changes of thymus were, in general, correlated well with gross findings. All seven age-matched control mice showed normal thymic architecture with preservation of cortico-medullary architecture (Fig. 2A). Group I (3–5 weeks) : Four mice with slightly enlarged thymus showed irregularity of arrangement in the cortex and medulla(Fig. 2B). However, the corticomedullary junction was clear and distinct. In these cases, cortical lymphocyte zone was relatively expanded, when compared to their normal littermates. The the large lymphoid cells (lymphoblasts) were the main element of the expansion, mixed with small thymocytes, showed occasional mitoses. Epithelial elements in cortex and medulla remained normal in these four cases. However, one case showed an increased number of epithelial cells in the medulla but still with well preserved cortico-medullary architecture.

Group II (6–7 weeks): The cortico-medullary architecture was disturbed and showed irregular arrangement as in group I. thymus in this group showed irregularly expanded medulla particularly compared to group I (Fig. 2C). The number of epithelial cells in the medulla increased considerably.

Group III (9–10 weeks): The striking features in this group were several. First, the cortico-medullary junction became indistinct mainly because of irregularly proliferated epithelial cells (Fig. 2D). The second characteristic finding was scattered foci of small epithelial cell clusters. Each cluster was composed of 5 to 30 bland-looking epithelial cells. (Fig. 3). These epithelial cells having large vesicular nuclei were also seen individually in both epithelial predominant zone and non-epithelial area.

Group IV (12–14 weeks) : Emergence of malignant epithelial foci was the most prominent finding in this group. It occurred in 2 out of 10 mice examined. The malignant foci were made up of tumor cells with large ovoid vesicular nuclei showing more than 10 mitotic figures per high power field (Fig. 4). The tumor cells noted organoid pattern in areas. The epithelial zone expanded markedly (Fig. 5A) and reached subcapsular portion of

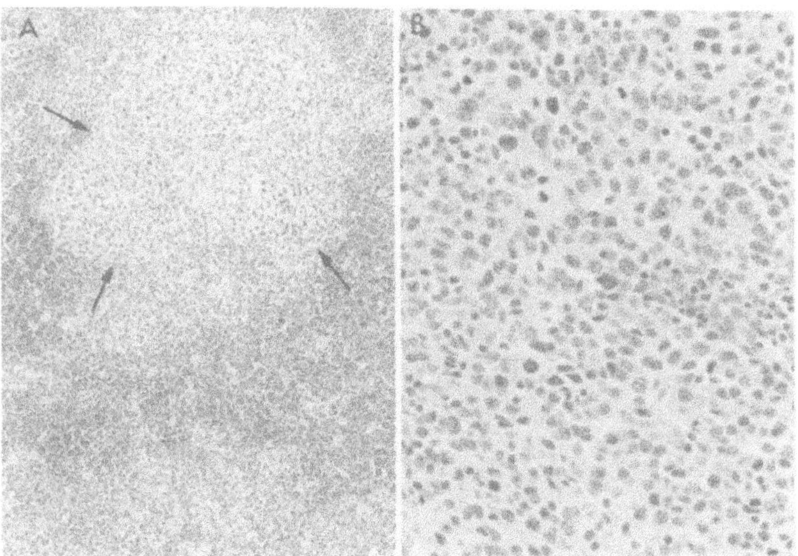

Figure 4. A: Malignant epithelial cell focus (arrows) is noted in the background of thymoma (H & E, x33). B: High magnification of malignant focus. It is made up of tumor cells having a large ovoid vesicular nucleus and occasional mitoses (H & E, x100).

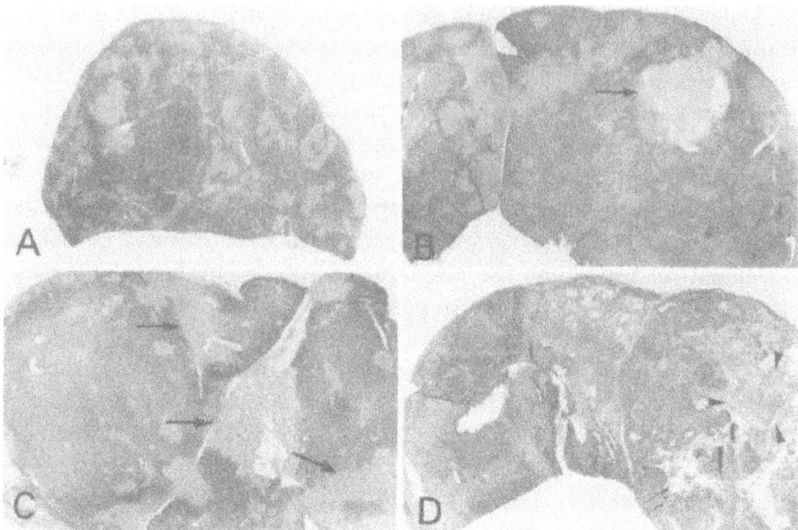

Figure 5. Low-power view of thymus after 12 weeks of age (H & E, x2.5). A: Epithelial zone expanded markedly in Group IV (12–14 weeks). B: Group V & VII (after 15 weeks); malignant epithelial foci (arrows) in the background of thymoma. C: Mass-forming carcinomas are noted in the background of thymoma at 18 weeks. D: Thymic carcinoma is well demarcated from benign thymoma portion (BT). Note central necrosis (arrowheads) in the carcinoma at 21 weeks.

the thymus. (Fig. 6A). The expanded epithelial zone consisited of bland-looking epithelial cells and thymocytes (Fig. 6B).

Occasionally mitosis could be detected in the expanded epithelial zone. This lesion was interpreted to be a benign thymoma. The cortico-medullary junction remained indistinct in this group and the epithelial cell population increased further. Scattered large epithelal cells were found not only in the expanded epithelial zone but also through the lymphocyte pre-

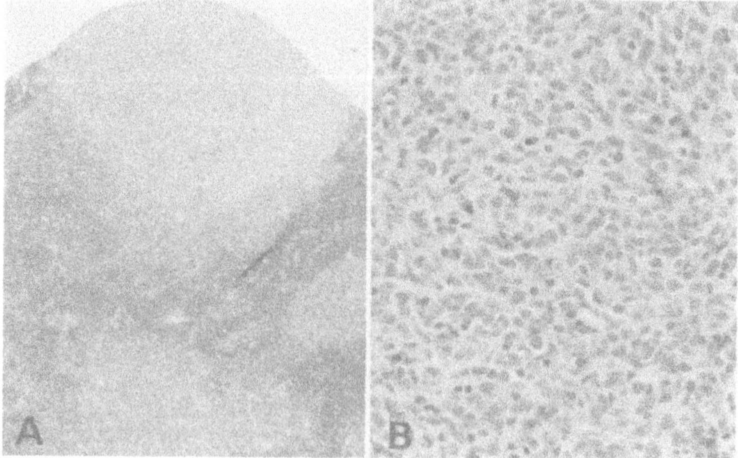

Figure 6. A: Epithelial zone reaches to the thymic surface, subcapsular area, in group IV (H & E, x16). B: The expended epithelial zone consists of bland-looking epithelial cells and a few lymphocytes (H & E, x100).

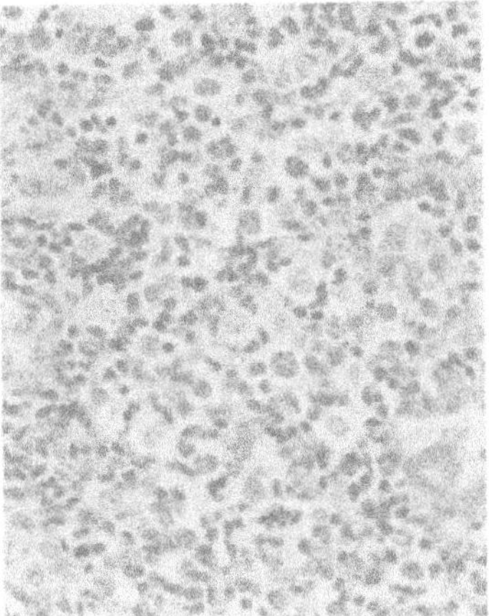

Figure 7. In benign thymoma portion, expanded epithelial zone showed increase of cortical-type epithelial cells (H & E, x100).

dominant area. Small epithelial cell nests seen in group III were found more often, even in lymphocyte-predominant area. Immature IV lymphocytes persisted in the lymphocyte- rich area, and showed occasional mitoses. Group V (15–16 weeks) : In four of ten mice in this group, mass-forming thymic carcinoma was found. The extent of the thymic carcinomas was different in each case. It varied from near-total involvement to a small focus of malignant cells in the background of benign thymoma (Fig. 5B,C). Three were high-grade thymic carcinomas with extensive necrosis, replacing most thymic mass. Their cut surfaces were yellow-gray and granular. Two of three high-grade carcinomas coexisted with cortical thymoma and WDTC in part, respectively. The other one of four mass-forming carcinoma cases was composed of WDTC component (30%) and cortical thymoma. The thymi having no carcinoma and the thymus tissue around the thymic carcinoma, showed a marked blurring of the corticomedullary junction, epithelial zone expansion, and a diffuse and marked increase of the epithelial cell population (Fig. 7). The proliferated epithelilal cells often showed bizarre cells. Two cases showed multifocal malignant foci in the expanded epithelial zone. Group VI (17–19 weeks) : One case was benign thymoma, and seven cases were carcinomas that included four WDTCs and three mixed type carcinomas (WDTC and high-grade carcinoma). Group VI (20–21 weeks) : Sixteen mice out of 20 in this group showed definite thymic carcinoma in the background of thymoma. Six were mainly high-grade carcinoma, and three were mainly WDTC. Seven showed mixed pattern of WDTC and high-grade carcinoma(Fig.5D). The other one case showed focal carcinoma in the background of benign thymoma. The remaining three cases had only benign thymoma. Group VII (23–32 weeks): All eight cases in this group showed massive thymic carcinoma occupying most of the thymic tissue. The histologic pattern of thymic carcinoma was similar to that of earlier groups. Benign thymoma component, however, remained as a small component usually at the periphery of the thymus.

Summary of Sequential Changes. Following facts became clear after these observations. First, the thymic size had a tendency to increase with aging in SV40T TG mice, second, while younger mice have benign thymoma older mice have thymic carcinoma. When SV40 T TG mice 248 line reached a certain age, their thymi had thymic carcinoma in

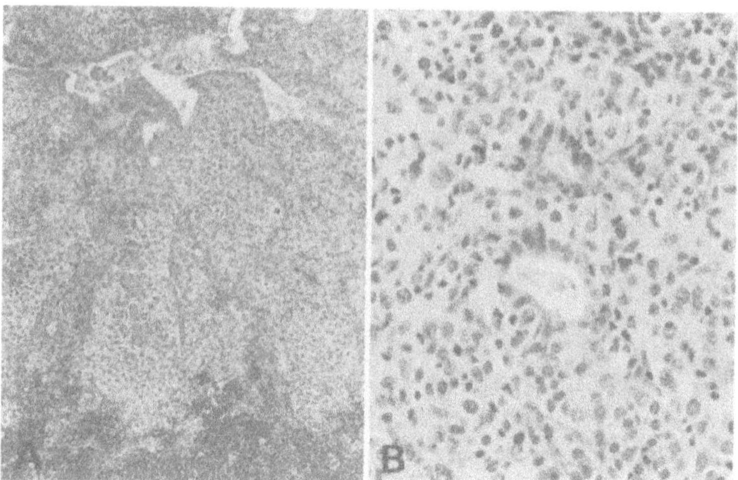

Figure 8. Gland-like palisade pattern in the solid sheet of ovoid epithelial cells in WDTC. (A: H & E, x25, B: H & E x100).

all(100%). Third, the benign lesion of the thymus became malignant within a predictable time span, strongly suggestive of thymoma-carcinoma sequence.

Histologic Classification of Thymic Carcinoma in TG Mice. Thymic carcinoma could be largely classified into two groups, i.e., well differentiated thymic carcinoma (WDTC) and high-grade thymic carcinoma. WDTCs were composed of large ovoid cells having large vesicular nuclei with one or two nucleoli and abundant pale eosinophilic cytoplasm. They showed a characteristic feature of gland-like epithelial palisading (Fig. 8). In some cases, they also showed lobulating margin (Fig. 9) and focal epidermoid feature (Fig. 9). WDTC showed

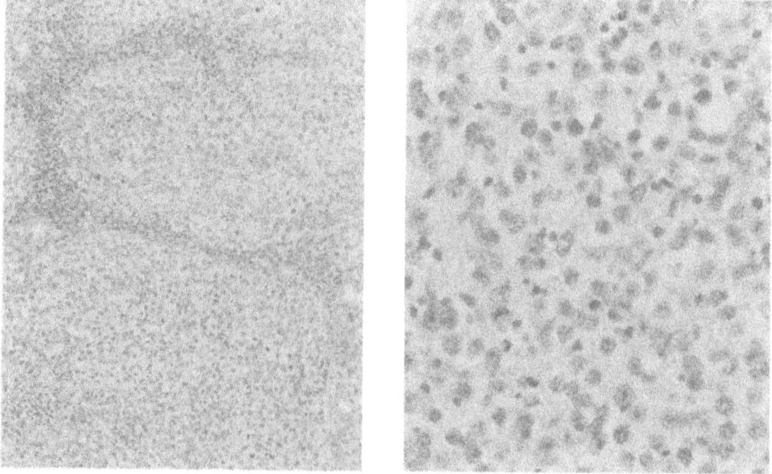

Figures 9 and 10. Lobulating pattern surrounded by lymphocytes in WDTC (H & E, x40). Cells having large ovoid vesicular nucleus in WDTC (H & E, x100).

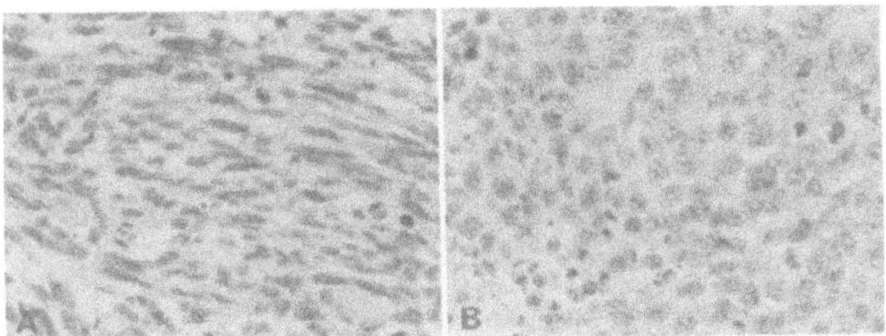

Figure 11. A: High-grade carcinoma with extremely hypercellular spindle cells having elongated or fusiform nuclei and small amount of cytoplasm (H & E, x100). B: High-grade thymic carcinoma aith large ovoid cell type (H & E, x100).

less pleomorphism, relatively low nuclear/cytoplasmic ratio, and less mitotic figures, 5–10/10HPF. However, high mitotic areas were frequently encountered in WDTCs of our series of TG mice (Fig. 10). High-grade thymic carcinoma showed two cell types; one is composed of extremely hypercellular spindle cells having elongated or fusiform nuclei and small amount of cytoplasm (Fig. 11A), and the other is ovoid large cell type mimicking thymic cortical epithelial cell (Fig. 11B). The latter overlaped with WDTC but it showed high mitotic counts and always necrosis. Most thymic carcinomas were combination types, i.e.,composed of more than one histologic type. Some showed squamous differentiation on focal area. In the large cell ovoid type, the tumor cell masses appeared merging into benign thymic epthelial cell proliferating zone or WDTC area, while in spindle cell type the carcinoma showed a clear demarcation from the surrounding benign area.

II. Expression of SV40 Large T Antigen in Thymic Tissue

Expression of the SV40 T transgene in tissues was determined by northern blot analysis. Relatively high level of expression of the 5.7kb transcript was detected in the thymic mass and the kidney of mice in all groups. The expression level was low in the spleen. The level of SV40 Tag expression in the thymic carcinoma was higher than in benign thymoma by northern blot ananlysis (Fig. 12, from submitted papers). By northern blot analysis, SV40 Tag expression in the thymic tumor was weaker than that of choroid plexus tumor which was found to be another consistent tumor from other TG line(125 line) harbouring SV40Tag (Data not shown). The choroid plexus tumor (125 line) and dysplastic tubules in the kidneys (248 line) revealed strong expression of SV40 Tag in the nuclei of tumor cells and dysplastic tubules by

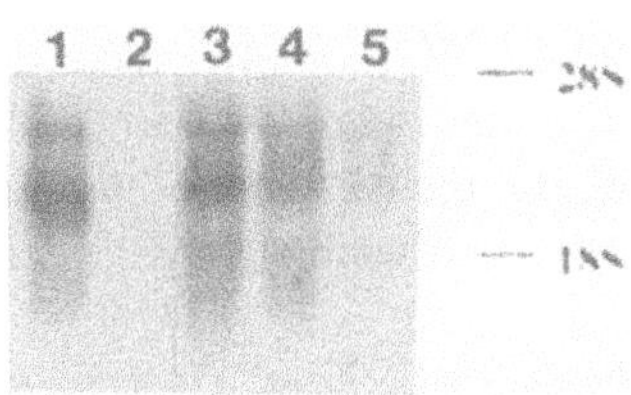

Figure 12. Northern blot analysis of TG SVT248 mice. Total RNAs from RHEK (lane 1) or liver (lane 2), spleen (lane 4), and kidney (lane 5) of TG SVT248 transgenic mice were analyzed by northern blot analysis with an SV40 DNA fragment probe.

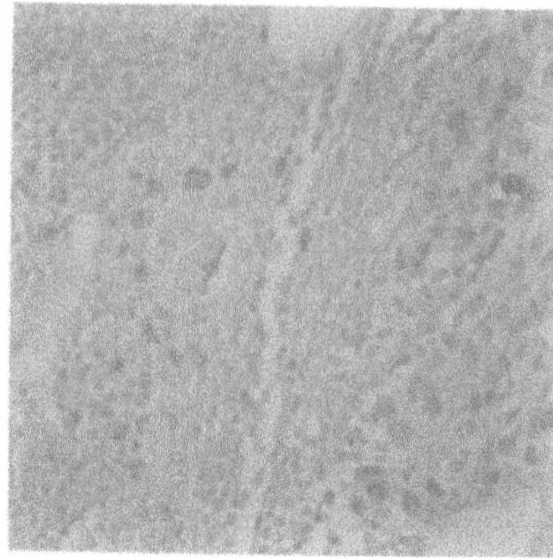

Figures 13 and 14. PCNA immunostaining of 7 weeks TGs. Cortical thymocytes shows high percentage of nuclear staining but medullary epithelial zones exhibit very low PCNA index (x13). PCNA in the epithelial expansion area of benign thymoma (left) and thymic carcinoma (right) (x40).

immunohistochemistry. The SV40 Tag expression was tested immunohistochemically in thymus and thymic tumors in this series. It was repeatedly negative in the thymus and thymic tumors through all experimental groups.

III. Results of PCNA Immunostaining

Mean percentage of cells positive for PCNA in each group was as follows; group II (7wks) cortical thymocyte zone (13.81), group II medullary zone (1..89), group IV epithelial zone (4.89) in group IV lymphoid zone (8.77), undifferentiated ovoid cell type (38.45spindle) cell type (52.11U̇) According to the above results, in the group I and II, cortical thymocytes seemed to be actively proliferating and after 12 weeks of age, thymocyte proliferation decreased and the PCNA positive epithelial cells gradually increased. The expanded epithelial areas showed moderately increased proliferating activity, and the carcinomatous area revealed high PCNA index (Fig. 14).

Above results of gradually increasing proliferating index coincided with those of sequential histological change of the thymus in various experimental groups.

IV. Cellular Characterization by Immunohistochemical Study and Flow Cytometry

1. Cytokeratin. Cytokeratin was positive for scattered clusters of epithelial cells in the benign thymoma. As the age of the mice increased, the cytokeratin-positive cells increased gradually until frank carcinoma developed. In carcinomas, cytokeratin was stained in some tumor cells in small foci, but the majority of carcinoma cells revealed no staining. Gland-like structures in WDTC were invariably positive for cytokeratin.

2. Thymic Epithelial Antibody (Th-3, Th-4, Thymic Medullary Epithelium). Thymic carcinomas were negative on both Th-3 and Th-4 by immunohistochemistry and flow cytometry. Antibody for thymic medullary epithelium (Biosource, MS-017-SN) revealed no reaction in carcinoma. The cortical epithelial cell marker, Th-3, was diffusely expressed mainly in the lymphocyte-rich zone and the epithelial expanded area of benign thymoma. Th-4 was focally expressed in benign thymoma. Thymic carcinoma revealed no reaction on Thy1.1, Thy1.2, and CD4. In cultured cells of thymic carcinoma, J11d was expressed on flow cytometry, however, immunohistochemistry showed nonspecific nuclear staining. These results indicated the thymomas of the mice were of cortical and of not medullary epithelium origin, and also thymic carcinoma is no longer traceable for its original character.

V. Transmission Electron Microscopy

The ultrastructural features of thymic carcinoma were basically the same in all cases. They were characterized by a variable amount of Golgi complex, short RER, mitochondria, and membrane-bound electron dense granules in their cytoplasm, and small desmosomes with short tonofilalments. Membrane-bound electron dense granules were the characteristics of type II human thymic epithelial cells by Kendall's classification[41]. However, the number of granules were fewer and nuclear characteristics were different from cortical epithelial cells. Many polysomes were frequently observed in the carcinoma cells compared to benign cells. Although epithelial cells resembled type II cells in that electron-dense granules were present in cytoplasm, we could not conclude that tumor cells were derived from cortical epithelial cells ultrastructurally.

DISCUSSION

In the animal literature, the term thymoma is often used for a lymphoma involving the thymus.[30,42] In laboratory animals, spontaneously occurring thymic epithelial cell tumors are uncommon.[30,43–45] Both naturally and experimentally induced thymic epithelial tumors were used as models for dissecting intrathymic lymphocyte maturation steps.[30,45–48] Hoot and Kettman induced thymic epithelial tumors in C3H/Bittner mice by neonatal inoculation with polyoma virus.[49]

Histologically the tumors were similar to human spindle cell thymoma.[49] In transgenic mouse, only two reports on frank thymic epithelial tumors can be found in SV40 T transgenic mice under control of erythroid specific enhancer24 and Thy1-myc transgenic mice.[25] Thymic hyperplasia has been described in transgenic mice harboring SV40 T antigen[4,6,7,10,22,23]. However, thymic carcinoma in laboratory animals including transgenic mice has never been observed. In this report, we found a stable line of transgenic mice which consistently develop thymic carcinoma after 23 weeks of age. We thought that this mouse model of thymic carcinoma could be utilized for determining the progressive steps of tumor development from hyperplasia to frank carcinoma.

Transgenic mice expressing SV40 Tag gene with its own regulatory region have been reported to develop choroid plexus tumor, thymic hypertrophy and kidney dysplasia.4 These findings in SV40 T transgenic mice are comparable to ours. In our series, other than thymic carcinoma, renal abnormalities such as tubular dysplasia, polycystic change, adenoma of renal tubule and sometimes carcinoma, were consistently found although none showed choroid plexus tumor.

Characteristic sequence of thymic tumor development has never been reported in TG mice harbouring SV40 T antigen.[4,6,7,10,22,23] Thymic hyperplasia was the only abnormality of the thymus in these animals. Botteri et al described thymic hyperplasia in 19 of 33 founder mice at 5 to 14 weeks of age, and all these hyperplastic thymi showed no architectural and cellular abnormalities other than their large size. In Moll's series[23], all hyperplastic thymi retained normal morphological features of the organ irrespective of the degree of hyperplasia.

The number of thymocytes increased, sometimes up to100-folds without alteration of cortico-medullary architecture.[23] Most other reports on thymic lesions have been similar only with relatively low incidence.[4,6,7,10] Jat et al[50] developed transgenic mice harbouring SV40 T antigen gene using the mouse major histocompatibility complex H-2kb promoter. The thymi of these mice showed consistent hyperplasia. No extrathymic tumor was noted. Wildin et al[51] reported that transgenic mice bearing functional proximal promoter sequence juxtaposed with the SV40 large T antigen gene, that invariably developed lymphoid tumors confined to the thymus. The transgenic mice bearing a 2.6-kb fragment of the human distal promoter fused to the SV40 large T antigen gene expressed large T antigen in thymocytes and in peripheral lymphoid cells.[51] These animals developed lymphoid tumors in the thymus and peripheral lymphoid organs. Again no thymic carcinoma was encountered.

Although northern blot analysis of our mice for SV40 Tag expression was positive in thymus, kidneys and spleen, immunohistochemical staining failed to demonstrate SV40 T expression in thymic tissue and thymic tumor sections throughout whole experimental groups. On the other hand, renal lesions of our TG mice revealed strong immunohistochemical expression of SV40 Tag in the nuclei of dysplastic tubular cells and adenoma cells. Two explanations could be provided for the negativity of SV40 Tag in thymus. The first one is that SV40 Tag expression in the thymus was too weak to be reactive by immunohistochemical method. The second one is that, SV40 Tag could work only during intrauterine or early postnatal period. It finished its role after activation of thymic cells, which subsequently progressed into true neoplasm. Expression time and pattern of SV40 Tag may vary to diverse TG strains and used promoters. According to Moll et al[23], neonatal GRF-Tag mice expressed SV40 Tag specifically in a small subset of thymic epithelial cells that are highly enriched near the corticomedullary junction. The number of SV40 Tag positive thymic epithelial cells increased rapidly in the first two post-natal weeks and the mice developed thymic hyperplasia. Of two assumptions we made, the first assumption is more probable, considering flow cytometric assessment for SV40 Tag positive cells. On flow cytometry, SV40 Tag positive cells were present but the majority was very weak for SV40 Tag expression.

In GRF-Tag mice, immortal SV40 Tag+ KL mRNA+ thymic epithelial cells cause a dramatic expansion of thymopoiesis[22,23]. Transgenic studies of other tumor types have also tentatively concluded that the SV40 genes are not sufficient to induce tumors [10,51,52]. As for SV40-induced choroid plexus tumors, this suggestion has been stemmed from the observation of nonuniform T antigen expression in focal tumors.[51,52] By Chen and van Dyke[10], differences in the rate of choroid plexus tumorigenesis reflected differences in the control regions of the two viruses, SV40 and lymphotropic papovavirus, rather than differences in T antigen per se. While SV40 T expression under SV40 regulation was limited to a fraction of the choroid plexus cells prior to the formation of focal tumors, its expression under lymphotropic papovavirus control was generally uniformly expressed in the choroid plexus with rapid expansion of the tissue ensued[10]. In pancreatic beta cells, uniform expression of T antigen is not sufficient for the immediate induction of proliferation. It requires several weeks before abnormal proliferation begins[9]. This result indicates an interesting difference in the ability of some distinct cell types to respond to T antigen. Other testable possibilities include differences in T-antigen levels or in the state of cellular differentiation at the onset of T-antigen expression[10]. Why does SV40 Tag gene specifically target thymus and renal tubules, in spite of using its own promoter and enhancer?

We cannot explain this organ-specificity. However, there is a common point among tumor-developing organs in TG mice harbouring SV40 Tag. Pancreatic islet cells, choroid plexus, thymic epithelial cells, and renal tubular cells are somewhat similar in that sense of having secretory function in a variable degree.

Although tissue expression of SV40 Tag by immunohistochemistry failed to be localized in the thymus in our series, our study showed that SV40 Tag by its own enhancer and promoter immediately induced proliferation of thymic cells in early neonatal period, and it takes several months for malignant transformation. Considering 100% penetration of thymic carcinoma production and the time period of 23 weeks, we could reasonably presume the sequence of thymic hyperplasia, thymoma and thymic carcinoma in the direct effect of SV40 Tag. Although the role of SV40 Tag in carcinogenesis still remains unclear, recent studies show that SV40 Tag binds the tumor suppressor gene products p53 and Rb, resulting in uncontrollable cellular proliferation. The thymic hyperplasia refers to an actual increase of thymic mass leaving the basic framework and histological appearance intact.[30,42] Thymoma is defined as an epithelial tumor of the thymus with a variable amount of reactive lymphocytes.[30] The thymomas are traditionally classified with regard to the ratio between epithelial cells and lymphocytes.[54] This classificaton system has no advantage to clinicopathological correlation and failed to point out that only epithelial cells are neoplastic. An alternative classification based solely on the morphological features of the epithelial components was proposed by Marino and Muller-Hermelink(1985)[55], and thymomas are histologically subtyped into three major groups: cortical, medullary, and mixed. And organoid thymoma, as a distinct variant of cortical thymoma mimicking the architecture of normal thymus, was proposed by Pescarmona et al[56]. There are some reports that this classification has prognostic significance, independent of tumor stage.[34–37] That is, medullary and mixed thymomas are benign tumors with no risk of recurrence, whereas organoid and cortical thymoma showed intermediate invasiveness and a low but significant risk of late relapse.[57] Five-year and 10-year survival rates of the patients with stage I thymoma have been reported to be 96.2% and 66.7%, respectively.[58] This result suggests that noninvasive thymoma may progress into invasive/metastatic thymoma if left untreated. The cell proliferation study supports the view that thymoma is essentially a low-grade malignant lesion regardless of stage.[59]

Thymic carinoma is a relatively rare neoplasm with a wide variety of morphologic appearance.[28] Thymic carcinoma and thymoma have been classified as distinct entities on the basis of morphology. Thymic carcinoma consists of large cells with marked cytological atypia, prominent nucleoli, a high N/C ratio, and abundant mitoses. It is frequently accompanied by multifocal or confluent necrosis, bearing no resemblance to normal thymic epithelium. On the other hand, thymoma has many organotypical features, such as perivascular space, epithelial palisading, medullary differentiation, and Hassall's corpuscles.[26–28,32,60] In a number of thymic epithelial tumors there is a degree of cytological atypia intermediate between conventional thymoma and thymic carcinoma, together with the signs of organo-typical differentiation. Such tumors have been recently defined as well-differentiated thymic carcinoma (WDTC).[33–37,61] The term WDTC at present refers to a distinctive subgroup of thymic neoplasm previously classified as cortical thymoma[55] or predominantly epithelial thymoma[42]. Its morphology is defined by a predominance of epithelial cells, epidermoid differentiation, slight to moderate cytological atypia, presence of few interepithelial cortical thymocytes, lobular growth, and perivascular epithelial palisades. Clinically it is frequently associated with myasthenia gravis and invades contiguous structures, frequently causes endothoracic metastasis, and rarely kills the patient by local recurrence and progressive endothoracic spread.[35] On account of the existence of so many intermediate histological forms and the paucity of clinical discrimination, Pan et al[36] proposed the suclassification of cortical thymoma as a morphological continuum rather than a distinct histological variants.

Our results showed that thymi of SV40 Tag TGs developed thymic carcinoma through a unique process. While nontransgenic control mice had normal thymus throughout the observation period, transgenic mice showed a variety of histopathological changes including increase of a lymphoid cell population, epithelial zone expansion, multifocal malignant transformation of the epithelial cells, and mass-forming carcinoma. Interestingly enough, these changes occurred in sequence. In our series, the thymi at 3 to 5 weeks of age were slightly larger than the control thymi and showed an irregular arrangement of cortical zone and medullary epithelial zone. However, the corticomedullary junction was distinct. At 6 to 7 weeks of age, the size and weight of thymi increased five times of control thymi. The corticomedullary architecture became more irregular than the previous group (3 to 5 weeks of age), and the cortical thymocyte zone became expanded. By the age of 9 to 10 weeks, the thymi were markedly enlarged up to twenty folds due to mass formations. Microscopically, the cortico-medullary junction became no longer distinct due mainly to the increased number of epithelial cells forming sheets. Medullary epithelial zone became expanded together with a few small nests of epithelial cells. Foci of malignant epithelial cell were noted in the thymus of 12 to 14 weeks of age. Based on grossly visible masses, effacement of original architecture and haphazard proliferation of thymic epithelial cells, we assumed that these lesions are thymoma rather than simple thymic hyperplasia. Most proliferating epithelial cells resembled cortical epithelial cells and they were regarded as cortical thymoma, and many of them were reminiscent of organoid thymoma of human, characterized by pale medullary foci surrounded by a neoplastic cortex-like tissue and a 'starry-sky' appearance. At 15 to 18 weeks of age, the cellular constituents of the masses were those of carcinoma. The malignant epithelial nature of the tumor cells could be confirmed histopathologically. At 20 to 21 weeks of age, the majority (16/20) of the animals revealed mass-forming carcinomas in the background of thymoma. After 23 weeks of age, all mice were found to have thymic carcinomas.

The thymic carcinomas in our series were characterized by mixture of benign thymoma element in various proportion. The simultaneous presence of these two components in TG mice has never been described in the literature, and certainly suggest causal relationship between benign thymoma and thymic carcinoma. In human there had been a few case reports of thymic carcinoma in the background of long standing thymoma.[26–28] From the largest series of 60 cases of human thymic carcinoma by Suster and Rosai[28], two patients had a history of myasthenia gravis associated with biopsy proven cytologically benign thymomas on which thymic carcinoma developed subsequently. Kuo et al [60] described two cases of that were presumed to come from thymoma. The carcinomatous portion was squamous cell carcinoma in one and another was undifferentiated (lymphoepithelioma-like) carcinoma. Similar observations were made by Shimosato et al [27] and by Morinaga et al [26]. Above findings together with our data in animal strongly suggest that thymic carcinoma may arise in the background of benign thymoma. However, since thymic carcinoma is rarely associated with benign thymoma in human material as well as in experimental animals, it is difficult to conclude the thymoma-carcinoma sequence at this time. Nevertheless, we believe that our findings provided an evidence for the development of thymic carcinoma from benign thymic epithelial tumor. Our results of PCNA immunostaining and histological findings indicate that proliferation of cortical thymocytes is the initial process during 'thymoma-carcinoma sequence'. The next process is the epithelial cell proliferation, with subsequent expansion of epithelial zone. PCNA index showed a statistically significant difference between premalignant thymoma and thymic carcinoma, suggesting that carcinoma is conceivably derived either from the increased and activated epithelial cells scattered in the cortical zone or from the areas of the epithelial expansion. We conclude that the thymic tumors are consistently developed in SV40 T transgenic mice, and among these thymic tumors there is a sequence from benign thymoma to thymic carcinoma.

SUMMARY

Transgenic mouse harboring large T antigen of simian virus 40 (SV40T) has been used as an animal model of spontaneous carcinogenesis by regulating its expression with a variety of transcriptional elements. Although a thymic hyperplasia and thymoma have been reported as incidental findings in transgenic mice, there has been no report on thymic carcinoma in transgenic mice. We have established a specific line of SV40T transgenic mice that consistently produce thymic carcinoma at the age of 5 to 7 months in all cases. Using this animal model, thymic tumor progression was studied by means of a morphological approach with special reference to sequential change at different time points in animals from 3 to 32 weeks of age. The first abnormality of the thymus was noted at 3–5 weeks of age to show an expansion of thymocyte zone with a high PCNA index of cortical thymocytes. At 9 weeks of age, the thymi formed gross masses, and cortico-medullary junction became indistinct due to irregularly expanded epithelial cell areas. These findings were compatible with thymoma. Frank malignant pithelial foci appeared at 12 weeks of age in the background of benign thymoma. Mass-forming thymic carcinoma was found after 15 weeks. Thymic carcinoma was noted in 3 out of 10 mice between 15–16 weeks of age, and in 16 out of 20 mice between 20–21 weeks. After 23 weeks, all eight mice had thymic carcinoma with tumor necrosis. In most thymic carcinoma, there was a benign thymoma co-existed in the thymic masses in varying proportion. By electron microscopy (EM), malignant tumor cells revealed desmosomes with short tonofilaments and few membrane-bound granules. Immunohisto-chemical study(IHS) for cortical thymic epithelium(Th-3) was positive for thymomas, but it was negative for thymic carcinoma. EM and IHS findings suggested that thymic carcinomas lost their original character of cortical or medullary epithelium. It is concluded that thymic carcinoma develop consistently in SV40 T transgenic mice and thymic carcinoma is preceded by benign thymoma.

REFERENCES

1. Levine AJ: Oncogenes of DNA tumor viruses. Cancer Res 1988, 48:493–496
2. Cory S and Adams J: Transgenic mice and oncogenesis. Ann Rev Immmunol 1988, 6:25–48
3. Cuthbertson RA, Klintworth GK: Transgenic mice: a gold mine for furthering knowledge in pathobiology. Lab Invest 1988, 58:484–502
4. Brinster RL, Chen HY, Messing A, van Dyke T, Levine AJ, Palmiter RD: Transgenic mice harboring SV40T-antigen genes develop characteristic brain tumors. Cell 1984, 37:367–379
5. Hanahan D: Heritable formation of pancreatic beta-cell tumors in transgenic mice expressing recombinant insulin/simian virus 40 oncogenes. Nature 1985, 315:115–122
6. Small JA, Blair DG, Showalter SD, Scangos GA: Analysis of a transgenic mouse containing simian virus 40 and v-myc sequences. Mol Cell Biol 1985, 5:642–648
7. Palmiter RD, Chen HY, Messing A, Brinster RL: SV40 enhancer and large-T antigen are instrumental in development of choroid plexus tumors in transgenic mice. Nature 1985, 316:457–460
8. Efrat S, Baekkeskov S, Lane D, Hanahan D: Coordinate expression of the endogeneous p53 gene in cells of transgenic mice expressing hybrid insulin-SV40T antigen genes. EMBO J 1987, 6:2699–2704

9. Teitelman G, Alpert S, Hanahan D: Proliferation, senescence, and neoplastic progrssion of cells in hyperplasic pancreatic islets. Cell 1988, 52:97–105
10. Chen J, van Dyke T: Uniform cell-autonomous tumorigenesis of the choroid plexus by Papovavirus large T antigens. Mol Cell Biol 1991, 11:5968–5976
11. Mahon KA, Chepelinsky AB, Khillan JS, Overbeek PA, Piatigorsky J, Westphal H. Oncogenesis of the lens in transgenic mice. Science 1987;235:1622–1628
12. Suda Y, Aizawa S, Hirai S, Inoue T, Furuta Y, Suzuki M, Hirohashi S, Ikawa Y. Driven by the same Ig enhancer and SV40T promoter, ras induced lung adenomatous tumors, myc induced pre-B cell lymphomas and SV40 large T gene a variety of tumors in transgenic mice. EMBO J 1987; 6:4055–4065
13. Behringer RR, Peschon JJ, Messing A, Gartside CL, Hauschka SD, Palmiter RD, Brinster RL: Heart and bone tumors in transgenic mice. Proc Natl Acad Sci USA 1988, 85:2648–2652
14. Ceci JD, Kovatch RM, Swing DA, Jones JM, Snow CM, Rosenberg MP, Jenkins NA, Copeland NG, Meisler MH: Transgenic mice carrying a murine amylase 2.2/SV40 T antigen fusion gene develop pancreatic acinar cell and stomach carcinoma. Oncogene 1991, 6:323–332
15. Knowles BB, McCarrick J, Fox N, Solter D, Damjanov I: Osteosarcomas in transgenic mice expressing an alpha-amylase-SV40 T-antigen hybrid gene. Am J Pathol 1990,137:259–262.
16. Messing A, Chen HY, Palmiter RD, Brinster RL: Peripheral neuropathies, hepatocellular carcinomas and islet cell adenomas in transgenic mice. Nature (London) 1985, 316:461–463
17. Sandgren EP, Quaife CJ, Pinkert CA, Palmiter RD, Brinster RL: Oncogene-induced liver neoplasia in transgenic mice. Oncogene 1989, 4;715–724
18. Sepulveda AR, Finegold MJ, Smith B, Slagle BL, DeMayo JL, Shen RF, Woo SL, Butel JS: Development of a transgenic mouse system for the analysis of stages in liver carcinogenesis using tissue-specific expression of SV40 large T-antigen controlled by regulatory elements of the human alpha-1-antitrypsin gene. Cancer Res 1989, 49:6108–6117
19. Fox N, Crooke R, Hwang LH, Schibler U, Knowles BB, Solter D: Metastatic hibernomas in transgenic mice expressing an alpha-amylase-SV40 T antigen hybrid gene. Science 1989, 244:461–463
20. Bradl M, Klein Szanto A, Porter S, Mintz B: Malignant melanoma in transgenic mice. Proc Natl Acad Sci USA 1991, 88:164–168
21. Windle JJ, Albert DM, Obien JM, Marcus DM, Disteche CM, Bernards R, Mellon PL: Retinoblastoma in transgenic mice. Nature (London) 1990, 343:665–669
22. Botteri FM, van der Putten H, Wong DF, Sauvage CA, Evans RM: Unexpected thymic hyperplasia in transgenic mice harboring a neuronal promoter fused with Simian Virus 40 large T antigen. Mol Cell Biol 1987, 7:3178–3184
23. Moll J, Eibel H, Botteri F, Sansig G, Regnier C, van der Putten H: Transgenes encoding mutant simian virus 40 large T antigens unmask phenotypic and functional constraints in thymic epithelial cells. Oncogene 1992, 7:2175–2187
24. Teitz T, Chang JC, Kan YW, Yen TSB: Thymic epithelial neoplasms in transgenic mice expressing SV40 T antigen under the control of an erythroid- specific enhancer. J Pathol 1995, 177:309–315
25. Spanopoulou E, Early A, Elliott J, Crispe N, Layman H, Ritter M, Watt S, Grosveld F, Kioussis D: Complex lymphoid and epithelial thymic tumors in Thy 1-myc transgenic mice. Nature 1989, 342:185–189
26. Morinaga S, Sato Y, Shimosato Y, Sinkai T, Tsuchiya R: Multiple thymic squamous cell carcinomas associated with mixed type thymoma. Am J Surg Pathol 1987, 11:982–988
27. Shimosato Y, Kameya T, Nagai K, Suemasu K: Squamous cell carcinoma of thymus: an analysis of eight cases. Am J Surg Pathol 1977, 1:109–121
28. Suster S, Rosai J: Thymic carcinoma. A clinicopathologic study of 60 cases. Cancer 1991, 67:1025–1032
29. Suire RA, Goodmann DG, Valerio MG, Fredrickson T, Strandberg JD, Levitt MH, Lingeman GH, harshbarger JC, Dawe CJ. Tumors: hemopoietic system. In Benirschke K, Garner FM, Jones TC, eds. Pathology of Laboratory Animals. New York: Springer-Verlag, 1978:1091–1125.
30. Kornstein MJ, deBlois GG: Pathology of the thymus and mediastinum. MPP Vol 33,pp104 W.B. Saunders Company, Philadelphia
31. Hogan BLM, Constantini F, Lacy E: Manuplating the mouse embryo: a laboratory manual. Cold Spring Harbor Laboratory, Cold Spring Harbor, N.Y.,1991.
32. Troung LD, Mody DR, Cagle PT, Jackson-York GL, Schwartz MR, Wheeler TM: Thymic carcinoma: A clinicopathologic study of 13 cases. Am J Surg Pathol 1990, 14:151–166
33. Kirchner T, Muller-Hermelink HK: New approaches to the diagnosis of thymic epithelial tumors. Prog Surg Pathol 1989, 10:167–189
34. Pescarmona E, Rosati S, Rendina EA, Venuta F, Baroni CD: Well-differentiated thymic carcinoma: a clinico-pathological study. Virchows Archiv A Pathol Anat 1992, 420:179–183

35. Kirchner T, Schalke B, Buchwald J, Ritter M, Marx A, Muller-Hermelink HK: Well-differentiated thymic carcinoma. An organotypical low-grade carcinoma with relationship to cortical thymoma. Am J Surg Pathol 1992, 16:1153–1169
36. Pan CC, Wu HP, Yang CF, Chen WYK, Chiang H: The clinicopathological correlation of epithelial subtyping in thymoma: A study of 112 consecutive cases. Hum Pathol 1994, 25:893–899
37. Quintanilla-Martinez L, Wilkins EW, Choi N, Efird J, Hug E, Harris NL: Thymoma. Histologic subclassification is an independent prognostic factor. Cancer 1994, 74:606–617
38. Hirokawa K, Utsuyama M, Moriizumi E, Handa S: Analysis of the thymic microenvironment by monoclonal antibodies with special reference to thymic nurse cells. Thymus 1986; 8:349–360
39. Crispe IN, Bevan MJ: Expression and functional significance of the J11d marker on mouse thymocytes. J Immunol 1987, 138:2013–2021
40. Brombacher F, Lamers MC, Kohler G, Eibel H: Elimination of CD8+ thymocytes in transgenic mice expressing an anti-Lyt2.2 immunoglobulin heavy chain gene. EMBO J 1989; 8:3719–3726.
41. van de Wijngaert FP, Kendall MD, Schuurman H-J, Rademakers LHPM, Kater L: Heterogeneity of epithelial cells in the human thymus: an ultrastructural study. Cell Tissue Res 1984, 237:227–237
42. Rosai J, Levine GD: Atlas of Tumor Pathology. Second Series Facs.13. Tumors of the thymus. Washington Dc, Armed Forces Institute of Pathology, 1976, pp.153–161
43. Squire RA, Goodman DG, Valerio MG, Fredrickson T, Strandberg JD, Levitt MH,Lingeman CH,Harshbarger JC, Dawe CJ: Tumors: hematopoietic system. In Benirschke K, Garner FM, Jones TC, eds. Patholgy of Laboratory Animals. New York: Springer-Verlag, 1978, pp. 1091–1125
44. Masuda A, Ohtsuka K, Matsuyama M: Establishment of functional epithelial cell lines from a rat thymoma and a rat thymus. In Vitro Cell Dev Biol 1990, 26:713–721
45. Lu J, Sakai Y, Wajjawalku W, Isobe K-I, Saito M, Amo H, Kojima A, Utsumi KR, Takahashi M, Hiai H, Matsuyama M: Establishment of transplantable tumor lines and in vitro cell lines of malignant thymoma developed in a BUF/Mna rat. Jpn J Cancer Res 1992, 83:618–624
46. Boeckman DE, Stutman O: Fine structure of a transplanted chemically induced non-lymphoid thymoma. Cancer Res 1969, 29:1663–1668
47. Rosai J: "Lymphoepithelioma-like" thymic carcinoma: Another tumor related to Epstein-Barr virus? New Engl J Med 1985, 312:1320–1322
48. Mokhtar N, Hsu S-M, Lad RP, Haynes BF, Jaffe ES: Thymoma:Lymphoid and epithelial components mirror the phenotype of normal thymus. Human Pathol 1984, 15:378–384
49. Hoot GP, Kettman JR: Primary polyoma virus-induced murine thymic epithelial tumors: a tumor model of thymus physiology. Am J Pathol 1989, 135:679–695
50. Jat PS, Noble MD, Ataliotis P, Tanaka Y, Yannoutsos N, Larsen L, Kioussis D: Direct derivation of conditionally immortal cell lines from an H-2Kb-tsA58 transgenic mouse. Proc Natl Acad Sci USA 1991, 88:5096–5100
51. Wildin RS, Garvin AM, Pawar S, Lewis DB, Abraham KM, Forbush KA, Ziegler SF, Allen JM, Perlmutter RM: Developmental regulation of lck gene expression in T lymphocytes. J Exp Med 1991, 173:383–393
52. Messing A, Pinkert CA, Palmiter RD, Brinster RL: Developmental study of SV40 large T antigen expression in transgenic mice and choroid plexus neoplasia. Oncogene Res 1988, 3:87–97
53. Van Dyke TA, Finlay C, Miller D, Marks J, Lozano G, Levine AJ. Relationship between simian virus 40 large tumor antigen expression and tumor formation in transgenic mice. J Virol 1987;61:2029–2032.
54. Sayer WR, Eggleston JC: Thymoma: A clinical and pathological study of 65 cases. Cancer 1976, 37:229–249
55. Marino M, Muller-Hermelink HK: Thymoma and thymic carcinoma. Relation of thymoma epithelial cells to the cortical and medullary differentiation of thymus. Virchows Arch [Pathol Anat] 1985, 407:119–149
56. Pescarmona E, Pisacane A, Rendina EA, et al: Organoid thymoma: A well differentiated variant with distinct clinicopathological features. Histopathology 1991, 18:161–164
57. Pescarmona E, Rendina EA, Venuta F, Ricci C, Ruco LP, Baroni CD: The prognostic implication of the thymoma histologic subtyping. A study of 80 consecutive cases. Am J Clin Pathol 1990, 93:190–195
58. Masaoka A, Monden Y, Nakahara K, Tanioka T: Follow-up study of thymomas with special reference to their clinical stages. Cancer 1981, 48:2485–2492
59. Tateyama H, Mizuno T, Tada T, Eimoto T, Hashimoto T, Masaoka A: Thymic epithelial tumors: evaluation of malignant grade by quantification of proliferating cell nuclear antigen and nucleolar organizer regions. Virchows Arch A Pathol Anat 1993, 422:265–269
60. Kuo T, Chang JP, Lin FJ, Wu WC, Chang CH: Thymic carcinomas: Histopathological varieties and immunohistochemical study. Am J Surg Pathol 1990, 14:24–34
61. Kuo TT, Lo SK: Thymoma. A study of the pathologic classification of 71cases with evaluation of the Muller-Hermelink system. Hum Pathol 1993, 24:766–771

21

ANALYSIS OF A MURINE THYMIC CARCINOGENESIS MODEL INDUCED BY THE EXPRESSION OF LARGE T OF SV40

Thierry Molina,[1] Lucile Miquerol,[2] Geoffroy de Ribbains,[2] Mounir Bouleksibat,[1] Catherine Martinon,[3] Sophie Ezine,[3] Alain Vandewalle,[4] Jacques Diebold,[1] and Axel Kahn[2]

[1]Laboratoire Universitaire de Recherches en Histopathologie
Faculté Broussais-Hôtel-Dieu
15 rue de l'Ecole de médecine, 75006 Paris, France
[2]Unité INSERM U 129
ICGM, Paris
[3]Unité INSERM U 345
Faculté Necker, Paris
[4]Unité INSERM U 246
Faculté Bichat, Paris

Large T of SV40 is a viral protein involved in the lytic cycle of its natural host, the monkey, but has transforming properties after transfection in some murine and human cell lines. The targeting of this oncogene under the control of tissue-specific promotors in transgenic mice led to the creation of in vivo models of tumors : hepatocarcinomas, lymphomas, neuroendocrine carcinomas, choroid plexus carcinomas, thymic hyperplasia, hypoplasia, thymomas. The oncogenic function of this protein is mainly linked to the sequestration of tumor suppressor gene products, namely p53 and Rb.

We report the development of a thymic tumor occuring among 3 transgenic lines. The transgene consists of 2,7 Kb of the coding sequences of SV 40 large T and small t under the control of the regulatory sequences of the rat L-type pyruvate kinase and of the 72bp repeats of SV40 enhancer.

Macroscopic examination in the line SV12 showed an enlargement of the thymus starting at 6 weeks until 20 weeks, usual date of death in this transgenic line. Northern blot demonstrated an expression of the transgene in the thymus and immunohistochemistry showed an expression of the transgene mainly by epithelial cells.

Histopathological study showed between 4 and 6 weeks an expansion of the thymic medulla with an ill-defined corticomedullary junction and hypertrophic and hyperplastic Hassal's corpuscles. This pattern resembles to thymic hyperplasia. After 6 weeks, there is a disorganization of the thymic architecture with numerous perivascular spaces, predomi-

Epithelial Tumors of the Thymus, edited by Marx and Müller-Hermelink.
Plenum Press, New York, 1997

nance of cortical type areas associated with numerous small lymphocytes and areas of medullary differentiation with numerous Hassal's corpuscles. Some pseudoglandular patterns as well as microcystic areas are present. Immunohistochemistry data showed a disorganization of the normal cortical reticular pattern (MTS 44, Boyd) and of the medullar staining (MTS10, Boyd). Overall, this pattern suggests an organoid thymoma. FACS analysis showed that although double positive thymocytes are predominant, there is a slight increase in mature thymocytes. There is no clonal T cell population according to the the germ-line pattern rearrangement of TCR beta chain gene. After 17 weeks, associated with the thymoma, cohesive sheets of epithelial cells lying in a fibrous stroma are present. There are numerous cytonuclear atypia and squamous pearls. This pattern suggests an epidermoid carcinoma developing on a preexisting thymoma.

Overall, our model of murine thymic carcinogenesis shows clearly the development of a thymic carcinoma through a multistep mechanism starting from thymic hyperplasia. Moreover, in this model, organoid thymoma represents an intermediate neoplastic stage to the development of a thymic carcinoma. This sequence further supports to consider this type of thymoma (similar to predominantly cortical human thymoma) as a potential malignant thymoma. This observation underlines the powerful tool of transgenic mice in defining histopathological patterns of tumor progression.

22

INEFFICIENT POSITIVE SELECTION OF CD4+ T CELLS IN EPITHELIAL CELL TUMORS OF THE HUMAN THYMUS

Yukiyasu Takeuchi, Yoshitaka Fujii,* Meinoshin Okumura, and Hikaru Matsuda

Immunology Laboratory
First Department of Surgery
Osaka University Medical School
Osaka, Japan

1. SUMMARY

Human thymomas are epithelial tumors that are associated with a large number of non-neoplastic T cells of mainly immature phenotype, suggesting that epithelial cells of thymomas retain the function of thymic cortical epithelium. But it has not been reported that lymphocytes within thymoma are positively selected. We studied whether the single-positive cells in thymomas had been positively selected using three-color flowcytometly. A large proportion (16–85%, mean±SD 58±22%, n=17) of CD4+ single-positive T cells within the thymomas lack cell surface expression of CD3 and also of CD69, an early activation antigen that is expressed in positively selected thymocytes. Normal thymus had this CD4+CD8-CD3- population at much lower frequencies (12±7%, n=11). It has been reported that in the human, the CD4+CD8-CD3- cells are the predominant population that is intermediate between the CD4-CD8- double-negative and CD4+CD8+ double-positive stages. In contrast to CD4+ single-positive cells, most of CD8+ single-positive cells in the thymoma as well as in the normal thymus expressed CD69 and a high level of CD3. These observations could be explained partly if the epithelial cells of thymoma were unable to positively select all the immature thymocytes generated in the thymoma. This relative inefficiently of positive selection could not be attributed solely to the paucity of MHC class II expression in the thymoma.

* Correspondence: Yoshitaka Fujii, Immunology Laboratory, First Department of Surgery, Osaka University Medical School, 2-2 Yamadaoka, Suita, Osaka, 565 Japan.

Epithelial Tumors of the Thymus, edited by Marx and Müller-Hermelink.
Plenum Press, New York, 1997

2. INTRODUCTION

In the normal human thymus, T cell differentiation has been extensively studied and it is widely accepted that the CD3-CD4-CD8- thymocytes generate mature single-positive cells via double-positive cells. However we and others have recently reported that there is an intermediate stage between the double-negative and double-positive (1–3). In the human, these cells express CD4 but do not express CD3 or CD8 and thus they are called immature single-positive cells. In the human thymoma which is an epithelial cell tumor of the thymus, there are a large number of non-neoplastic T cells associated with the tumor (4–7). And Willcox *et al.* using immunohistology and we, using FACS, have shown that these associated T cells are double-positive and in every sense similar to thymic cortical T cells (7.8). This suggested that the epithelial cells of thymomas retain the function of thymic cortical epithelium. Willcox *et al.* have also reported that epithelial cells of thymomas had cortical phenotype and varying degrees of HLA-DR expression (8). We present an interesting difference between T cell maturation in thymoma and in normal thymus. We studied whether the single-positive cells in thymoma had been positively selected by means of analyzing expression of CD3 and CD69, an early activating antigen, using three-color flow cytometry (9–12) .

3. MATERIALS AND METHODS

3.1 Cell Preparation

Lymphocytes were prepared from the thymus or thymoma by mincing the tissue with scissors and pressing through a stainless steel mesh. Normal thymuses were obtained at cardiac surgery of patients with no apparent immunological disorder. Four patients had myasthenia gravis of moderate severity.

3.2 Flow Cytometry

Lymphocytes (2×106) were stained with FITC-conjugated anti-CD4, PE-conjugated anti-CD3 or anti-CD69, and biotin-conjugated anti-CD8 (Becton Dickinson, San Jose, CA) in 100μl of PBS for 20 min. Cells were washed twice and incubated with streptavidine Red 670 (Gibco, Gaithersberg, MD) for 20 min before washing once and analysis with FACScan (Becton Dickinson). Lymphocytes were gated according to the forward and side scatter pattern. Subpopulation of thymocytes (or lymphocytes in thymoma) of small population sizes were analyzed using data acquired using a gate for that particular phenotype (e.g. for CD8+CD4- cells). Data was analyzed and histograms were generated using Lysys program (Becton Dickinson).

3.3 Immunohistochemistry

Tissues were fixed in 10% formalin and then paraffin-embedded. Sections were stained using streptavidin-biotin-peroxidase kit (Dakopatts, Glostrup, Denmark) with diaminobenzidine as the chromogen. Sections were counter-stained with Hematoxylin. The primary antiserum, monoclonal mouse anti-human HLA-DR, CR3/43 (Dakopatts, Glostrup, Denmark) at a dilution of 1:100, rabbit anti-keratin/cytokeratin (pre-diluted, Nichirei, Tokyo, Japan) or rabbit anti-human lysozyme (pre-diluted, Dako, Carpinteria,

CA) were applied overnight at 4°C. For negative control specimens, normal mouse serum (1:100 dilution) or nonimmune rabbit serum (Dako, Carpinteria, CA) were used in place of the primary antibodies.

4. RESULTS

4.1 CD3 and CD69 Expression in Lymphocytes from Normal Thymus and Thymoma (Table 1 and Fig. 1)

Fig. 1 shows representative data from a normal thymus and a thymoma. In the normal thymus, 51 % of double-negative subset and 76 % of double-positive subset express CD3. All CD8+ single-positive subset expressed CD3, but quite consistently, about 8% of CD4+ single-positive subset did not express CD3 and 22% of the subset did not express CD69. This population was called immature single-positive cells. In the thymoma, this population was much larger and in this thymoma only 21% of CD4+ single-positive cells expressed CD3 and only 11% expressed CD69. In contrast to the CD4+ single-positive cells, almost all CD8+ single-positive cells in the tumor expressed CD3 and 82% of them expressed CD69. So for the CD8+ single-positive, they are quite similar to the normal thymus.

Table 1 summarizes the data from the three-color flowcytometric analysis of CD3 and CD69 expression in lymphocyte subsets in the 11 normal thymuses and 17 thymomas. The thymomas contained varying numbers of CD4+CD8+ double-positive cells. Thymomas have both CD4+ and CD8+ single-positive cells as many as normal thymus, but CD3- cells among CD4+ single-positive cells far exceeded those in the normal thymus. In another words, thymomas have fewer percentage of mature CD4+ single-positive cells than normal thymuses. The CD69 expression is correlated with CD3 expression. The frequencies of CD3- or CD69- cells among CD8+ single-positive population was consistently very low, as in the normal thymus. So this apparent block of T cell maturation in thymomas is limited to CD4+ T cells.

4.2 MHC Class II Expression in the Thymoma (Fig. 2)

The epithelial cells of thymomas have been reported to have varying degree of MHC class II expression (8). Therefore it is possible that the accumulation of immature CD4+ single-positive-cells have been caused by the inefficient positive selection of CD4+ T cells because of fewer MHC class II molecules available.

Fig. 2 shows the results of two thymomas. Case 7 thymoma contained 40% double-positive cells, 46% CD3- cells in CD4+ single-positive cells, and 42% CD69- cells in CD4+ single-positive cells, and case 15 thymoma contained 64%, 82% and 75% respectively. So the latter had a large number of immature, pre-selection CD4+ single-positive cells and the former had a moderate number of immature CD4+ single-positive cell. However, quite contrary to our expectations, the epithelial cells (keratin+ lysozyme-) of the latter thymoma expressed HLA-DR at a level comparable to that in the normal thymus but somehow failed to generate CD4+ single-positive cells efficiently. The former epithelial cells (keratin+ lysozyme-) did not have plenty of class II molecules. Table 1 shows that the result of a normal thymus and nine thymomas. Two thymomas were HLA-DR negative, three were some positive, and four were positive. There was no correlation between the level of HLA-DR expression and the frequency of immature CD4 single-positive cells in the thymoma.

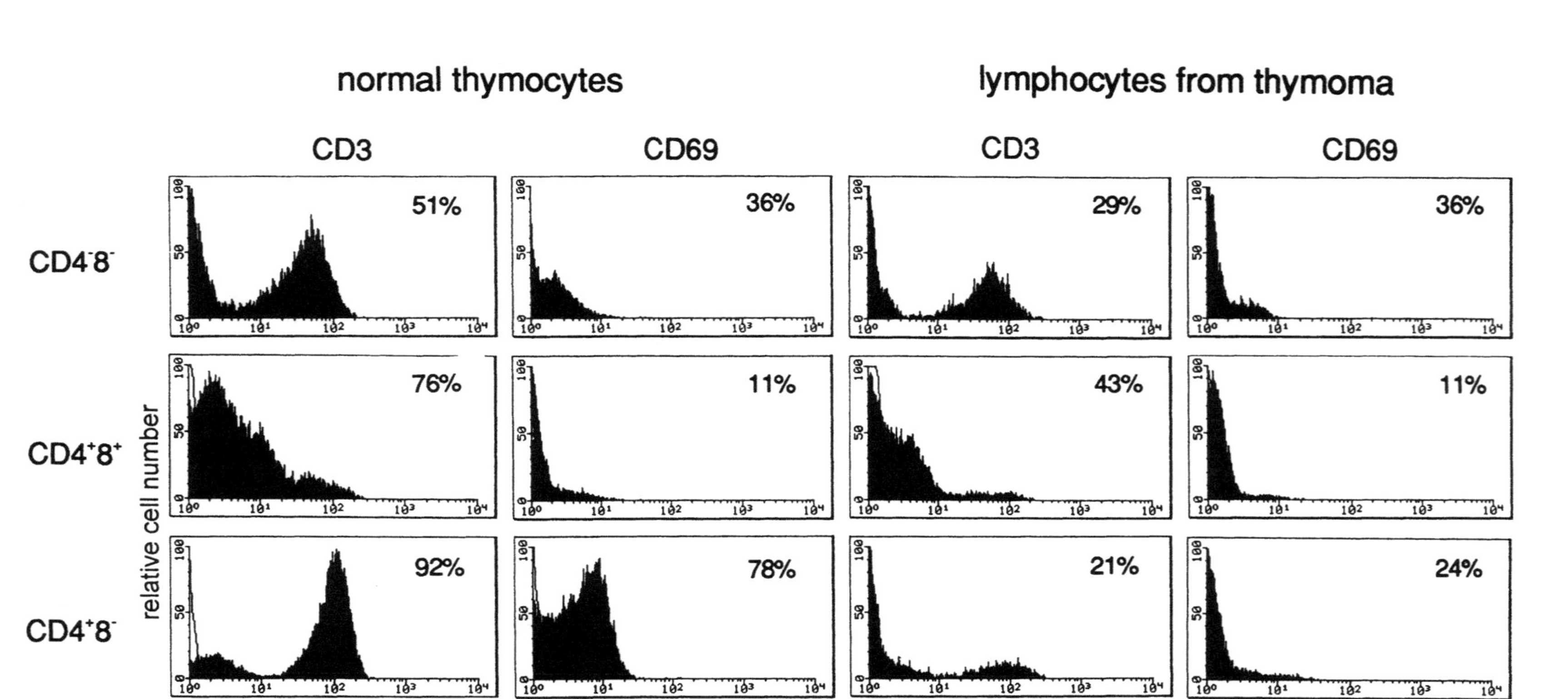
normal thymocytes
lymphocytes from thymoma
CD3
CD69
CD3
CD69
CD4-8-
CD4+8+
CD4+8-
relative cell number
51%
36%
29%
36%
76%
11%
43%
11%
92%
78%
21%
24%

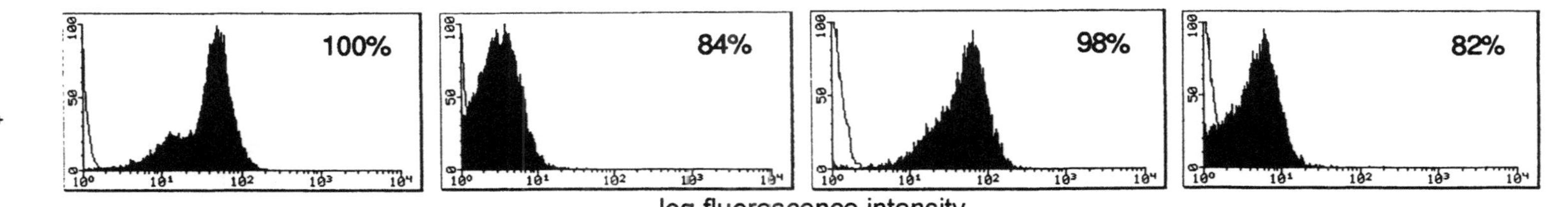

Figure 1. CD3 and CD69 expression of T cell subsets defined by CD4/CD8 expression in a normal thymus (from a 1-year-old donor) and a thymoma (case 11). Lymphocytes were stained with FITC-conjugated anti-CD4, PE-conjugated anti-CD3 or anti-CD69, and biotin-conjugated anti-CD8 (in combination with streptavidine-Red 670, Gibco, Gaithersberg, MD) and CD3 or CD69 expressions of lymphocyte subsets are shown in shaded histograms.Open histograms indicate cells stained with PE-conjugated control mouse IgG in place of anti-CD3 or CD69. Figures indicate percentages of cells stained above the control level. The proportions of CD3+ cells among CD4-CD8- Subpopulation in other samples were 39–65% (mean±SD, 52±8) for the normal thymus and 15–48% (32±9) for the thymoma.

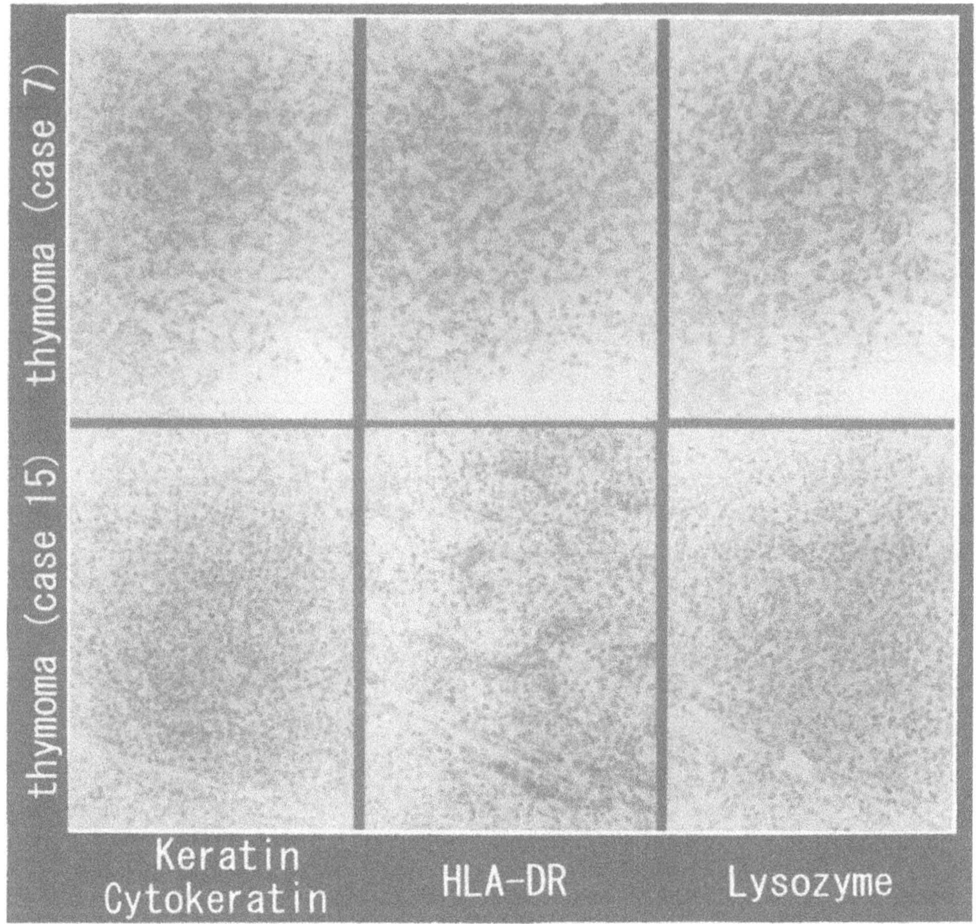

Figure 2. MHC class II expression in thymomas. Immunohistochemical staining with antibodies to keratin/cytokeratin, HLA-DR and lysozyme. Case 7 thymoma which contained relatively few immature CD4+ single-positive cells (47% of CD4+ single-positive cells), and case 15 thymoma which contained many immature CD4+ single-positive cells (82%). Original magnification; ×200.

5. DISCUSSION

We have shown that a large proportion of CD4+ single-positive lymphocytes lacked CD3 and CD69 in 17 human thymomas (Table and Fig. 1). The accumulation of CD4+CD8-CD3- T cells in thymomas has an interesting implication. The process of positive selection within the thymoma may be rate limiting. If more immature T cells are generated in the thymoma than in the normal thymus, T cells of pre-selection stages (stages at or before the CD4+CD8+ double-positive cells) may accumulate as a result of overload. We had speculated that the level of class II MHC expression on epithelial cells in thymomas may be relevant to their inefficiency in positive selection. However, an immunohistochemical study revealed a significant amount of class II MHC expressed even in thymomas with CD3- cells occupying as much as 80% of the CD4+ single-positive cells. Thus, the lack of class II MHC antigen is not the sole cause of the accumulation of imma-

Table 1. CD3 and CD69 expression of lymphocyte subsets defined by CD4/CD8 expression and HLA-DR expression of the epithelial cells

		CD4+8+/total	CD4+8-/total	CD4-8+/total	CD3-/CD4+8-	CD3-/CD4-8+	CD69-/CD4+8-	CD69-/CD4-8+	HLA-DR**
normal thymus (n=11)									
mean±SD		55±13(%)	27±10(%)	9±4(%)	12±7(%)	1.3±2.0(%)	17±11(%)	16±7(%)	+
thymoma	*1	20	29	26	16	2.3	25	10	−
	*2	50	12	22	35	1.2	17	12	ND
	3	66	29	9	36	1.5	41	9	+
	4	5	21	12	37	1.8	31	14	+
	5	60	14	16	38	0.7	47	16	ND
	*6	54	22	19	38	0.3	34	10	±
	7	40	18	40	46	0.1	42	6	−
	8	84	6	5	52	4.1	40	10	ND
	9	47	23	9	52	0.3	70	13	+
	10	76	14	9	73	0.5	65	20	±
	11	53	6	2	75	2.1	76	18	±
	12	52	26	7	75	2.0	72	31	ND
	13	28	30	23	77	1.9	68	33	ND
	*14	63	23	13	79	1.2	68	15	ND
	15	64	38	6	82	0.5	75	9	+
	16	68	31	2	83	0.5	79	9	ND
	17	64	26	5	85	0.9	86	10	ND
mean±SD		53±20	22±9	13±10	58±22	1.3±1.0	55±21	14±8	

The ages of the doners of the normal thymus were 4d - 39 y (median 10 m). The ages of the thymoma patients were 34 - 69y (mean±SD 51±10). Thymoma case 4 was classified as epithelial cell predominant ; others as lymphocyte predominant or mixed type. *: myasthenia gravis. **: HLA-DR expression of epithelial cells (keratin+, lysozyme-) were graded arbitrarily into - (negative), ± (some positive cells), and + (positive).
ND: not done.

ture CD4+ single- positive cells in the thymomas. In any case, it has to be stressed that thymomas do generate mature single-positive CD4+ or CD8+ cells because they contain CD69+ cells; the defect in positive selection is partial.

The present study indicates the positive selection of T cells in thymomas may be inefficient when compared with the normal thymus. Still, it should be stressed that a significant number of mature T cells are generated in the thymoma. Because thymomas lack the medulla, it is not known if negative selection operates efficiently in the thymoma (13). If the mature T cells generated in thymomas are allowed to seed the periphery without being censored by the negatively selecting element, it may well have relevance to the frequent association of thymoma with autoimmune diseases.

REFERENCES

1. Hori, T., Cupp, J., Wrighton, N., Lee, F., and Spits, H., J. Immunol. 146, 4078, 1991.
2. Kraft, D. L., Weissman, I. L., and Waller, E. K., J. Exp. Med. 178, 265, 1993.
3. Takeuchi, Y., Fujii, Y., Okumura, M., Inada, K., Nakahara, K., and Matsuda, H., Cellular Immunology 151, 481, 1993.
4. Rosai, J., and Levine, G. D., Atlas of Tumor Pathology 2nd Series Fascicle 13. US Armed Forces Institute of Pathology 1976.
5. Lauriola, L., Musiani, P., Ranelletti, F. O., Maggiano, N., and Piantelli, M., Clin. Exp. Immunol. 52, 477, 1983.
6. Palestro, G., Geuna, M., Novero, D., Godio, L., Ciccone, G., and Azzoni, L., Virchows Archiv B Cell Pathol. 59, 297, 1990.
7. Fujii, Y., Hayakawa, M., Inada, K., and Nakahara, K., Eur. J. Immunol. 20, 2355, 1990 .
8. Willcox, N., Schluep, M., Ritter, M. A., Schuurman. H. J., Newsom-Davis, J., and Christensson, B., Am. J. Pathol. 127, 447, 1987.
9. Bendelac, A., Matzinger, P., Seder, R. A., Paul, W. E., and Schwartz, R. H., J. Exp. Med. 175, 731, 1992.
10. Swat, W., Dessing, M., Von Boehmer, H., and Kisielow, P., Eur. J. Immunol. 23, 739, 1993.
11. Muller, K-P., and Kyewski, B. A., Eur. J. Immunol.23, 1661, 1993.
12. Brandle, D., Muller, S., Muller, C., Hengartner, H., and Pircher, H., Eur. J. Immunol. 24, 145, 1994.
13. Fujii, Y., Okumura, M., Inada, K., and Nakahara, K., Cell. Immunol. 137, 428, 1991.

23

ABNORMAL T LYMPHOCYTE DEVELOPMENT IN MYASTHENIA GRAVIS-ASSOCIATED THYMOMAS*

Regina Nenninger,† Anja Schultz, Bart Vandekerckhove, Thomas Hünig, Berthold Schalke, Hans Konrad Müller-Hermelink, and Alexander Marx

Institutes of Pathology and Virology, and Department of Neurology
University of Würzburg
Josef-Schneider-Str. 2, 97080 Würzburg, Germany
Institute of Bacteriology and Virology
University Hospital
9000 Gent, Belgium

ABSTRACT

To get an insight into the pathogenesis of thymoma-associated myasthenia gravis we studied intratumorous thymocyte maturation in different thymoma subtypes by three-colour flow cytometry. The thymocyte subset composition was characteristically altered in each histological thymoma subtype. A medullary thymoma was almost devoid of immature thymocytes and the mature intratumorous lymphocytes appeared to be mostly of peripheral origin. In contrast, mixed and cortical thymomas exhibited thymocyte development from the most immature precursor cells to cells with a pre-emigrant phenotype. These mature lymphocytes were of central origin. In mixed more than in cortical thymomas representation of immature $CD4^+$/ $CD8^-$/$CD3^-$ thymocytes was increased although the percentage of earlier precursors was normal. A decreased production of mature CD4+ SP T cells suggests inefficient positive selection. Supporting this view, MHC class II expression was reduced on neoplastic epithelium. Inefficient generation of mature T cells in thymomas could be one reason why thymoma patients have no general defect of central tolerance. Maintained but inefficient intratumorous T cell maturation supports the concept that abnormal positive selection of potentially autoaggressive T cells is the basis of

* Supported by grant Ma 1492/2–1 of the Deutsche Forschungsgemeinschaft (DFG) and by a grant from the "Förderungsschwerpunkt Autoimmunitätsforschung" of the German Ministry of Education and Science (BMBF)
† Correspondence: Regina Nenninger, MD, Institute of Pathology, University of Würzburg, Josef-Schneider-Str. 2, D-97080 Würzburg, Germany. Tel.: 0931/201 3786; fax : 0931/201 3440.

Epithelial Tumors of the Thymus, edited by Marx and Müller-Hermelink.
Plenum Press, New York, 1997

autoimmunization in mixed and cortical thymomas. Autoimmunity in medullary thymomas might have a different pathogenesis.

INTRODUCTION

Myasthenia gravis (MG) is an autoimmune disease characterized by muscle weakness due to an impairment of AChR function at the neuromuscular junction by anti-AChR autoantibodies[1,2]. $CD4^+$ AChR-specific T cells play a pivotal role in the production of these autoantibodies[2,3,4]. About 10 % of MG patients have a thymoma[6,7] and only these patients have also anti-striated muscle and anti-neuronal autoantibodies[8,9]. Thymomas are epithelial tumors[10]. Benign thymomas and category I malignant thymomas have thymus-like morphological and functional features and show paraneoplastic autoimmunity more often than any other human neoplasm[6,7]. In contrast, category II malignant thymomas have no thymus-like features and never exhibit autoimmune phenomena[7,10]. Interestingly, MG is encountered only in patients with benign and category I malignant thymomas that show intratumorous T cells with an immature phenotype, $CD1^+/CD4^+/CD8^+/CD3^{-/low}$[11–13], suggesting a defect of central T cell tolerance in paraneoplastic MG[2,4,7,14,15]. In fact, the lack of a well organized medulla and the rarity of dendritic cells, which mediate negative selection of the T-cell repertoire[16,17] are typical of MG-associated thymomas[6,18]. However, a defective negative selection alone would not explain why autoimmunity in paraneoplastic MG is not systemic but specifically directed against the AChR, striated muscle proteins and neuronal antigens. To reconcile these clinical observations with the constant pathological finding of thymus-like features in MG-associated thymomas an abnormal positive selection of antigen-specific autoaggressive T cells has been invoked[19]. The antigen-specificity of the abnormal selection process is thought to be driven by abnormally expressed thymoma epithelial proteins that share cross-reacting epitopes with the AChR, striational muscle proteins and neuronal antigens[7,9,14,19,20–22]. This hypothesis suggests that potentially autoaggressive T cells are generated inside thymomas and then exported to the periphery due to the paucity of negatively selecting intratumorous elements[19].

In order to investigate the presumed intratumorous mechanisms of tolerance breakdown in thymoma patients two-colour flow cytometric analyses of thymoma lymphocytes have been performed previously[13,23–27]. These studies found either no or inconsistent abnormalities. A recent three-colour flow cytometric analysis of the expression of CD4, CD8, CD3 and CD69 in thymoma lymphocytes demonstrated a higher percentage of immature $CD4^+/CD8^-/CD3^-$ thymocytes and suggested that intratumorous positive selection was inefficient[18]. The small panel of differentiation markers investigated in this study did, however, not allow conclusions about the mechanisms underlying these alterations.

Furthermore, the question has not been addressed whether mature T cells in thymomas are generated in situ or result from the recirculation of peripheral T cells. Finally, the different histological phenotypes of MG-associated thymomas were not taken into account, although clinical findings suggest distinct phenotype-associated mechanisms of tolerance breakdown[7,14,28].

We therefore undertook a three-colour flow cytometric analysis of different thymoma subtypes with a large panel of monoclonal antibodies to differentiation antigens expressed by the most immature to the most mature intrathymically generated lymphocytes[11,29–33]. Our findings suggest different mechanisms of maturational disturbances that are characteristic for each histologically defined thymoma subtype. The detection of mature T cells with features of "pre-emigrant thymocytes" in mixed and cortical thymomas implies that mature and potentially autoaggressive T cells arise in situ, demonstrating a prerequisite for the "false-positive selection model" of paraneoplastic MG in these tumors[7,19].

MATERIALS AND METHODS

Patients and Tumors

The clinical and pathological findings in the patients included in this study are given in Table 1. The diagnosis of MG was based on clinical findings, the demonstration of a decrement in electrophysiological investigations and the detection of anti-AChR autoantibodies by a radio immunoassay based on human muscle derived ^{131}J-labelled AChR. The tumors were subtyped according to the classification of Müller-Hermelink and co-workers as medullary, cortical or mixed thymomas[6,7].

Cell Preparation

Thymocytes were prepared from thymuses and thymomas by passing minced tissue through a stainless-steel seeve followed by Ficoll-Hypaque density gradient centrifugation and 2 washings in cold phosphate buffered saline (PBS). Normal thymuses were obtained at cardiac surgery of patients with no apparent immunological disorders. Lymph nodes and the residual thymus tissue adjacent to the thymomas were carefully separated from the tumor.

Table 1. Clinical and pathological findings in the thymoma patients and controls investigated in this study

Case no.	Tumor type/ diagnosis	Age	Sex	MG	Anti-AChR -autoantibody titer (mmol/l)
1006/96	MDT	73 y	female	+	> 30
24864/94	MXT	75 y	female	+	19
17821/94	MXT	38 y	female	+	> 5
14839/95	MXT	54 y	male	—	n.a.
12211/95	MXT	62 y	female	—	—
2516/95	CT	48 x	male	+	3.2
3792/95	CT	59 y	female	+	< 20
15173/94	CT	58 y	male	—	1.0
4858/95	CT	60 y	male	+	> 5
1	NT	2 y	female	—	—
2	NT	32 y	male	—	—
3	NT	2 y	female	—	—
4	NT	3 y	male	—	—

MG= Myasthenia Gravis
n.a. = not available
MDT = Medullary Thymoma
MXT = Mixed Thymoma
CT = Cortical Thymoma
NT = Normal Thymus

Cell Surface Markers

Staining of surface antigens was performed using the following monoclonal antibodies (mAbs) obtained from Becton Dickinson (Heidelberg, Germany): CD1a (PE-labeled), anti CD3 (PerCP-labeled), anti CD4 (PerCP-labeled), anti CD69 (FITC-labeled), obtained from Dako (Hamburg, Germany): anti CD3 (FITC-, PE-labeled), anti CD4 (FITC-labeled), anti CD8 (PE-labeled), anti CD14 (unlabeled), anti CD19 (FITC-labeled), anti CD34 (unlabeled), anti CD45RO (unlabeled); obtained from Dianova (Hamburg, Germany): anti CD8 (FITC-labeled), anti CD27 (unlabeled), anti CD45RA (FITC-labeled), anti CD56 (unlabeled), anti CD71 (FITC-labeled); obtained from Sigma (Deisenhofen, Germany): isotype controls, anti CD3 and anti CD4 (Quantum-Red labeled). Gamma/delta TCR-1 was purchased from Biermann GmbH (Bad Nauheim, Germany).

Immunohistochemistry

MHC class II (HLA-DR) was detected on frozen sections by a three-step immunoperoxidase technique as described in detail previously[21]. Staining intensity was assessed independently by two of the authors (H.-K. Müller-Hermelink and A. Marx) as either negative, weak, intermediate or strong.

Flow Cytometry

Data sampling and analysis were performed on a Becton Dickinson FACScan flow cytometer equipped with a 15-mW air-cooled 488-nm Argon-ion laser. By suitable gating of lymphoid populations (forward versus sideward scatter) dot-plots for 3-colour fluorescence analysis of $2x10^5$ cells were obtained. All immunofluorescence profiles are plotted on a 4-decade log scale. Data were analyzed and histograms generated using the Lysis II software (Becton Dickinson).

RESULTS

Identification of the Main Lymphocyte Subsets in Thymomas

Thymoma- and thymus-derived thymocytes were analyzed for the expression of CD34, CD2, CD3, CD4 and CD8 in order to characterize triple negative (TN), immature $CD4^+$ SP, $CD4^+/8^+$ double positive (DP) and mature SP T cells as the main T cell subsets. The results of these investigations are summarized in Table 2. There was no significant difference in the percentage of the earliest immature thymocytes, i. e. cells expressing CD34 or CD2 but neither CD4 nor CD8. By two-colour analysis of CD4 and CD8 expression only the medullary thymoma appeared clearly abnormal due to a substantial lack of DP thymocytes while cortical thymomas showed a slight reduction of $CD4^+$ SP thymocytes and mixed thymomas appeared virtually normal (Table 2 and Fig. 1). Three-colour flow cytometric analysis, however, revealed that an abnormally high proportion of $CD4^+$ SP thymocytes had an immature $CD4^+/CD8^-/CD3^-$ phenotype in mixed and cortical thymomas (Table 2 and Fig. 2). In fact, these thymomas contained immature $CD4^+/CD8^-/CD3^-$ thymocytes at a 5–10 fold higher frequency than controls while mature $CD4^+/CD8^-/CD3^+$ SP cells were reduced. The increase in $CD4^+/CD8^-/CD3^-$ SP thymocytes in mixed and cortical thymomas was accompanied by a slight increase in the immature $CD4^+/CD8^+/CD3^-$ DP thymocyte subset that is thought to be

Table 2. Thymocyte subset composition (given as percentages of all mononucleus cells) in thymomas and normal thymus, and MHC class II expression (DR) by epithelial cells

Phenotype *(Tumor type/case no.)*	$CD34^+$	$CD4^-8^-2^+$	$CD4^+8^-3^-$	$CD4^+8^+3^-$	$CD4^+8^+3^+$	$CD4^+8^-3^+$	$CD4^-8^+3^+$	MHCII[a]
Medullary thymoma								
1006/95	n.d.	4.0	1.0	1.0	3.0	17.0	66.0	+
Mixed thymoma								
24864/94	2.0	2.0	7.0	34.0	38.0	1.0	4.0	+
17821/94	1.0	3.0	9.0	44.0	9.0	1.0	6.0	+
14839/95	0.1	2.0	12.0	62.0	8.0	1.0	1.0	–
12211/95	0.0	1.0	14.0	37.0	40.0	2.0	2.0	+
Cortical thymoma								
2516/95	n.d.	7.0	4.0	23.0	45.0	4.0	11.0	–
27942/95	0.2	2.0	4.0	26.0	50.0	3.0	9.0	+
15173/94	n.d.	0.3	2.0	30.0	31.0	2.0	26.0	–
858/95	0.3	0.7	2.0	25.0	42.0	4.0	11.0	+
Normal thymus								
1	1.0	3.0	1.0	10.0	51.0	16.0	9.0	+++
2	0.3	9.0	2.0	19.0	37.0	13.0	11.0	++
3	0.1	2.0	1.0	27.0	41.0	10.0	10.0	+++
4	10.1	3.0	0.7	29.0	35.0	14.0	10.0	+++

[a] Intensity of epithelial MHC class II expression was estimated in immunoperoxidase-stained frozen sections as negative (-), weak (+), moderate (++) or strong (+++), n.d. not done.

the immediate progeny of $CD4^+/CD8^-/CD3^-$ cells[34–36] (Table 2 and Fig. 3). In contrast, the mature $CD4^+/CD3^+$ SP thymocytes were decreased in mixed and cortical thymomas. The proportion of mature $CD8^+/CD3^+$ SP thymocytes was significantly diminished in mixed but not cortical thymomas. An immature $CD8^+/CD4^-/CD3^-$ population was not detected in thymomas or thymuses. The percentages of $CD19^+$, $CD56^+$ and $CD14^+$ cells were each below 1 % (not shown).

Characterization of Immature $CD3^-$ Thymocytes in Thymomas

A higher frequency of $CD4^+/CD8^-/CD3^-$ thymocytes and $CD4^+/CD8^+/CD3^-$ thymocytes among the $CD3^-$ thymocytes was one of the main findings in mixed and cortical thymomas. A panel of differentiation and activation markers characterized these thymocytes as immature cells comparable to the $CD3^-$ cells in the normal thymus[34–36]. As shown in Fig. 3, $CD3^-$ thymocytes in mixed and cortical thymoma were all $CD1^{high}$ and $CD44^{low}$ but did not express CD69, CD27 or CD45RA. This implies that the $CD4^+/CD8^-/CD3^-$ subpopulation in mixed and cortical thymomas is indeed immature as it is in the normal thymus[34–36]. The only difference was a higher number of $CD71^+$ cells in $CD4^+/CD8^-/CD3^-$ cells of mixed and cortical thymomas (not shown).

Characterization of Mature $CD3^{high}$ Thymocytes in Thymomas

The vast majority of $CD3^{high}$ thymocytes has obtained a differentiation signal during positive selection which results in a change of cell surface marker expression[37–40]. Given the significantly decreased percentage of $CD3^+$ thymocytes in mixed and cortical thy-

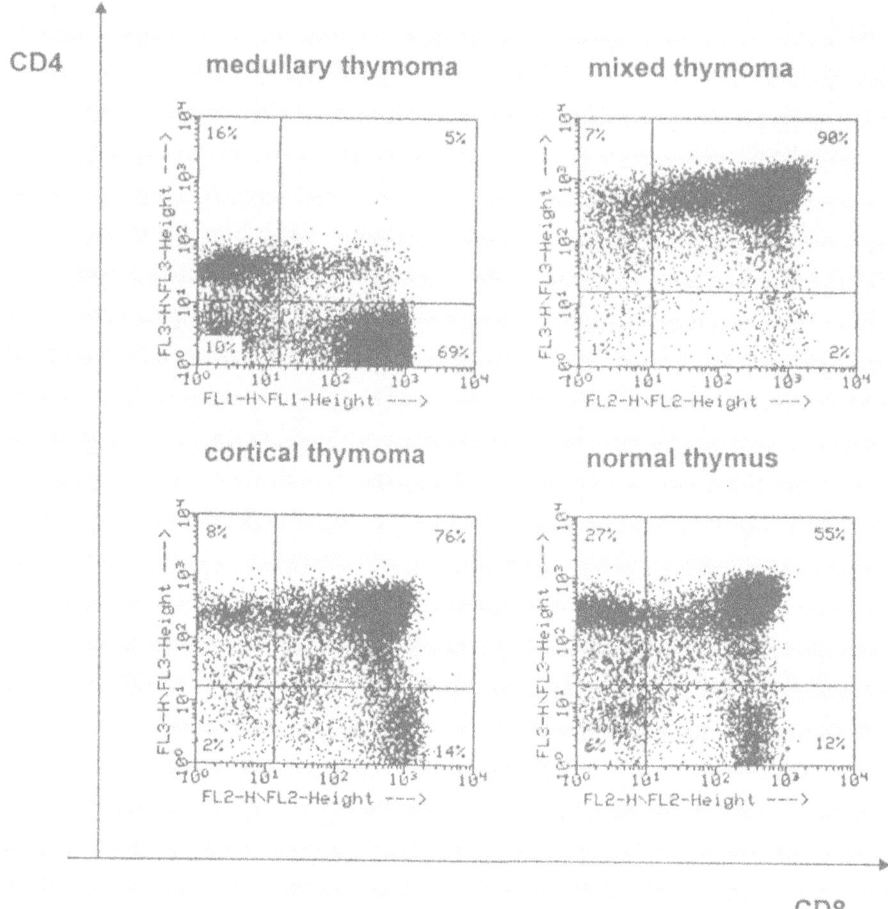

Figure 1. Typical thymocyte subset composition in terms of CD4 and CD8 expression in normal human thymus and the various histological thymoma subtypes of myasthenia gravis patients. Characteristic reduction of CD4+/8+DP thymocytes in a medullary thymoma and of SP T cells in cortical and mixed thymomas.

momas (concerning the DP and SP subsets) (Table 2) we determined a detailed antigenic profile of $CD3^{+high}$ intratumorous lymphocytes. As shown in Table 3 there were striking differences between the mixed and cortical thymomas on the one hand and the medullary thymoma on the other hand.

In all mixed and cortical thymomas there was a significant reduction in cells expressing CD69, CD27 and CD45RA. As the expression of these markers follows positive selection in the normal thymus[41] we conclude that in mixed and cortical thymomas positive selection is inefficient. However, the occurrence of $CD3^{high}$/CD27/$CD45RA^{+}$ thymocytes suggests that the most mature intrathymic product of positive selection[41] is also present in mixed and cortical thymomas though at low frequency. To investigate whether these mature cells are generated in the tumor or represent recirculated T cells we analyzed whether thymomas harbour the same $CD3^{high}$ subsets that in the normal thymus develop sequentially after positive selection[33,42,43]. As shown in Table 3 all these thymocyte subsets which are delineated by the sequential acquisition or loss of differentiation markers were present. In particular, the presence of CD69^{+}/CD1^{-}/CD45RA^{+} thymocytes that are all SP cells[42] and of their CD69^{+}/CD1^{+}/CD45R0^{+} precursors suggests that the most mature pre-emigrant thymocyte subset[41,44] is generated in mixed and cortical thymomas.

In the medullary thymoma, a very rare tumor type constituting only 5 % of the MG-associated thymomas[6,7], the situation was completely different because there was an enormously increased proportion of CD3^{high} cells expressing CD27^{+} and CD45RA^{+} and not CD69^{+} (Table 3). Almost all of these cells were SP T cells with a predominance of CD8^{+} T cells (Table 2). Given the very low percentage of DP (Table 2) in the medullary thymoma we suggest that the majority of mature T cells in this thymoma subtype results from the recirculation of peripheral T cells. However, a long lasting block of thymocyte export from the tumor and/or a sustained proliferation of SP thymocytes in situ can not completely be excluded (see Discussion below).

MHC Class II Expression on Neoplastic Epithelial Cells

Since a reduced or variable expression of MHC class II molecules on thymoma epithelial cells has been reported previously[45], we investigated whether a reduced expression of HLA-DR might be associated with the inefficient positive selection especially of CD4^{+}/CD8^{-} T cells in mixed and cortical thymomas. As given in Table 2 there was a general reduction of MHC class II molecules in the majority of thymomas investigated as compared to the normal thymus. The expression of MHC class I on epithelial cells was not significantly different (not shown).

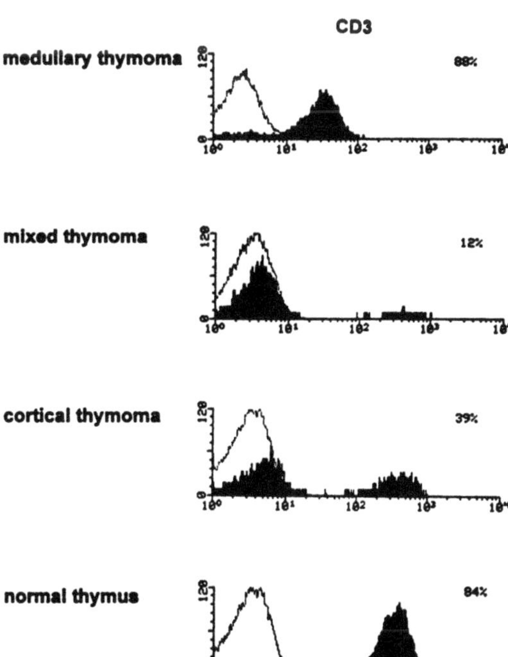

Figure 2. CD3 profiles of CD4+/8-SP T cells in normal human thymus and the various histological thymoma subtypes of MG patients. Increased percentage of immature CD3^{-} thymocytes among CD4+/8- cells in a cortical and mixed but not a medullary thymoma.

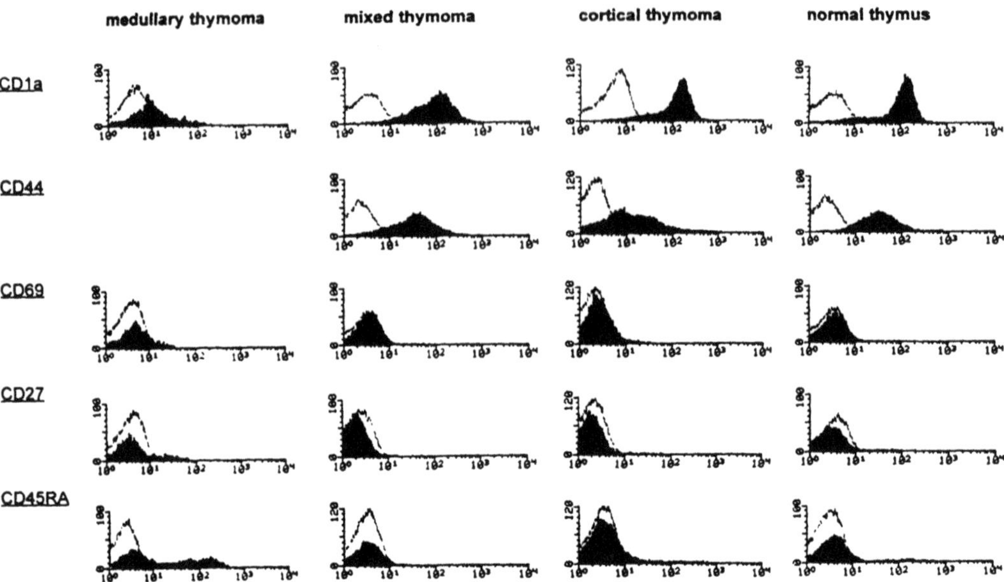

Figure 3. Marker distribution in immature CD3⁻ T-cells in normal human thymus compared to cortical thymoma, mixed thymoma and medullary thymoma. CD3⁻ thymocytes were all CD1a high and CD44 low, but did not express CD69, CD27, CD45RA except in medullary thymoma.

DISCUSSION

It is the main finding of the present study that all MG-associated thymomas contain the main thymocyte subsets also found in normal thymuses, but that each histologically distinct thymoma subtype is associated with very characteristic quantitative alterations of the subset composition. Furthermore, evidence is provided that substantial numbers of mature and potentially autoaggressive T cells arise inside mixed and cortical thymomas while this process does not substantially contribute to the number of mature T cells in medullary thymoma.

The most striking alteration in subset composition was encountered in the one medullary thymoma investigated that was almost devoid of DP and $CD1^+$ thymocytes in accordance with previous immunohistochemical investigations. Mixed and cortical thymomas on the other hand resembled the normal thymus with respect to a predominance of DP thymocytes[13,23–27].

Previous two-colour flow cytometric analyses had reported a virtually normal or increased percentage of intratumorous $CD4^+$ thymocytes presumed to be mature[13,23–27]. In contrast a recent three-colour flow cytometric study[18] reported that the $CD4^+$ SP T cell population in thymomas exhibits an increased percentages of its immature $CD4^+/CD8^-/CD3^-$ subset and that this immature subset predominates over the mature $CD4^+/CD8^-/CD3^+$ subset in 40 % of thymoma cases. As we show here, this heterogeneity of the $CD4^+$ T cell population with respect to its mature ($CD3^+$) versus immature ($CD3^-$) subsets can be explained by the heterogeneity of histologically defined thymoma subtypes: While a clear predominance of immature $CD4^+/CD8^-/CD3^-$ over mature $CD4^+/CD8^-/CD3^+$ thymocytes is typical of mixed thymomas, an almost balanced ratio of mature versus immature CD4+ SP thymocytes is characteristic for cortical thymomas (Ta-

Table 3. Percent of CD3 cells expressing the respective phenotype

Phenotype *Tumor type/case no.*	$CD3^{high}CD69^{+}$	$CD3^{high}CD69^{+}CD1^{+}$	$CD3^{high}CD69^{+}CD27^{+}$	$CD3^{high}CD1^{-}$, $CD45RA^{+}$	$CD3^{high}CD27^{+}$ $CD45RA^{+}$
Medullary thymoma					
1006/95	16	0,6	28	70	64
Mixed thymoma					
24864/94	15	3	6	0,4	3
17821/94	9	5	7	1	0,5
14839/95	3	1	2	0,5	0,8
12211/95	10	6	3	0,3	0,5
Cortical thymoma					
2516/95	14	10	7	4	3
27942/95	14	6	8	5	3
15173/94	15	5	5	2	2
858/95	17	6	6	6	6
Normal thymus					
1	28	15	20	10	17
2	29	12	10	8	4
3	22	7	18	15	18
4	29	8	20	6,4	16

ble 2 and Figure 2). On the contrary, the mature $CD4^{+}$ SP T cells outnumbered the $CD4^{+}/CD8^{-}/CD3^{-}$ subset in the medullary thymoma by far. The predominance of mature $CD4^{+}$ SP cells over mature $CD8^{+}$ SP cells that is typical of non-neoplastic thymuses was inverted in all thymomas (Table 2).

As we show here for the first time the subset of $CD4^{+}/CD8^{-}/CD3^{-}$ T cells in thymomas resembles its counterpart in the normal human thymus by the absence of CD69, CD28, CD27 and CD45RA[34,35]. Although the $CD4^{+}/CD8^{+}/CD3^{-}$ immediate progeny of the $CD4^{+}/CD8^{-}/CD3^{-}$ subset[34,35] is increased in mixed and cortical thymomas (Table 2) the ratio of $CD4^{+}/CD8^{-}/CD3^{-}$ to $CD4^{+}/CD8^{+}/CD3^{-}$thymocytes is highly elevated. In contrast to a previous interpretation[18] this finding suggests that the transition of $CD4^{+}/CD8^{-}/CD3^{-}$ SP T cells to $CD4^{+}/CD8^{+}$ DP T cells is less efficient in thymomas than in the normal thymus. In support of this idea previous studies reported that the spontaneous transition from the $CD4^{+}/CD8^{-}/CD3^{-}$ SP to the $CD4^{+}/CD8^{+}$ DP stage in vitro and in the absence of stroma is incomplete, resulting in DP cells with an immature CD8 alpha/alpha phenotype[35,46]. Therefore, microenvironmental mechanisms that normally accelerate maturation at the $CD4^{+}/CD8^{-}/CD3^{-}$ stage may be either less efficient in thymomas or unable to handle the 5–15 times higher input of $CD4^{+}/CD8^{-}/CD3^{-}$ cells (Table 2). A more efficient homing of immature progenitors as another possible explanation for the large $CD4^{+}/CD8^{-}/CD3^{-}$ subset in thymomas is unlikely due to the normal number of CD34+ and of TN thymocytes (Table 2).

The mature $CD4^{+}/CD8^{-}/CD3^{+}$ subset was reported to be smaller in thymomas in a previous study and this was interpreted as the result of inefficient positive selection[18]. Our findings confirm these results and their interpretation for mixed and cortical but not medullary thymomas (Table 2). The inefficiency of positive selection mirrored by the paucity of $CD3^{high}/CD69^{+}$ SP T cells was most pronounced in mixed thymomas while cortical thymomas were in between mixed thymomas and non-neoplastic thymuses (Table 3). This finding supports conclusions from morphological analyses that the neoplastic epithelium of cortical thymomas is more akin to normal cortical epithelial cells than the epithelium of mixed thymomas[7,47] although the homing capacity and the capacity to produce immature double positive thymocytes are not diminished (Table 2).

With respect to the mechanism producing inefficient positive selection in mixed and cortical thymomas an overload of the selection process by immature DP precursors has been considered[18]. This possibility seems unlikely given the capacity of normal thymic epithelium to increase the output of mature T cells by a factor of 10–15 after an increased load of selectible T cells[48]. We, therefore, favour the alternative that epithelial cells of mixed and cortical thymomas are less efficient than normal cortical epithelial cells to positively selected immature T cells. Considering that the mature $CD4^+$ but not the $CD8^+$ SP T cell subset is substantially diminished in thymomas, we checked whether a reduced MHC class II expression might be associated with the inefficiency of positive selection. While a previous study found no correlation between a reduced number of $CD4^+$ mature T cells and a reduced epithelial expression of MHC class II[18] such an association was obvious in our study (Table 2). However, this association does not exclude the possibility that factors other than the reduction in MHC II expression[49] contribute to the inefficiency of positive selection of $CD4^+$T cells in thymomas.

The occurrence of $CD3^+$ mature $CD4^+$ or $CD8^+$ single positive (SP) thymocytes in thymomas was reported previously[18,23–27]. With respect to different models for the pathogenesis of paraneoplastic MG we asked whether these cells are generated in situ[19] or represent recirculated peripheral T cells[45,50]. As shown in Table 3 mixed and cortical thymomas contain the same post-selection thymocyte subsets as normal thymuses[41,44] leading from one of the most immature products of positive selection ($CD3^{high}/CD69^+$)[51] via intermediate stages of maturation ($CD3^{high}/CD27^+/CD45RA^-$) to the most mature pre-emigrant subsets ($CD3^{high}/CD27^+/CD45RA^+$, $CD3^{high}/CD1^-/CD69^+$ and $CD3^{high}/CD1^-/CD45RA^+$ thymocytes). Since all $CD3^{high}/CD1^-$ thymocytes are either mature single positive TCR alpha/beta$^+$ T cells or $CD4^-/CD8^-$ gamma/delta$^+$ T cells[42] we conclude that mature single positive T cells are produced by intratumorous thymopoiesis. However, CD69 is not only a marker of pre-emigrant thymocytes[43,44] but also an activation antigen of peripheral T cells. To exclude that $CD69^+/CD1^-$ or $CD69^+/CD27^+$ cells are activated peripheral T cells, further activation markers were investigated. ICAM-1 and CD25 that are expressed with similar or slower kinetics, respectively, than CD69 on stimulated peripheral T cells[52] were not detected on thymocytes of mixed and cortical thymomas.

In the medullary thymoma intratumorous thymopoesis takes place as well with generation of positively selected $CD69^+$ T-cells (Table 3). However, as SP T cells outnumber DP T cells by a factor of about 20 it seems unlikely that the mature SP cells in the medullary thymomas are the progeny of the intratumorous DP thymocytes. To explain the preponderance of mature T cells an isolated block of thymocyte export is not likely because the majority of all SP cells in the medullary thymoma were $CD69^-$ cells, while SP T cells of non-neoplastic thymuses are typically $CD69^+$[41,44] as were the mature SP T cells in mixed and cortical thymomas (not shown). Furthermore, a sustained intratumorous proliferation is also not likely because more than 90 % of mature T cells in the medullary thymoma lack late activation antigens and are $CD45R0^-/CD25^-/CD71^{low}$. We therefore favour the view that the vast majority of SP T cells in the medullary thymoma represent recirculated peripheral T cells.

How could the inefficient positive selection in mixed and cortical thymomas be related to anti-AChR autoimmunity while not increasing the risk of systemic autoimmune disease in paraneoplastic MG ? We speculate that the inefficiency of thymomas to generate mature T-cells may counterbalance the potential hazard of a general defect of central tolerance conferred by the intratumorous lack of well developed medullary structures and the paucity of tolerogenic dendritic cells. To explain the specific anti-AChR autoimmunity in thymoma patients an abnormal intratumorous positive selection has been invoked[19]. This process is thought to depend on the abnormal expression of crossreacting AChR-like epitopes in thymomas as described previously[14,21] and on the development of immature thymocytes into potentially autoaggressive mature T cells in an abnormal microenvironment (Table 2). The enigma has been so far, why an abnormally hyperexpressed protein in thymoma epithelial cells[6,21] should not result in epithelium-mediated negative selection as observed in mice[54–56]. We propose from our present findings that an inefficient thymocyte/stroma interaction as indicated by an inefficient positive selection may contribute to the generation of antigen-specific autoaggressive T cells in mixed and cortical thymomas: while a high dose or affinity of abnormally expressed crossreacting peptide may rescue antigen-specific thymocytes[57,58] from "neglect"[59], inefficient thymocyte/epithelial cell interaction may preclude epithelium-mediated negative selection.

This hypothesis is in perfect agreement with recent findings in a TCR transgenic mouse demonstrating the dependence of epithelium-mediated negative selection on the level of MHC class II expression by thymic epithelial cells[60].

This scenario of a false-positive selection[19] implies the testable prediction that mature thymocytes produced in mixed and cortical thymomas are enriched for T cells with a specificity for abnormally expressed epithelial cell antigens. Autoimmunity in medullary thymomas probably has a different pathogenesis and may involve the intratumorous activation of peripheral T cells.

REFERENCES

1. Lindstrom J, Shelton D, Fujii Y: Myasthenia gravis. Adv. Immunol. 42:233–284, 1988
2. Willcox N: Myasthenia gravis. Current Opinion in Immunology 5:910–917, 1993
3. Hohlfeld R, Toyka KV, Heininger K, Gross-Wilde H, Kalies I: Auto-immune Human T Lymphocytes Specific for Acetylcholine Receptor. Nature 310:244–246, 1984
4. Hohlfeld R: Editorial: Myasthenia gravis and thymoma: Paraneoplastic failure of neuromuscular transmission. Lab. Invest. 62:241–243, 1990
5. Protti MP, Manfredi AA, Horton RM, Bellone M, Conti-Tronconi BM: Myasthenia Gravis: Recognition of a Human Autoantigen at the Mole-cular Level. Immunol. Today 14:363–368, 1993
6. Kirchner Th, Schalke B, Buchwald J, Ritter M, Marx A, Müller-Hermelink HK: Well-differentiated thymic carcinoma. An organotypic low-grade carcinoma with relationship to cortical thymoma. Am. J. Surg. Pathol. 16:1153–1169, 1992
7. Müller-Hermelink HK, Marx A, Kirchner Th: Advances in the diagnosis and classification of thymic epithelial tumors. In Anthony PP and MacSween RNM, Eds. Recent Advances in Histopatho-logy, Fascicle 16: 49, Edinburgh, Churchill Livingstone, 1994
8. Aarli JA, Stefansson K, Marton LSG, Wollmann RL: Patients with myasthenia gravis and thymoma have in their sera IgG autoantibodies against titin. Clin. Exp. Immunol. 82:284–288, 1990
9. Marx A, Kirchner Th, Greiner A, Schalke B, Müller-Hermelink HK: Myasthenia gravis-associated thymic epithelial tumors express neurofilaments and are associated with antiaxonal autoimmunity. Ann. N.Y. Acad. Sci. 681:107–109, 1993
10. Rosai J, Levine GD: "Atlas of Tumor Pathology", 2nd Series Fascicle 13, US Armed Forces Institute of Pathology, 1976
11. Lauriola L, Musiani P, Ranelletti FO, Maggiano N, Piantelli M: Human thymoma lymphocyte mitogenesis: glucocorticoid inhibitory capacity as a function of the size of the more mature T cell subset. Clin. Exp. Immunol. 52:477–484, 1983
12. Palestro G, Geuna M, Novero D, Godio L, Ciccone G, Azzoni L: Immunophenotype of thymoma-associated lymphoid cell component of T-cell type. A new analytic procedure in keeping with structural heterogeneities. Virchows Arch. B Cell Pathol. 59:297–304, 1990

13. Fujii Y, Hayakawa M, Inada K, Nakahara K: Lymphocytes in thymoma: association with myasthenia gravis is correlated with increased number of single-positive cells. Eur. J. Immunol. 20:2355–2358, 1990
14. Marx A, O'Connor R, Geuder KI, Hoppe F, Schalke B, Tzartos S, Kalies I, Kirchner Th, Müller-Hermelink HK: Characterization of a protein with an acetylcholine receptor epitope from myasthenia gravis-associated thymomas. Lab. Invest. 62:279–286, 1990
15. Marx A, Kirchner Th, Greiner A, Müller-Hermelink HK, Schalke B, Osborn M: Neurofilament epitopes in thymomas and antiaxonal autoantibodies in myasthenia gravis. Lancet 339:707–708, 1992
16. Carlow DA, Ten SJ, Teh HS: Altered Thymocyte Development Resulting from Expressing a Deleting Ligand on Selecting Thymic Epithelium. J. Immunol. 148:2988–2995, 1992
17. Jenkinson EJ, Anderson G, Owen JJT: Studies on T cell maturation on defined thymic stromal cell populations in vitro. J. Exp. Med. 176:845–853, 1992
18. Takeuchi Y, Fujii Y, Okumura M, Inada K, Nakahara K, Matsuda H: Accumulation of immature $CD3^-$ $CD4^+CD8^-$ single-positive cells that lack CD69 in epithelial cell tumors of the human thymus. Cellular Immunology 161:181–187, 1995
19. Marx A, Geuder KI, Schoepfer R, Tzartos S, Kristofferson U, Schalke B, Kirchner Th, Müller-Hermelink HK: Analysis of the acetylcholine receptor epitope-bearing protein p153 in thymomas favours "false-positive T-cell selection" as a mechanism of paraneoplastic myasthenia gravis. In: Lymphatic Tissues and In Vivo Immune Responses, Marcel Decker: pp. 577–583, 1991
20. Dardenne M, Savino W, Bach JF. Thymomatous epithelial cells and skeletal muscle share a common epitope defined by a monoclonal antibody. Am. J. Pathol. 126:194–198, 1987
21. Kirchner Th, Tzartos S, Hoppe F, Schalke B, Wekerle H, Müller-Hermelink HK: Pathogenesis of Myasthenia Gravis. Acetylcholine Re-ceptor-Related Antigenic Determinants in Tumor-Free Thymuses and Thymic Epithelial Tumors. Am. J. Pathol. 130:268–280, 1988
22. Marx A, Kirchner Th, Hoppe F, O'Connor R, Schalke B, Tzartos S, Müller-Hermelink HK: Proteins with epitopes of the acetylcholine receptor in epithelial cell cultures of thymomas in myasthenia gravis. Am. J. Pathol. 134:865–877, 1989
23. Lauriola L, Maggiano N, Marino M, Carbone A, Piantelli M, Musiani P: Human thymoma: Immunologic characteristics of the lymphocytic component. Cancer 48:1992–1995, 1981
24. Aisenberg AC, Wilkens B, Harris NL, Frist WH: The predominant lymphocyte in most thymomas and in non-neoplastic thymus from pa-tients with myasthenia gravis is the cortical thymocyte. Clin. Immunol. Immunopathol. 35:130–136, 1985
25. Sato Y, Watanabe S, Mukai K, Kodama T, Upton MP, Goto M, Shimosato Y: An immunohistochemical study of thymic epithelial tumors. II. Lymphoid component. Am. J. Surg. Pathol. 10:862–870, 1986
26. Machi M, Itoyama Y, Goto I, Kuroiwa Y: Surface phenotypes of lymphoid cells altered in the human myasthenic thymus. Neurology 38:592–596, 1988
27. Ichikawa Y, Shimizu H, Yoshida M, Arimori S: Two-color flow cytometric analysis of thymic lymphocytes from patients with myasthenia gravis and/or thymoma. Clin. Immunol. and Immunopath. 62:91–96, 1992
28. Chilosi M, Iannucci A, Fiore-Donati L, Tridente G, Pampanin M, Pizzolo G, Ritter M, Bofill M, Janossy G: Myasthenia gravis: Immunohistological heterogeneity in microenvironmental organization of hyperplastic and neoplastic thymuses suggesting different mechanisms of tolerance breakdown. J. Neuroimmunol. 11:191–204, 1986
29. Reinherz EL, Kung PC, Goldstein G, Levey RH, Schlossman SF: Discrete stages of human intrathymic differentiation: Analysis of normal thymocytes and leukemic lymphoblasts of T-cell lineage. Proc. Natl. Acad. Sci. USA 77:1588–1592, 1980
30. Janossy N, Tidman N, Parageorgiou ES, Kung PC, Goldstein G: Distribution of T lymphocyte subsets in the human bone marrow and thymus: An analysis with monoclonal antibodies. J. Immunol. 126:1608–1613, 1981
31. Haynes BF, Martin ME, Kay HH, Kurtzberg J: Early events in human T cell ontogeny. Phenotypic characterization and immuno-histologic localization of T cell precursors in early human fetal tissues. J. Exp. Med. 168:1061–1080, 1988
32. Haynes BF, Denning S, Singer KH, Kurtzberg J: Ontogeny of T cell precursors: a model for the initial stages of human T cell development. Immunol. Today 10:87–91, 1989
33. Terstappen WMM, Huang S, Picker LJ: Flow Cytometric Assessment of Human T-cell Differentiation in Thymus and Bone Marrow. Blood 79:666–677, 1992
34. Hori T, Cupp J, Wrighton N, Lee F, Spits H: Identification of a novel human thymocyte subset with a phenotype of CD3-CD4+CD8 alpha+ beta-1. Possible progeny of the CD3-CD4-CD8- subset. J. Immunol. 146:4078–4084, 1991
35. Kraft DL, Weissman IL, Waller EK: Differentiation of CD3–4–8- human fetal thymocytes in vivo: characterization of a CD3–4+8- intermediate. J. Exp. Med. 178:265–277, 1993

36. Takeuchi Y, Fujii Y, Okumara M, Inada K, Nakahara K, Matsuda H: Characterization of CD4+ single positive cells that lack CD3 in the human thymus. Cell Immunol. 151:481–490, 1993
37. Penit C: Positive selection is an early event in thymocyte differentiation: high TCR expression by cycling immature thymocytes precedes final maturation by several days. Int. Immunol. 2:629–638, 1990
38. Shortman K, Vremec D, Egerton M: The kinetics of T cell antigen receptor expression by subgroups of CD4+8+ thymocytes: delineation of CD4+8+3(2+) thymocytes as post-selection intermediates leading to mature T cells. J. Exp. Med. 173:323–332, 1991
39. Swat W, Dessing M, v. Boehmer H, Kisielow P: CD69 expression during selection and maturation of CD4$^+$8$^+$ thymocytes. Eur. J. Immunol. 23:739–746, 1992
40. Petrie HT, Hugo P, Scollay R, Shortman K: Lineage relationships and developmental kinetics of immature thymocytes: CD3, CD4, and CD8 acquisition in vivo and in vitro. J. Exp. Med. 172:1583–1588, 1990
41. Vanhecke D, Leclercq G, Plum J, Vandekerckhove B: Characterization of Distinct Stages During the Differentiation of Human CD69$^+$CD3$^+$ Thymocytes and Identification of Thymic Emigrants. J. Immunol. (in press)
42. Sotzik F, Boyd A, Shortman K: Surface antigens of human thymocyte populations defined by CD3, CD4 and CD8 expression: CD1a is ex-pressed by mature thymocytes but not peripheral T cells. Immunology Letters 36:101–106, 1993
43. Plum J, De Smedt M, Defresne MP, Leclercq G, Vandekerckhofe B: Human CD34$^+$ Fetal Liver Stem Cells Differentiate to T Cells in a Mouse Thymic Microenvironment. Blood 84:1587–1593, 1994
44. Vanhecke D, Verhasselt B, Debacker V, Leclercq G, Plum J, Vandekerckhofe B: Differentiation to T helper cells in the thymus: gradual acquisition of T helper cell function by CD3+CD4+ cells. J. Immunol., 1995
45. Willcox N, Schluep M, Ritter MA, Schuurman HJ, Newsom-Davis J, Christensson B: Myasthenic and non-myasthenic thymoma. An expansion of a minor cortical epithelial cell subset ? Am. J. Pathol. 127:447–460, 1987
46. Galy A, Verma S, Barcena A, Spits H: Precursors of CD3+CD4+CD8+ cells in the human thymus are defined by expression of CD34. Delineation of early events in human thymic development. J. Exp. Med. 178:391–401, 1993
47. Marino M, Müller-Hermelink HK: Thymoma and thymic carcinoma. Relation of thymoma epithelial to the cortical and medullary differentiation of thymus. Virchows Arch. (Pathol. Anat.) 407:119–149, 1985
48. Huesmann M, Scott B, Kisielow P, v. Boehmer H: Kinetics and effi-cacy of positive selection in the thymus of normal and T cell receptor transgenic mice. Cell 66:533–540, 1991
49. Petrie HT, Strasser A, Harris AW, Hugo P, Shortman K: CD4$^+$8$^-$ and CD4$^-$8$^+$ mature thymocytes require different post-selection pro-cessing for final development. J. Immunol. 151:1273–1279, 1993
50. Sommer N, Willcox N, Harcourt GC, Newsom-Davis J: Myasthenic thymus and thymoma are selectively enriched in acetylcholine receptor-reactive T cells. Ann. Neurol. 28:312–319, 1990
51. Swat W, Dessing M, Baron A, Kisielow P, v. Boehmer H: Phenotypic changes accompanying positive selection of CD4$^+$8$^+$ thymocytes. Eur. J. Immunol. 22:2367–2372, 1992
52. Aversa GG, Hall BM: Activation panel antigen expression of PBL activated by PHA or in MLR (pp. 498–502) in: Leucocyte Typing IV ed. by W. Knapp et al., Oxford University Press, 1992
53. Agus DFB, Surh CD, Sprent J: Reentry of T cells to the adult thymus is restricted to activated T cells. J. Exp. Med. 173:1039–1046, 1991
54. Pircher H, Brduschka K, Steinhoff U, Kasai M, Miouchi T, Zin-kernagel RM, Hengartner H, Kyewski B, Müller KP: Tolerance induc-tion by clonal deletion of CD4$^+$CD8$^+$ thymocytes in vitro does not require dedicated antigen-presenting cells. Eur. J. Immunol. 23:669–674, 1993
55. Bonomo A, Matzinger P: Thymus Epithelium Induces Tissue-Specific Tolerance. J. Exp. Med. 177:1153–1164, 1993
56. Hugo P, Kappler JM, Godfrey DJ, Marrack PC: Thymic epithelial cell lines that mediate positive selection can also induce thymocyte clonal deletion. J. Immunol. 152:1022–1031, 1994
57. Ashton-Rickardt PG, Van Kaer L, Schumacher TNM, Ploegh HL, Tonegawa S: Peptide contributes to the specifity of positive selection of CD8$^+$ T cells in the thymus. Cell 73:1041–1049, 1993
58. Hogquist KA, Jameson SC, Haeth WR, Howard JL, Bevan MJ, Carbone FR: T cells receptor antagonist peptides induce positive selection. Cell 77:18–27, 1994
59. von Boehmer H, Teh HS, Kisielow P: The thymus selects the useful, neglects the useless and destroys the harmful. Immunol. Today 10:57–61, 1989
60. Spain LM, Berg LJ: Quantitative analysis of the efficiency of clonal deletion in the Thymus. Dev. Immunol. 4:43–53, 1994

24

OLIGOCLONAL PERIPHERAL T-CELL LYMPHOCYTOSIS AS A RESULT OF ABERRANT T-CELL DEVELOPMENT IN A CORTICAL THYMOMA

Daphne De Jong,[1*] Dick Richel,[2] Cees Schenkeveld,[3] Lucie Boerrigter,[1] and Laura van 't Veer[1]

[1]Department of Pathology
Netherlands Cancer Institute/Antoni van Leeuwenhoekziekenhuis
Amsterdam, The Netherlands
[2]Department of Internal Medicine
[3]Clinical Chemistry, Medisch Spectrum Twente
Enschede, The Netherlands

SUMMARY

A 42 year old man presented with a locally invasive cortical thymoma. Before chemotherapy was commenced 36 months after presentation, a peripheral lymphocytosis of 19×10^9/l had slowly developed over time. After the first course of chemotherapy, the lymphocytosis showed a sharp decline to normal absolute cell numbers and subsequently remained at normal levels. Currently, the patient is in stable partial remission and doing well.

Immunophenotypic analysis showed 95% $CD3^{+ve}$ cells; 36% $CD4^{+ve}$ and 56% $CD8^{+ve}$ cells with a mature T-cell phenotype. 78% of the T-cells expressed TcR-aß and 16% TcR-γδ as assessed by immunocytochemistry. No CD4/CD8 double positive population was detected. 4% $CD16/CD56^{+ve}$ NK-cells could be demonstrated. Southern blot analysis of peripheral blood mononuclear cells before chemotherapy showed a striking oligoclonal pattern with 13–20 rearranged fragments of different intensity for theTcRß-gene. TcRγ also showed a pattern compatible with a oligoclonal proliferation with 6 of the 8 theoretically possible rearranged fragments in EcoRI-digested DNA. After treatment, when absolute blood counts had returned to normal, the distribution of subsets still showed a slightly

* Correspondence: Daphne De Jong, Dept. of Pathology, The Netherlands Cancer Institute/Antoni van Leeuwenhoek-ziekenhuis, Plesmanlaan 161, 1066 CX Amsterdam, The Netherlands, tel: 31-20-5122752; fax: 31-20-5122759.

aberrant pattern with a CD4/CD8 ratio of 3.25 and 80%TcR-aß and 16% TcR-γδ expressing cells. Immunophenotypic analysis of a blood sample taken 6 months later, also at normal absolute cell counts, showed an aberrant phenotype of late thymocytes (CD34$^-$, TdT$^-$ CD1$^+$, CD4/CD8 single positive) and of mature T-cells (CD1$^-$). TcRß- and TcRγ-gene rearrangment of the same sample showed a polyclonal pattern.

Thymomas may rarely be associated with peripheral lymphocytosis. Immunophenotypic analysis showed a T-cell phenotype in all reported cases. We describe a patient with a locally invasive cortical thymoma, who presented with an oligoclonal peripheral lymphocytosis of mature T-cell phenotype and subsequent polyclonal emergence of late thymocytes. These findings may be interpreted as the result of aberrant positive and negative selection and development of thymocytes in the microenvironment of neoplastic thymic epithelial cells and clonal selection through continuous peripheral stimulation.

INTRODUCTION

Thymomas are neoplasms of thymic epithelium that are thought to mimic to a certain extent the organization and microenvironment of normal thymic compartments. Based on this model, Müller-Hermelink and co-workers have proposed a new classification of thymic epithelial tumors[1–3]. Several studies have now shown, that this classification is of prognostic value, predicting local invasiveness and metastatic potential[4–6]. Moreover, a distinct association of auto-immune diseases such as myasthenia gravis with cortical types of thymoma and well differentiated thymic carcinoma has been demonstrated in contrast to medullary and mixed thymomas[3]. A characteristic feature of thymomas associated with auto-immune disorders is the presence of a dense, non-neoplastic infiltrate of CD1-expressing thymocytes. There are indications that the microenvironment of these thymomas may be involved in aberrant differentiation and selection of thymocytes resulting in auto-immune disorders e.g. myasthenia gravis[3,7,8].

Thymomas may rarely be associated with peripheral lymphocytosis. Immunophenotypic analysis has shown a T-cell phenotype in all reported cases. The reported cases behaved in general as benign proliferations that were responsive to remission of the primary (thymic) tumor[9–15]. several cases of highly aggressive lymphoblastic proliferations have also been described, however[16,17].

We describe a patient with a locally invasive cortical thymoma, who presented with an oligoclonal peripheral lymphocytosis of mature T-cell phenotype and a polyclonal pattern with immature T-cell phenotype during partial remission. We attribute these findings to aberrant positive and negative selection and development of thymocytes in the microenvironment of neoplastic thymic epithelial cells and clonal selection through continuous peripheral stimulation.

MATERIALS AND METHODS

Histologic sections of the tumor biopsy material were stained with hematoxylin-eosin and reticulin. Bone marrow biopsies were obtained.

Paraffin immunoperoxidase studies were performed using LCA (CD45), L26 (CD20), CD3, UCHL-1 (CD45RO) (All obtained from Dako, Golstrup, Denmark) and CAM5.2 (Becton Dickinson, Mountain View, Ca, USA) monoclonal antibodies in a three-stage indirect immunoperoxidase method with pronase pre-treatment or microwave-based antigen-retrieval. Mononuclear cells from heparinized peripheral blood samples before (September, October and December 1993, April, June, July 1994) and after chemotherapy (November 1994, January, May 1995) were isolated with Ficoll/Hypaque gradient centrifugation and analyzed according to standard procedures by fluorescence-activated flow cytometry using the following antibodies: CD10, CD19, CD20, CD21, CD22, immunoglobulin kappa and lambda, CD2, CD3 (membranous and intracytoplasmic staining), CD4, CD8, CD16, CD25, CD13, CD14, CD11c, CD34, TdT, HLA-DR, TcR-αß and TcR-γδ.

DNA was isolated according to standard methods from peripheral blood leukocytes of the patient prior to chemotherapy (April 1994) and during complete remission (May 1995). Peripheral blood leukocytes from a healthy donor and a peripheral T-cell non-Hodgkin's lymphoma samples were used as controls. DNA was digested to completion with BamHI, EcoRI, KpnI and HindIII. Southern blots were hybridized with ^{32}P labelled probes. The T-cell receptor ß-chain was assessed with a mix of JßI and JßII probes, the T-cell receptor γ-chain with a Jγ probe, reactive to the homologous region of the Jγ1.3 and Jγ2.3 genes. The immunoglobulin genes were assessed with a JH probe. (All probes obtained from Oncor, Gaithersburg, MD, USA).

CASE REPORT

In 1990, a 42 year old man presented with an anterior mediastinal mass, multiple left pulmonary nodules involving the pleural and diaphragmatic surfaces, and a pleural effusion. CT-scan showed a lobulated mediastinal mass with cyst formation and calcifications extending into the left pleura. The pleural thickening extended into the upper abdomen to the level of the renal arteries. There was no bone destruction and no evidence of lymphadenopathy. Biopsies of the pleural mass showed islands of large epithelial tumor cells in a dense background of small lymphocytes of T-cell phenotype. A diagnosis of cortical thymoma was made (according to the classification of Müller-Hermelink and Marino[1]) (fig. 1) At presentation the blood count and other laboratory findings were unremarkable. No initial therapy was instituted. A peripheral lymphocytosis developed over the following months, reaching levels of $19x10^9/l$. In September 1994, chemotherapy was commenced with 6 cycles of CAP (cyclophosphamide, adriamycin and cisplatin), resulting in partial remission. After the first course of chemotherapy, the lymphocytosis showed a sharp decline to normal absolute cell numbers and subsequently remained at normal levels. Presently, the clinical status is unaltered and the patient is doing well.

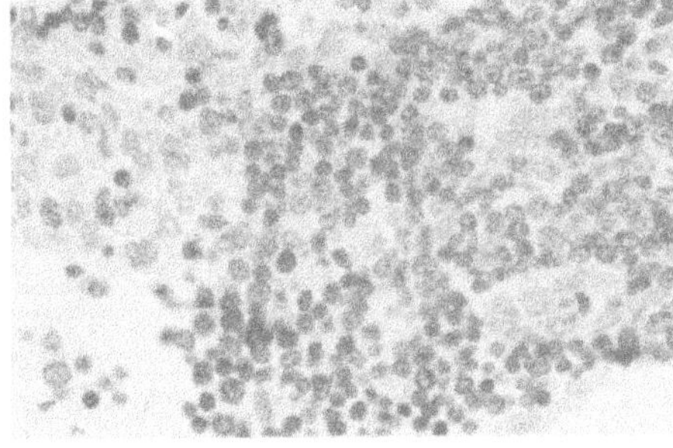

Figure 1. Pleural biopsy showing localization of cortical thymoma with large vesicular nuclei and admixture of lymphocytes and lymphoblasts.

Table 1. Immunophenotype of peripheral blood cells using FACS-analysis

	Pre-treatment 3/12/93	Post-treatment 8/11/94	Post-treatment 29/5/95
lymphocytosis	$19x10^9/l$	$1.9x10^9/l$	$2.3x10^9/l$
CD3	95	97	91
cy-CD3	neg	neg	neg
CD4	36	20	31
CD8	56	65	68
CD4/CD8	7	0	6
CD7	96	97	98
CD1a	8	1	68
TdT	neg	neg	neg
CD34	3	0	1
CD16/CD56	4	4	4
TcR-αβ	78	80	n.d.
TcR-γδ	16	16	n.d.
CD21	95	93	28

RESULTS

Before chemotherapy was commenced in December 1993, a peripheral lymphocytosis of $19x10^9/l$ was found. Immunophenotypic analysis showed 95% $CD3^{+ve}$ cells; 36% $CD4^{+ve}$ and 56% $CD8^{+ve}$ cells without expression of CD1, TdT and intracytoplasmic CD3, indicating a mature T-cell phenotype. 78% of the T-cells expressed TcR-αß and 16% TcR-γδ as assessed by immunocytochemistry. No CD4/CD8 double positive population was detected. 4% $CD16/CD56^{+ve}$ NK-cells could be demonstrated (table 1). Southern blot analysis of peripheral blood mononuclear cells before chemotherapy showed that the immunoglobulin heavy chain genes were in germline configuration. The TcRß-gene showed a striking oligoclonal pattern with 13–20 rearranged fragments of different intensity (Fig. 2). TcRγ also showed a pattern compatible with a oligoclonal proliferation (fig. 3). The

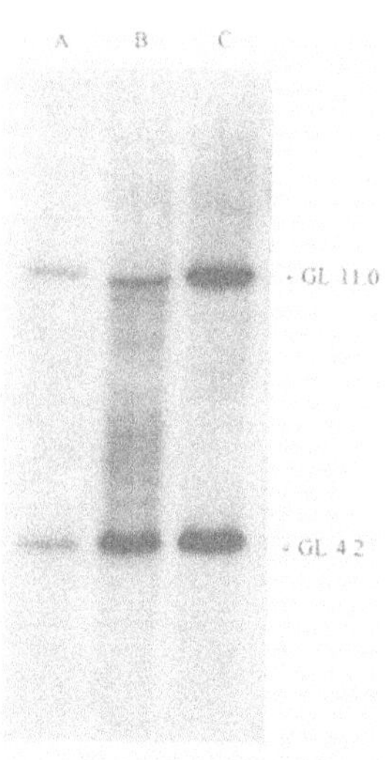

Figure 2. Southern blot analysis of a peripheral blood samples of the patient before (lane B) and after (lane A) chemotherapy together with a germline control of peripheral blood cells of an unrelated healthy individual (lane C). TcRβ shows an oligoclonal pattern of rearrangment. GL= germ line, fragment lenghts are indicated in kilo-basepairs (kb).

Table 2. Reported germline fragments with the used probes and expected rearranged fragments TcRγ-genes as detected with the used probes

Probe	EcoRI	BamHI	HindIII	KpnI
JH	18	18	11	
JßI/JßII	11/4.2	24	7.7/4.1	
Jγ	3.3/1.8	20/15	5.4/2.2*	16/9
	Possible Jγ rearranged fragments			
Vγ11	9.5			6.0
Vγ10	0.6			1.8
Vγ9	2.4			7.5
Vγ8	4.2			1.8
Vγ5	2.2			1.8
Vγ4	0.9			1.8
Vγ3	5.4			1.8
Vγ2	0.9			1.8

* polymorphic in the J γ2.3 region.

limited recombinational diversity of the TcRγ–gene results in only 8 possible rearranged fragments sizes in EcoRI-digested DNA. Six of these were demonstrated in the EcoRI-digested patient DNA, indicative of an oligoclonal process (table 2).

After treatment, when absolute blood counts had returned to normal, the distribution of subsets still showed a slightly aberrant pattern with a CD4/CD8 ratio of 0.325 and 80%TcR-αß and 16% TcR-γδ expressing cells (table 1). Immunophenotypic analysis of a blood sample taken 6 months later, also at normal absolute cell counts, showed a phenotype of late thymocytes (CD34$^-$, TdT$^-$, CD1$^+$,CD7$^+$, CD4/CD8 single positive) and of mature T-cells (CD1$^-$) (table 1). TcRß- and -γ-gene rearrangment of the same sample did not show clonally rearranged fragments and was interpreted as a polyclonal pattern.

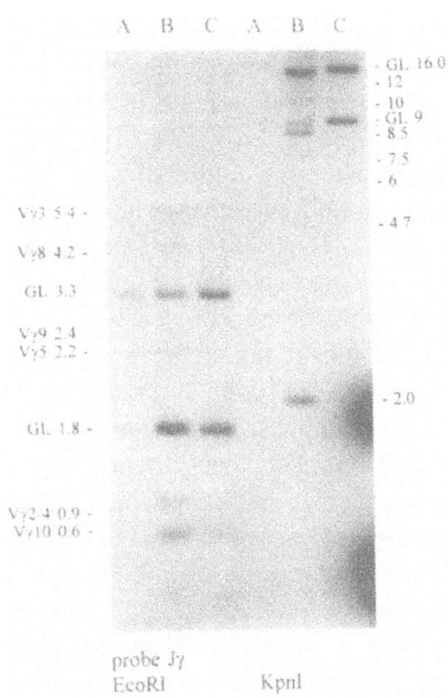

Figure 3. Southern blot analysis of a peripheral blood samples of the patient and a control individual as in figure 2. TcRγ also shows an oligoclonal pattern of rearrangment with 6 of 8 theoretically possible TcRγ-fragments. GL= germ line, Vγ2–10= rearranged fragments, fragment lenghts are indicated in kilo-basepairs (kb).

DISCUSSION

One of the striking characteristics of thymomas is their association with a large number of T lymphocytes of immature CD1+/CD4+/CD8+/CD3- phenotype. Cortical thymomas in particular show this infiltrate, suggesting that the function of normal cortical thymic epithelium is at least partially retained in neoplastic cortical epithelium. This concept is supported by the virtual absence of thymocytes in well-differentiated thymic carcinoma, which is a less differentiated proliferation of thymic epithelium. There are several lines of evidence to suggest, that the functional properties for T-cell developmental regulation of the malignant cortical epithelium are disturbed, however. Firstly, a variety of thymoma-associated auto-immune diseases, including myasthenia gravis, red-cell aplasia and hypogammaglobulinemia are known to be associated with thymoma. These auto-immune disorders are thought to be related to abnormal selection within the malignant thymic environment and in interaction with auto-antigen presented on malignant cells to T-cell clones reactive to these auto-antigens[3,7,18,19]. Defective function of neoplastic thymic epithelium has also been suggested as the basis of thymoma-associated T-cell proliferations[20].

A few cases of T-cell lymphocytosis, both of mature and immature phenotypes, associated with thymoma have been reported. In the majority of cases, a lymphocytosis with a mature phenotype, sometimes of large granular lymphocytes, was reported at first diagnosis of thymoma or associated with relapse of disease[10–14]. In the peripheral blood, these proliferations were shown to be polyclonal by molecular biological techniques in 4 of 5 cases and resolved upon remission of the thymoma in 5 of 6 reported cases[10,12,14]. A monoclonal T-lymphocytosis of mature TcR-γδ phenotype reported by Lisher at al., showed a monoclonal pattern with additional clonal genetic aberrations (delY) and behaved progressive with the features of malignant lymphoma[13]. Friedman et al. reported a monoclonal, T-lymphoblastic proliferation in relation with a locally invasive thymoma that clinically behaved as high grade leukemia/lymphoma[17]. In a similar case, reported by Macon et al., clonality was not investigated[16].

Taken together with the presently presented patient, the described cases of association of a benign behaving polyclonal or oligoclonal mature T-lymphocytosis with a cortical thymoma, are in strong support of a mechanism of deregulation of T-cell selection in the thymic neoplastic environment. In normal thymic epithelium, thymocytes are involved in a process of positive and negative selection. In positive selection, direct interactions of CD4+CD8+ thymocytes and epithelial cell surface molecules are essential , whereas in induction of tolerance to self-antigens, medullary interdigitating cells are involved[21,22]. Perturbations of the positive selection process in the neoplastic cortical environment may result in accumulation of aberrantly selected or unselected clones. Absence of a medullary environment may be responsable for inadequate neagtive selection. The net result can present as the emergence from the neoplastic thymic environment of mature T-cells possibly directed towards self-antigens, but may also present as a polyclonal lymphoblastic/thymocytic spill-over as may be the cases in the later phase of disease in our patient. As a more general explanation for thymoma-associated lymphocytosis direct spill-over from the thymoma may not be a likely mechanism, since the reported lymphoblastic proliferations all behave in a distinctly malignant fasion and are not responsive to elimination of the primary thymic neoplasm. These proliferations may rather be the result of induction of malignancy by cumulative genomic alterations in an expanded lymphoid target population in the thymic neoplastic environment. Depending on the type of oncogenic event and/or the differentiation stages of the target cells involved the resulting malignancy may either present as lymphoblastic leukemia/lymphoma or as a mature peripheral T-cell lymphoma/leukemia.

REFERENCES

1. Marino M, Müller-Hermelink HK. Thymoma and thymic carcinoma. Relation of thymoma epithelial cells to the cortical and medullary differentiation of thymus. Virchows Arch. (Pathol.Anat) 1985;407:119–149.
2. Müller-Hermelink HK, Marino M, Palestro G. Pathology of thymic epithelial tumors. In Müller-Hermelink HK ed. *Current Topics in Pathology*: The human thymus. Berlin: Springer-Verlag 1986:208–268.
3. Kirchner T, Müller-Hermelink HK. New approaches to the diagnosis of thymic epithelial tumors Prog.Surg.Pathol. 1989;10:167–189
4. Pescarmona E, Rendia EA, Venuta F, Ricci C, ruco LP, Baroni CD. The prognostic implication of thymoma histologic subtyping. Am.J.Clin.Pathol. 1990;93:190–195.
5. Quintanilla-Martinez L, Wilkins EW, Ferry JA, Harris NL. Thymoma-morfologic subclassification correlates invasiveness and immunohistologic features. A study of 122 cases. Hum.Pathol. 1993;24:958–969.
6. Kuo TT, Lo SK. Thymoma: astudy of the pathologic classificaion of 71 cases with evaluation of the Müller-Hermelink system. hum.Pathol. 1993;24:766–771.
7. Müller-Hermelink HK, Marx A, Geuder K, Kirchner T. The pathological basis of thymoma-associated myasthenia gravis. Ann N Y Acad Sci. 1993;681:56–65.
8. Gilhus NE, Willcox N, Harcourt G, Nagvekar N, Beeson D, Vincent A, Newsom-Davis J. Antigen presentation by thymoma epithelial cells from myastenia gravis patients to potentially pathogenic cells. J.Neuroimmunol. 1995;56:65–76.
9. Arntzenius AB, Bieger R. Disappearance of autoantibody-induced haemolysis after excision of a malignant thymoma. Neth J Med. 1991;38:117–21.
10. Doll DC, Landreneau RJ, List AF. Malignant thymoma associated with peripheral T-cell lymphocytosis. Med.Pediatric Oncol. 1991:19;496–498.
11. Medeiros LJ, Bhagat SKM, Naylor P, Fowler D, Jaffe ES, Stetler-Stevenson M. Malignant thymoma associated with T-cell lymphocytosis. Arch.Pathol.Lab.Med. 1993;117:279–283.
12. Handa SI, Schofield KP, Sivakumaran M, Short M, Pumphrey RS. Pure red cell aplasia associated with malignant thymoma, myasthenia gravis, polyclonal large granular lymphocytosis and clonal thymic T cell expansion. J Clin Pathol. 1994;47:676–9.
13. Lishner M, Ravid M, Shapira J, Radnay J, Amiel A, Leytn V, Shapiro C, Klein A. Delta-T lymphocytosis in a patient with thymoma. Cancer 1994;74:2924–2929.
14. Smith GP, Perkins SL, Segal GH, Kjeldsberg CR. T-cell lymphocytosis associated with invasive thymomas. Am.J.Clin.Pathol. 1994;102:447–453.
15. Yoshioka K, Terasaki J. CD7+, CD5+, CD4-, CD8-, and CD3- T-cell malignancy of the spleen after remission of invasive thymoma. Am.J.Hematol. 1995;48:141–142.
16. Macon WR, Rynalski TH, Swerdlow SH, Cousar JB. T-cell lymphoblastic leukemia/lymphoma presenting in a recurrent thymoma. Mod Pathol. 1991;4:524–8.
17. Friedman HD, Inman DA, Hutchison RE, Poiesz BJ. Concurrent invasive thymoma and T-cell lymphoblastic leukemia and lymphoma. A case report with necropsy findings and literature review of thymoma and associated hematologic neoplasm. Am J Clin Pathol. 1994; 101:432–7.
18. Fujii Y, Okumura M, Inada K, Nakahara K. Lymphocytes in thymomas are tolerant to self-MHC. Cell Immunol. 1991;137:438–47.
19. Willcox N, Baggi F, Batocchi AP, Beeson D, Harcourt G, Hawke S, Jacobson L, Matsuo H, Moody AM, Nagvekar N et al. Approaches for studying the pathogenic T cells in autoimmune patients. Ann N Y Acad Sci. 1993;681:219–37.
20. Takeuchi Y, Fujii Y, Okumura M, Inada K, Nakahara K, Matsuda H. Accumilation of immature CD3-CD4+CD8- single positive cells that lack CD69 in epithelial cell tumors of the human thymus. Cell.Immunol. 1995;161:181–187.
21. Spits H, Lanier LL, Phillips JH. Development of human T and natural killer cells. Blood 1995;85:2654–2670.
22. Anderson G, Owen JJT, Moore NC, Jenkinson EJ. Thymic epithelial cells provide unique signal for positive selection of CD4+CD8+ thymocytes in vitro. J.Ex.Med. 1994;179:2027–2031.

25

ESTROGENS MODULATE IL-6 PRODUCTION BY CULTURED NORMAL AND PATHOLOGICAL HUMAN THYMIC EPITHELIAL CELLS

A. P. Riviera,[1] F. Scuderi,[2] C. Provenzano,[2] M. P. Marino,[2] S. Gallucci,[2] E. Bartoccioni,[2] F. O. Ranelletti,[3] and G. Tridente[1]

[1]Institute of Immunology and Infectious Diseases
University of Verona
Verona, Italy
[2]Institute of General Pathology
[3]Department of Histology
Catholic University
Rome, Italy

INTRODUCTION

Interleukin-6 (IL-6) is a multifunctional cytokine, which regulates the immune response by polyclonal B cell activation and differentiation; it enhances peripheral T lymphocyte responses, thymocyte growth and induction of cytotoxic T cell differentiation [1]. Many clinical and experimental observations suggest that IL-6 could be involved in pathogenetic processes; in fact, elevated levels of IL-6 have been detected during autoimmune diseases, infections, and tissue injury. It has been shown that cultured human thymic epithelial cells (TECs) are able to secrete IL-6 both constitutively and after stimulation with interleukin-1ß (IL-1ß) and/or LPS [2]. Some authors have suggested that TEC IL-6 production may be related to the thymic abnormalities found with a high frequency in Myasthenia Gravis (MG) [3]. Thymoma is found in about 10% of the MG patients, while hyperplastic thymus is often observed in MG female patients with young-age at onset. The thymus has estrogen receptors [4]; these steroids modulate IL-6 production in different tissues, such as bone marrow-derived stromal cells, osteoblasts and blood mononuclear cells in vitro [5,6,7] and are able to increase secretion of thymic hormones by TECs in vitro [8].

In this study we investigated the relationship between estrogens and the intrathymic immune response by IL-6 secretion in cultured human TECs from normal subjects, under basal conditions and after addition of 17-ß-estradiol (E2) alone or associated to IL-1ß. We found that E2 is able to stimulate the IL-6 secretion in normal human TECs, an effect that

Epithelial Tumors of the Thymus, edited by Marx and Müller-Hermelink.
Plenum Press, New York, 1997

is enhanced by the association with IL-1β. Furthermore, we evaluated the presence of type I and type II E2 receptors on TECs from normal and pathological subjects and the effect of E2 on IL-6 release from TECs of myasthenic hyperplastic thymus and thymoma.

MATERIALS AND METHODS

Patients

Normal thymuses were obtained from seven children undergoing corrective cardiac surgery (sex: 2 male, 5 female; age ranging from 2 months to 6 years). Fresh thymic tissue was obtained from nine MG patients (age: 15–65 years; MG Osserman's grade: I-III; anti-AChR antibody titer: 0.2->30 nM; thymic pathology: 5 hyperplasia, 4 thymoma) undergoing therapeutic thymectomy.

Establishment of TECs Culture

Primary cultures of human TECs were established according to the method of De Luca [9]. Briefly, thymic specimens were minced into small pieces and treated with a 0.05% trypsin and 0.01% EDTA solution for 90 min at 37°C, in a three steps incubation procedure. The cell suspension was plated on lethally irradiated 3T3-J2 cells (a gift of Prof. H. Green, Harvard Medical School, Boston, MA) in DMEM/Ham's F12 medium (2:1 mixture) containing FCS (10%), insulin (5 μg/ml), transferrin (5 μg/ml), adenine (0.18 mM), hydrocortisone (0.4 μg/ml), cholera toxin (0.1 nM), triiodothyronine (20 pM), EGF (10 ng/ml), glutamine (4 mM) and penicillin-streptomycin (50 IU/ml). Confluent primary cultures were split by trypsin treatment. In stimulation experiments the cells were seeded (1.3 to 1.7 x 10^5/well) in 24-wells plates in DMEM/ Ham's F12 (2:1) medium containing only 4 mM glutamine and 10% charcoal/dextran-treated FCS, without 3T3-J2 feeder layer; after 18–24 h incubation, fresh medium containing IL-1ß (from 3 to 12 U/ml) and/or 17-ß-estradiol (10^{-6}M-10^{-8}M, Sigma) were added to the cells. When used, the inhibitors ICI 182–270 or tamoxifen (10^{-4}M-10^{-6}M, Sigma) were added together to E2. The supernatants were collected after 12/24/48/72 hours and frozen at -80°C until cytokines determination.

The epithelial nature of primary cultures was routinely controlled by immunostaining with a monoclonal anti-keratin antibody (Becton-Dickinson).

IL-6 Determination

IL-6 activity in the supernatants was measured by the hybridoma growth factor biological activity [10] on B9 cells (a gift of Dr. L. Aarden). Results were expressed as U/ml, using human recombinant IL-6 (Genzyme) as the standard, the detection limit of the test being 1 U/ml. In addition, some samples were analyzed by a commercial ELISA test (DuoSet, Genzyme) which has a detection limit of 31 pg/ml, as reported by the manufacturer.

The values of IL-6 were constanly related to the number of viable TECs at the end of the test, to obtain the U/ml value of IL-6 secreted by 10^5 cells.

IL-1ß Determination

The presence of IL-1ß in the tested samples was analyzed by a commercial ELISA test (Genzyme) with a detection limit of 3 pg/ml, as reported by the manufacturer.

Type I Estrogen Receptor (ER) Analysis

Cells were analyzed for type I ER by a whole cell assay. TECs in 24-well plates ($4x10^4$ cells/well) in medium without serum were incubated with 2nM [2,4,6,7–^{3}H]-estradiol (Amersham) alone or in the presence of 300-fold molar excess of unlabeled diethylstilbestrol (Sigma) for 30 min at 37°C in 5% CO_2. At the end of incubation the cells were washed 3 times with ice-cold Hank's Balanced Salt Solution (HBSS) and then resuspended in 1 ml 80% (vol/vol) absolute ethanol, to extract bound steroid. Radioactivity was measured by a liquid scintillation spectrometer. The specific binding was calculated as the difference between total binding and non specific binding . The results were expressed as the number of binding sites per cell. Each result represents the mean of triplicate determinations.

Type II Estrogen Binding Sites (EBS)

Cells were analyzed for type II EBS by a whole cell analysis. TECs in 24-well plates ($4x10^4$cells/well) were incubated for 2.5 h with 40–50 nM of [6,7–^{3}H]-estradiol (Amersham) alone or in the presence of a 300-fold molar excess of unlabeled quercitine (Carlo Erba). The cells were washed 3 times with ice-cold HBSS and then resuspended in 1 ml 80% (vol/vol) absolute ethanol. The specific binding was calculated as the difference between total and non specific binding. The results were expressed as the number of binding sites per cell.

Statistical Elaboration

We used Student's t Test for paired samples to analyze data.

RESULTS

The epithelial origin of TECs primary cultures from normal and pathological thymuses was previously checked and confirmed by the positive staining (>95%) with anti-keratin antibody (data not shown).

In the first step of this study we evaluated the presence of E2 receptors in human cultured TECs from three normal and six myasthenic thymuses (3 hyperplasia and 3 thymoma). Data reported in Tab. 1 show that human TECs exhibited appreciable amounts of type I and type II estrogen receptors, with no difference in the number and distribution of both receptor types in all conditions tested.

The assessed basal production of IL-6 in all normal TEC cultures ranged from 100 to 2300 U/ml after 24h of culture. Subsequently, we evaluated the effect of E2 on IL-6 secretion in TECs from four normal subjects, performing time-course experiments (12, 24, 48, 72 h) and assaying different concentrations of E2 (10^{-6}, 10^{-7}, 10^{-8} M). Figure 1 shows a time-course experiment, obtained with 10^{-6} M and 10^{-8} M E2, of one representative patient. E2 was constantly able to stimulate the secretion of IL-6 in our model. The stimula-

Table 1. Human thymic epithelial cells express Type I estrogen receptors (ER) and Type II estrogen binding sites (Type II EBS)

Patients	Sex	Age	Thymus	ER Sites /cell x 10^{-4}	Type II EBS Sites /cell x 10-4
RS	F	5	normal	7.4	315.1
MM	F	1	normal	2.9	138.6
BE	M	4	normal	5.8	n.d.
VA	F	32	hyperplasia	5.2	160.4
AB	M	15	hyperplasia	5.4	140.2
FE	F	29	hyperplasia	2.4	133.2
RA	M	27	thymoma	4.3	80.1
ZD	F	60	thymoma	7.6	200.6
VC	M	74	thymoma	5.7	140.3

n.d.: not done.

tory effect was more evident with an E2 concentration of 10^{-8} M than 10^{-6} M. This effect was always evident at 48h, while at 24h showed not to be constant (ranging from 0% to 176%). Therefore, we used an E2 concentration of 10^{-8} M for the following experiments, at time-points of 24 and 48h.

To confirm the specificity of E2 action on IL-6 secretion by TECs, we used two specific estrogen inhibitors: ICI 182–270 and tamoxifen. Fig. 2 shows the effect of E2 on IL-6 secretion by TECs from six normal subjects, stimulated for 24 and 48 h. As already found in time-course experiments, we observed a non significant stimulation at 24 h (basal vs. stimulated, $p=0.085$) and a statistically significant increment at 48h ($p=0.012$), up to 5.8 fold increase. This effect was blocked by both estrogen inhibitors used. On the contrary, the basal secretion was not modified by the two inhibitors (Fig. 3) (basal versus ICI-additionated: $p=0.47$; basal versus tamoxifen-additionated $p=0.90$). In order to verify whether the estrogen effect on IL-6 production was mediated by IL-1, we looked for the presence of IL-1β in some basal and E2 stimulated media at 24 and 48h. We found no detectable IL-1β in any of the tested samples (data not shown).

In order to evaluate the hypothesis that estrogens might also modify the known stimulating effect of IL-1β on IL-6 secretion, we performed time-course experiments in TECs from four normal subjects with different concentrations of IL-1β (12, 6, 3 U/ml), to

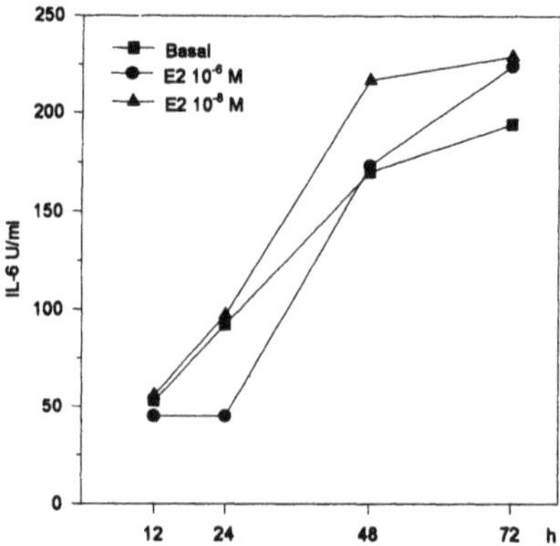

Figure 1. Time-course of effect of E2 on IL-6 production from TEC of a normal thymus.

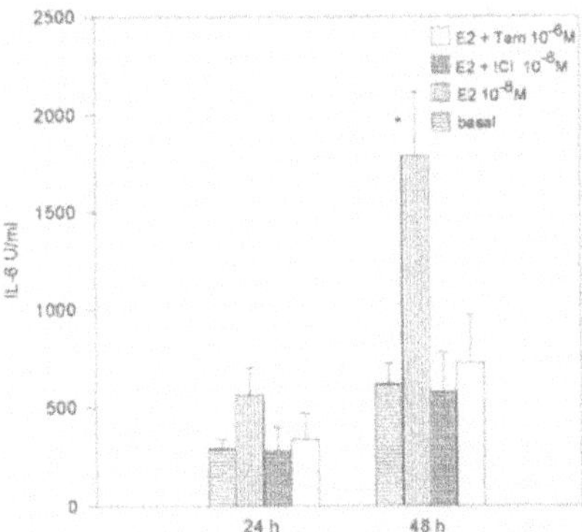

Figure 2. E2 effect on IL-6 secretion by TEC from seven normal subjects. (*p=0.012)

identify eventually a sub-maximal dose able to stimulate IL-6 secretion. Constitutive production of IL-6 was increased by IL-1β in all samples, with a secretion index ranging from 7 to 23 at 24 h with 3 U/ml of IL-1β. Fig. 4 shows a representative time-course graph of such experiments. Since similar results were obtained with IL-1β concentrations of 6 and 3 U/ml, the latter was used in further experiments in which E2 was associated to IL-1β.

Figure 5 shows the effect of E2 and IL-1 on IL-6 secretion. The association of E2 and IL-1β gives a higher stimulation than IL-1β alone at 24 h but not at 48 h (IL-1β versus IL-1β + E2: p=0.002).

In order to evaluate possible different behaviours in secretion patterns of normal and pathological thymuses and between different pathological thymic tissues, we performed preliminary experiments in which TECs from five patients with hyperplasia and four with thymoma were stimulated with E2 10^{-8} M for 24 h (fig. 6a and 6b). E2 induced a slight decrease of IL-6 secretion in TECs from hyperplastic thymuses, with significant values in two out of five cases. This positive effect was inhibited by tamoxifen. However, a statistically significant increment of IL-6 secretion was detected in three out of four samples of thymoma TECs.

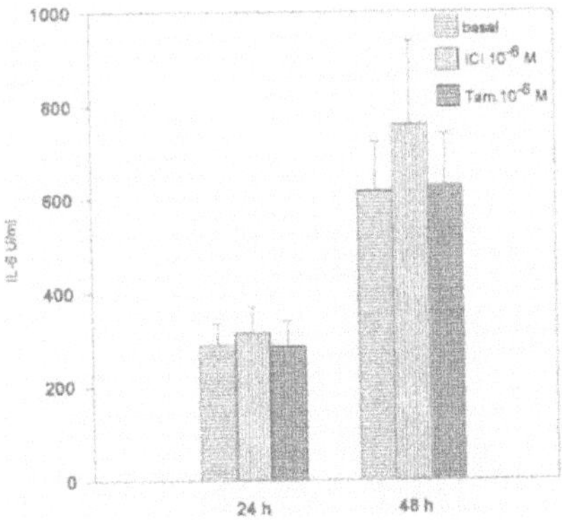

Figure 3. Effect of E2 inhibitors on basal IL-6 secretion from TEC of seven normal subjects at 24 and 48 h of incubation.

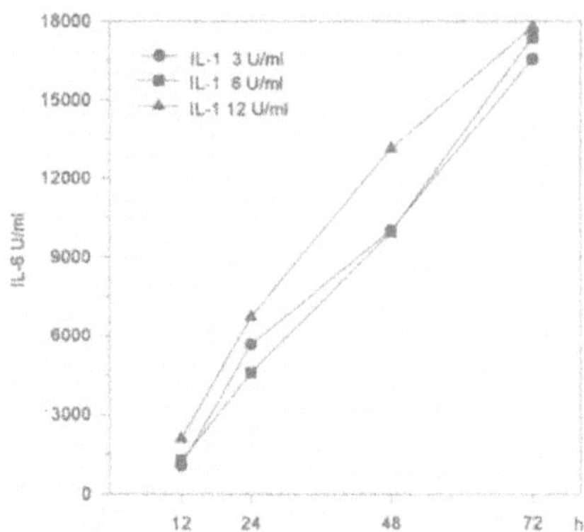

Figure 4. Time-course of IL-6 secretion stimulated by IL-1 in TEC from a normal thymus.

DISCUSSION

This study clearly shows that human thymic epithelial cells in our in vitro model are constitutively able to secrete IL-6 in a time-dependent way, confirming previous reports [11]. As the culture medium was devoid of endotoxin, IL-1β, E2 and growth factor, the basal production of IL-6 was attributed to a spontaneous release from the cultured cells. In this model estrogens increase the basal secretion of IL-6 from all the TECs of normal subjects, regardless of sex and age. This effect appears to be mediated by the type I estrogen receptor, as the entity of rise is not modified by the increase of E2 concentration and is blocked by the specific inhibitors ICI 182–270 and tamoxifen, used at 100 fold the concentration of E2. The stimulatory effect on IL-6 secretion was more marked after 48 hours of incubation, suggesting that it could be mediated by the secretion of some IL-1β in the medium [12, 13]. However, IL-1β was not detectable either in the culture medium, nor in the supernatants of unstimulated and E2-stimulated cells. We believe that our different cell culture conditions (lower cell density and a non stimulant medium) can explain the difference between these results and other reports [12, 13].

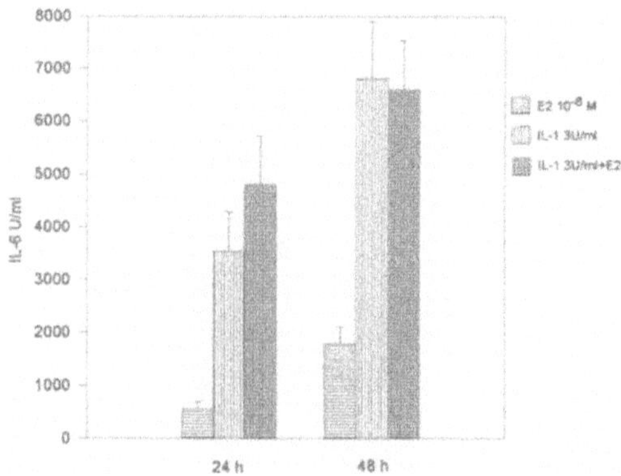

Figure 5. Effect of association of E2 and IL-1 on IL-6 secretion from TEC of normal thymuses.

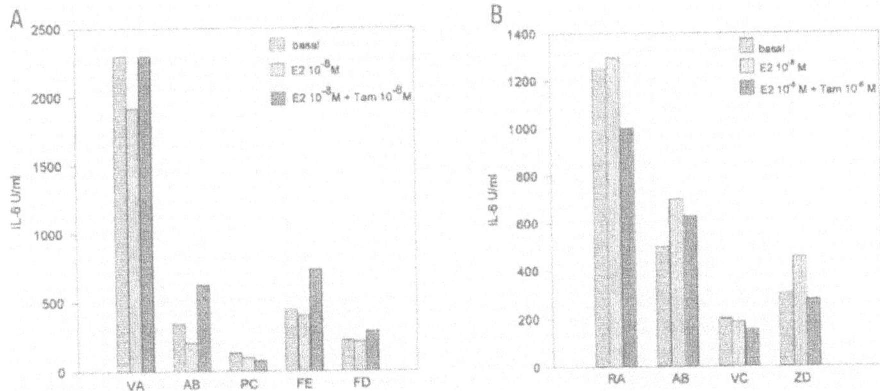

Figure 6. IL-6 activity measured by hybridoma growth factor assay and by ELISA commercial kit gave comparable results (data not shown). Effect of E2 on IL-6 secretion from TECs of (A) hyperplastic thymuses and (B) thymoma.

The basal IL-6 production was unaffected by the specific inhibitors of ER we used, while the E2-stimulation was blocked by them. These findings suggest that IL-6 secretion can be modified by E2, and that its basal production is not mediated by ER.

Estrogen receptors have been shown in thymic tissue, but data on human epithelial cells are limited [4]. We have shown that TECs from normal and pathological tissues have estrogen receptors, both of the classical type I and of the type II. Our results underline that the E2 effects are mediated by type I receptors.

The present data are in agreement with those reports showing a stimulatory action of estrogens on IL-6 production [7, 14], and are in contrast with reports showing that estrogens can inhibit IL-6 secretion [6, 15]. This discrepancy may derive again from the cell type and/or the experimental conditions employed.

Preliminary observations on pathological TECs indicate that thymomas and hyperplastic thymuses have different behaviors. Both of them show a basal secretion of IL-6. In three out of four samples of thymoma TECs, we could observe an increase of this basal secretion after a 24 hours of E2 stimulation. Basal production of IL-6 from hyperplastic thymus TECs, on the contrary, was inhibited by E2 addition.

More experiments on a greater number of patients are needed to establish whether abnormal estrogen-induced IL-6 production by TECs may have implications in the development of follicular hyperplasia or thymoma in myasthenic thymus, as our preliminary results, showing a different pattern of behaviour between hyperplastic and thymomatous myasthenic TECs, may suggest.

ACKNOWLEDGMENTS

This work was supported by funds from MURST 40% "Neuroimmunologia" and from Telethon Italy (grant #590).

REFERENCES

1. Kishimoto T: The biology of interleukin-6. Blood, 1989, 74(1):1–10

2. Galy A.H.M., Dinarello C.A., Kupper T.S., Kameda A., Hadden. J.W.: Effects of cytokines on human thymic epithelial cells in culture. Cell Immunol,1990, 129: 161–175
3. Emilie D., Crevon M.C., Cohen-Kaminsky S. , Peuchmaur M., Devergne O., Berrih-Aknin S., Galanaud P. In situ production of interleukins in hyperplastic thymus from myasthenia gravis patients. Hum Pathol, 1991, 22:461–468
4. Kawashima I., Sakabe K., Seiki K., Fujii-Hanamoto H., Akatsuka A., Tsukamoto H. Localization of sex steroid receptor cells, with special reference to thymulin (FTS)-producing cells in female rat thymus. Thymus, 1991, 18:79–93
5. Jacobs A.L., Sehgal P.B. , Julian J., Carson D.D. Secretion and hormonal regulation of interleukin-6 production by mouse uterine stromal and polarized epithelial cells cultured in vitro. Endocrinology, 1992, 131(3):1037–1046
6. Girasole., Jilka R.L., Passeri G., Boswell S., Boder G., Williams D.C., Manolagas S.C. 17ß-Estradiol inhibits interleukin-6 production by bone marrow-derived stromal cells and osteoblasts in vitro: a potential mechanism for the antiosteoporotic effect of estrogens. J Clin Invest, 1992, 89:883–891
7. Li Z.G., Danis V.A., Brooks P.M.: Effect of gonadal steroids on the prodution of IL-1 and IL-6 by blood mononuclear cells in vitro. Clin Exp Rheumatol, 1993, 11:157–162
8. Savino W., Bartoccioni E., Homo-Delarche F., Gagnerault M.Cl., Itoh T., Dardenne M.: Thymic hormone containing cells-IX. steroids in vitro modulate thymulin secretion by human and murine thymic epithelial cells. J Steroid Biochem, 1988, 30: 479–484
9. De Luca M., Cancedda R.: Culture of human epithelium. BURNS, 1992, 18: S5–10.
10. Aarden LA, De Groot R, Schaap OL, Landsorp PM: Production of hybridoma growth factor by human monocytes. Eur J Immunol, 1987, 17: 1411–1416.
11. Cohen-Kaminsky S, Delattre RM, Devergne O, Klingel-Schmitt I, Emilie D, Galanaud P, Berrih-Aknin S: High IL-6 gene expression and production by cultured human thymic epithelial cells from patients with myasthenia gravis. Ann NY Acad Sci, 1993, 681: 97–98
12. Le P.T., Singer K.H.: Human thymic epithelial cells: adhesion molecules and cytokine production. Int J Clin Lab Res, 1993, 23: 56–60.
13. Aime C, Cohen-Kaminsky S, Berrih-Aknin S: In vitro IL-1 production in thymic hyperplasia and thymoma from patients with myasthenia gravis. J Clin Immunol, 1991, 11: 268–278.
14. Mamata DE, Sanford TR, Wood GW: IL-1, IL-6 and TNF-α are produced in the mouse uterus during the estrous cycle and are induced by estrogen and progesterone. Dev. Biol, 1992, 151: 297–305.
15. Jacobs AL, Sehegal PB, Julian J, Carson DD: Secretion and ormonal regulation of IL-6 production by mouse uterine stromal and polarized epithelial cells cultured in vitro. Endocrinology, 1992, 131: 1037–1046.

26

THYMOMA AND AUTOIMMUNE NEUROLOGICAL DISORDERS

A Search for Missing Links in Pathogenesis

Angela Vincent, Nick Willcox, Ioannis Roxanis, John Newsom-Davis, Cal McLennan, and David Beeson

Neuroscience Group
Institute of Molecular Medicine
John Radcliffe Hospital
Oxford OX3 9DU

1. THE ASSOCIATED DISORDERS

It has long been recognised that autoimmunity may be associated with particular tumours, and the regular co-occurrence of myasthenia gravis (MG) with thymoma is well established. In this brief review we will summarise some of the evidence for thymoma-associated antibodies in myasthenia, and in other neurological disorders, and discuss the possible relationship between the tumour, these antibodies and the initiation of the disease.

Autoimmunity and associations with thymoma were reviewed by Souadjian et al[1]. Almost 50% of the 47 thymoma patients had MG, though other estimates vary from 20–60%. Other autoantibody mediated diseases were rare. There were no cases of autoimmune neuromyotonia or Stiff-Man syndrome, but these have since been recognised in association with thymic tumours (see below). It is worth pointing out that at least some of the diseases thought by Souadjian et al to be associated with thymoma, eg. polymyositis and rheumatoid arthritis, are considered to be T cell rather than antibody-mediated conditions.

2. MYASTHENIA GRAVIS

2.1. The Acetylcholine Receptor (AChR)

The typically fatiguable weakness in MG is mediated by autoantibodies that bind to the acetylcholine receptors (AChR) at the neuromuscular junction (reviewed by Drachman[2]). The antibodies have a high affinity and are heterogeneous in their light chain, subclass and reactivity with different extracellular epitopes on the AChR[3]. The AChR is

Epithelial Tumors of the Thymus, edited by Marx and Müller-Hermelink.
Plenum Press, New York, 1997

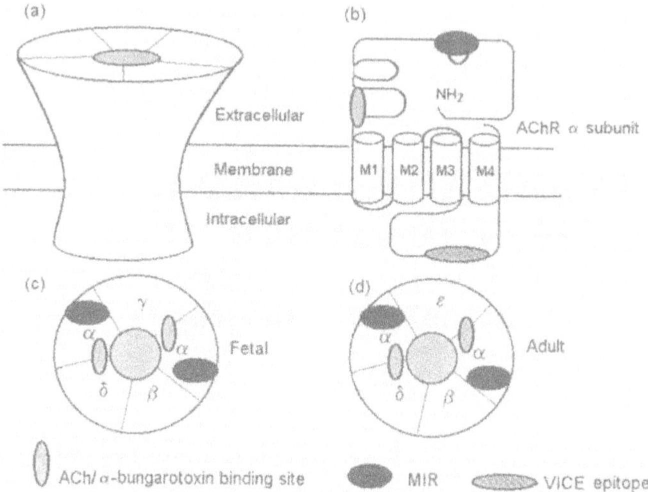

Figure 1. Diagram of the AChR showing the intact molecule sitting in the membrane (a), the topology of each subunit, illustrated for the α which contains the ACh/α-Bungarotoxin binding site, the MIR and the VICE epitope (b), and the adult and fetal subtypes (c and d).

particularly well characterised and is a cylindrical protein consisting of five subunits (each about 50kd) arranged around a central ion channel (Fig 1; see[4]). Each subunit has an N-terminal extracellular domain of about 210 aminoacids, three transmembrane segments and a cytoplasmic loop before a final C terminal transmembrane segment. The α neuro-toxins such as a-BuTx are targeted at the two α subunits, principally to α185–199, and they can be used to label the AChR for localisation studies and immunoprecipitation assays. Also located on the α subunits are the main immunogenic regions (MIR) that are thought to represent the dominant epitopes for antibody binding[5–7]. The MIR is very conformation-dependent, but with a major contribution from the sequence α67–76.

In general, the antibodies in MG only recognise the conformation of the extracellular AChR domain including the MIR, and bind weakly if at all to denatured AChR subunits or synthetic peptides, suggesting that the immune response is generated against the whole native AChR, probably in its membrane environment. Production of these high affinity IgG antibodies to this protein antigen almost certainly depends on 'T cell help' which, as we discuss below, could arise in the thymoma.

2.2. Patient Characteristics

Caucasian patients with generalised MG fall into three main subgroups. Those with onset before 40 years of age are frequently female, have a high incidence of the HLA antigens B8 and DR3, and typically have a 'hyperplastic' thymus with medullary T cell areas and germinal centres[8]. AChR is present on rare myoid cells in the thymic medulla[9], and plasma cells within the thymus spontaneously synthesise anti-AChR antibodies[10,11] which show some preference for the fetal AChR expressed by the myoid cells[11]. These patients often respond well to thymectomy, and anti-AChR levels may fall substantially within 1–2 years after the operation[12] (Fig 2 and Cornelio, these proceedings). Therefore, it is generally considered, though not proven, that AChR within the thymic medulla provides at least some of the stimulus for generation of both T and B cells.

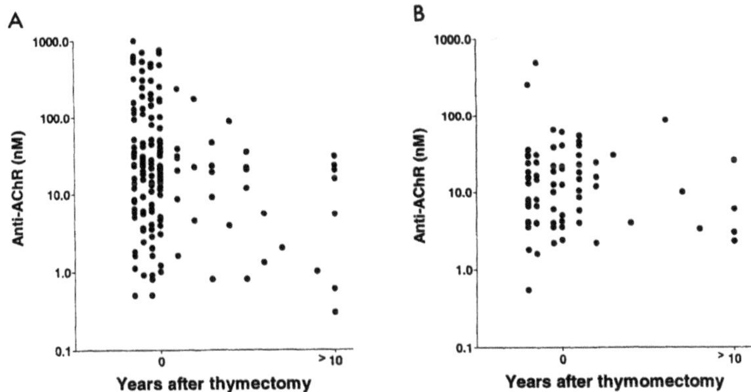

Figure 2. Anti-AChR levels in MG patients before and at various time points after thymectomy. None of the patients was on immunosuppression at the time of sampling. a. Young onset patients with thymic hyperplasia. b. Thymoma cases.

Late onset patients (arbitrarily >40 years at presentation) do not show a strong sex bias, have a moderate association with HLA B7 and/or DR2, and commonly have an involuted thymus[8]. Thymectomy is not usually performed in this age group, but they respond well to immunosuppressive therapy. It is not clear why and how they develop an immune response to AChR, but in some of these patients antibodies to other muscle antigens are also present (see Aarli, for further discussion).

Patients with thymoma usually present in middle age with no major sex or HLA biasses. Thymoma lymphocytes rarely synthesise even traces of anti-AChR antibodies in culture[10,13], but cells from the adjacent thymic remnant may do so, in keeping with the 'hyperplasia' that it frequently shows[14]. The patients respond poorly to thymomectomy; indeed, their MG often deteriorates or begins afterwards, and anti-AChR levels seldom fall unless immunosuppressive therapy is introduced[15] (Fig 2). On the other hand, these patients almost always have high titres of antibodies to other muscle antigens, particularly actin, myosin, troponin, ryanodine receptor and especially titin (see Aarli, this volume). Some of these antigens have epitopes that are shared by the AChR but, so far, there is little evidence that these are recognised by the patients' antibodies.

2.3.1 The Role of the Thymoma in Autosensitisation. Thymoma epithelial cells express undefined striated muscle antigens and one epitope of titin[16,17,18]. They are moderately efficient antigen presenting cells when in culture[19]. If they also expressed AChR epitopes, they might well immunise some of the abundant infiltrating T cells[14] - either those developing in the tumours or others entering from the circulation. These could either be CD8+ or CD4+, and must presumably activate specific B cells elsewhere, since the latter are usually rare in thymomas.

Many groups have therefore searched for AChR expression. In some thymomas, rare myoid-like inclusions are present (see Henry, this volume) and contain striated muscle fibrils. It is extremely likely that these cells do express AChR. However, in general, complete AChR has not been detected in thymoma tissue (eg.[20]). A few studies have looked at binding of ^{125}I-α-BuTx to extracts of thymoma tissue, but these have been negative too (see [21]).

Immunohistochemistry with monoclonal anti-AChR antibodies to the MIR also failed to detect AChR, but one monoclonal antibody (Mab 155) to a very immunogenic cytoplasmic epitope (VICE) (α 371–378) showed marked epithelial cell staining[17] that was largely restricted to thymomas associated with MG and labelled very few epithelial cells in the normal thymic medulla. This is an unusually stable and conformation-independent epitope, and antibodies raised against the peptide sequence bind well to the intact molecule (see Fig 1), as should any similar antibodies in the patients'sera. However, there is no evidence that MG patients with or without thymoma have an antibody response to this sequence, and moreover, T cell responses to this region have not been obvious in MG thymoma patients[22], although AChR-reactive T cells have been found against extracellular sequences of the AChR[23] (Nagvekar et al in preparation). Recently, it has become clear that while this epitope is shared with fast Troponin (I)[24], the 153kd protein expressing it in thymomas may be Neurofilament M[25]; there is also evidence that a titin-like epitope may be expressed in thymoma[18], perhaps on the same protein (Willisch, these proceedings), and B cells secreting IgM antibodies to striational antigens have been cloned from thymoma[26]. Thus the epitopes for some of the thymoma-associated anti-muscle antibodies are present, and T cell responses to these epitopes should be sought.

Extremely sensitive PCR techniques have detected low levels of expression of individual AChR subunits in thymoma (eg[27]). We have used less sensitive but more quantitative RNAase protection assays. Only the ε subunit was detected in eight of 15 thymomas at levels comparable with human amputated leg muscle; the other thymomas showed no significant expression of any AChR subunit (MacLennan, Beeson, Willcox, Vincent and Newsom-Davis in preparation). Obviously, expression at the protein level needs to be tested now.

The expression of the AChR ε subunit is potentially interesting because this subunit replaces the γ subunit during development and defines the adult form of the AChR (Fig 1). It was important, therefore, to see whether patients with thymoma reacted more strongly to adult AChR than to fetal AChR. Quite to the contrary, anti-AChR antibodies in thymoma cases mostly bind more strongly to fetal AChR (as previously reported[28]). Only two sera showed greater binding to adult AChR; one of these came from a patient with strong ε expression in his thymoma. Perhaps in the others, the responses to fetal AChR reflect subsequent determinant spreading after initiation by the ε epitopes. T cell responses to these subunits therefore need to be studied.

2.3.2 Determinant Spreading and Myasthenia. Over the last few years it has become increasingly clear that autoimmune responses may 'spread', either to different epitopes on a single protein (intramolecular spreading, eg.[29]) or to different proteins expressed by the same tissue (intermolecular spreading). Until recently, determinant spreading was not well-recognised in MG. However rabbits immunised against three synthetic peptides, representing α137–199 of the human α subunit, subsequently developed high affinity antibodies specific for rabbit AChR in its native conformation including the MIR and ^{125}I-α-BuTx binding site[30]. Interestingly, the anti-peptide antibodies, that appeared soon after the first immunisation and did not bind detectably to soluble AChR, could be separated on a peptide-affinity column from the anti-AChR antibodies which passed straight through the column. This suggests that the peptides somehow initiated a quite separate immune response against the whole receptor molecule. The mechanism(s) by which this occurs have not been elucidated; possibly early antibodies against α137–199 reacted with the AChR at the neuromuscular junction (where the high concentration of antigen would favour binding even of low-affinity antibodies) and initiated muscle damage resulting in release of postsynaptic membrane or antibody-AChR complexes with subsequent stimulation of antibodies specific for autologous rabbit AChR. Alternatively, the peptide immunisation might have induced specific cytotoxic T cells that attacked the muscle endplates. In either case, one might expect immune responses to other muscle antigens as well as the AChR, and a search for these is in progress.

3. OTHER THYMOMA-ASSOCIATED NEUROLOGICAL DISORDERS

Several other disorders have been reported in association with thymoma. Acquired neuromyotonia (NMT) is a rare condition in which hyperexcitability of peripheral motor axons leads to spontaneous muscle activity with cramps, fasciculations and myokymia[31]. It is now thought to be due to antibodies to the voltage-gated potassium channels (VGKC) that regulate neuronal excitability[32]. Low levels of antibodies to ^{125}I-α-dendrotoxin-labelled (human brain) VGKC can be detected in about 50% of patients, and interestingly about 20% of NMT patients also have anti-AChR antibodies and MG with or without thymoma. In two such cases examined recently the tumour was an atypical carcinoid in appearance with strikingly fewer lymphocytes than in a typical MG thymoma; however, one also had small areas of cortical thymoma (Fig 3). Interestingly, they also expressed ε subunit, and did so even more strongly in another atypical thymic carcinoid from a patient with neither MG nor NMT. Perhaps, the epithelial cells in these rather different tumours immunise mature recirculating T cells rather than nascent thymocytes.

The stiff-man syndrome (SMS) is another rare condition in which defects in central inhibitory pathways lead to muscle stiffness and cramps. It associates with a variety of tumours (eg of breast and colon) as well as with insulin-dependent diabetes mellitus. Antibodies to glutamic acid decarboxylase (GAD) were first detected by Solimena and his colleagues[33] by immunohistochemistry and immunoprecipitation of ^{35}S-labelled recombinant GAD. A new immunoprecipitation assay employing ^{125}I-GAD promises to provide a rapid and sensitive technique for measuring these antibodies (Vincent, Grimaldi, Martino, Davenport and Todd, in preparation).

The associations of these other antibody-mediated neurological diseases with thymoma, and the presence of more than one antibody in some sera, suggests that there may be overlap between several of these syndromes. Fig 4 shows antibodies to VGKC, GAD and RAPsyn (a postsynaptic skeletal protein that is thought to be responsible for clustering AChRs at the neuromuscular junction) in 13 MG cases with thymic tumours, two of whom also had neuromyotonia. Anti-VGKC antibodies were found in two MG/thymoma patients without obvious neuromyotonia, and one of the patients with neuromyotonia also had anti-GAD antibodies. None of these antibodies have been found in healthy controls.

3.1. Small Cell Lung Cancer and Autoimmune Neurological Disorders

The first disorder to be labelled paraneoplastic is the Lambert Eaton myasthenic syndrome (LEMS); about 60% of cases have a small cell lung cancer (SCLC). In these and the patients without tumours, antibodies to voltage-gated calcium channels on motor and parasympathetic nerve terminals lead to reduced ACh release and a combination of myasthenic and autonomic symptoms (see[34]). The associated SCLC cells express functional VGCC, and culture in LEMS serum or IgG reduces the number of functioning VGCC[35]. Antibodies to VGCC can be measured by immunoprecipitation of ^{125}I-ω-cono-

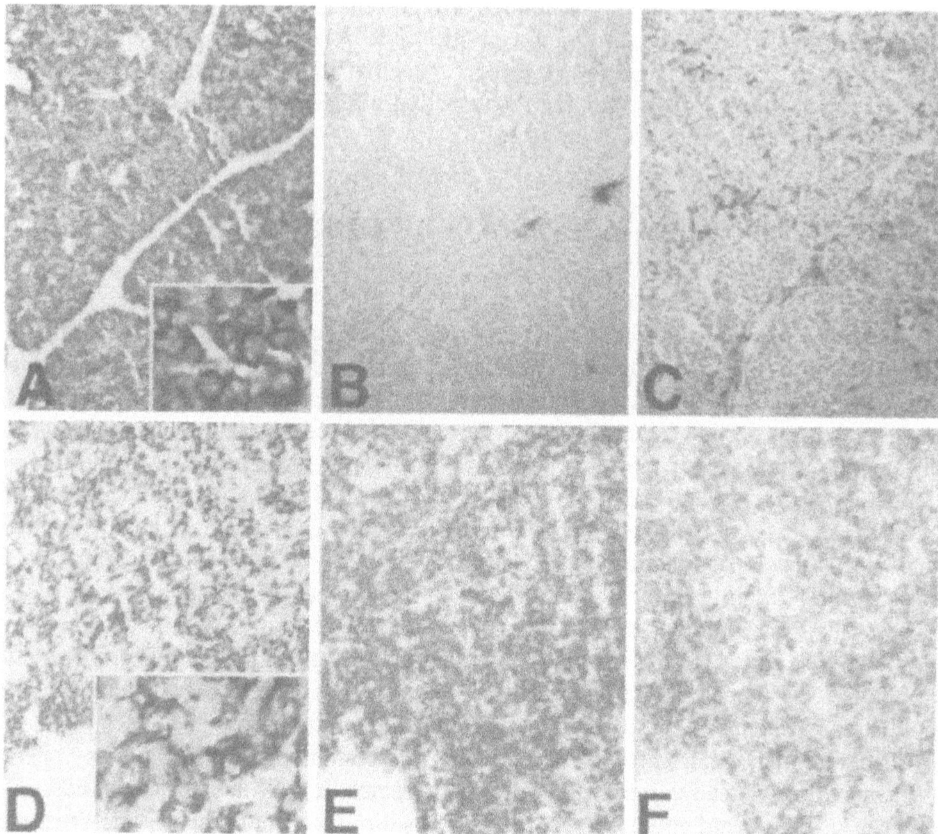

Figure 3. A thymic tumour from a patient with neuromyotonia and myasthenia gravis (not pretreated with corticosteroids). The appearances are mainly of an atypical thymic carcinoid (a-c) strongly expressing chromogranin (not shown) and cytokeratin (Mab LP34,(a)), and cortical (MR6+) and subcapsular medullary (MR19+) thymic epithelial markers (as in ref 14; not shown). CD1+ cells are rare (b) and most appear (at higher magnification) to be dendritic cells rather than cortical thymocytes, but there is sparse infiltration by CD3+ T lymphocytes (c). There were also small areas of typical cortical thymoma (d-f) with a cytokeratin+ epithelial network (d) enmeshing abundant CD1+ (e) and CD3+ thymocytes (f). In the carcinoid areas, by contrast, the epithelial cells appear polygonal with more cytoplasm and fewer processes (Compare insets of (a) and (d)).

toxin MVIIC labelled P-type VGCC extracted from human cerebellum[36]. These antibodies are highly specific for LEMS, but are also occasionally found in patients with other SCLC-associated paraneoplastic disorders of the central nervous system[37] some of whom also have LEMS (Lang, Moll, Vincent et al in preparation)). These patients, especially those with a particular anti-neuronal nuclear antibody, termed anti-Hu or anti-ANNA2, may have subacute sensory neuropathies (SSN) or limbic encephalitis. The tumours usually also express the neuronal antigens (eg Hu in SCLC), again implicating them in autosensitisation. In contrast with the MG in thymoma patients, those with LEMS tend to improve if the SCLC can be removed or destroyed, which is strong circumstantial evidence that the tumour provokes the antibody response[38].

In general the CNS symptoms in the other syndromes do not respond similarly, possibly because of irreversible damage at an early stage. Recently, antibodies to other central nervous system antigens have been detected by immunohistochemistry in cases of

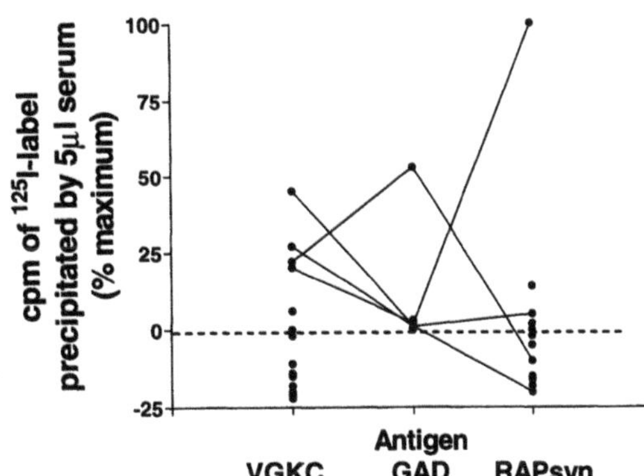

Figure 4. Antibodies to VGKC, GAD and RAPsyn in sera from patients with thymic tumours. Sera from 13 MG patients were assayed by immunoprecipitation using ^{125}I-α-dendrotoxin-labelled VGKC, ^{125}I-GAD (obtained from RSR Ltd), and ^{125}I-RAPsyn (expressed in E.coli by Ms Alex Buckel).

thymoma-associated limbic encephalitis. These antibodies stain different cell layers and can be anti-nuclear or anti-cytoplasmic (eg.[39]). Interestingly, some of these conditions improved after thymomectomy, and antibody titres fell.

4. CONCLUSIONS

The strong associations with thymic and SCLC tumours in these varied autoimmune neurological disorders must hold vital clues to their aetiology. By contrast, apparently identical disorders and autoantibodies can exist without any evidence of a tumour, when their origins are just as hard to explain as in most other autoimmune diseases.

The role of SCLC in inducing antibodies to VGCC in LEMS appears to be the clearest example. The SCLC cells express complete functional VGCC, and these tumours are probably the site of initial immunisation of both T and B cells[40]. The resulting autoantibodies may be part of a natural and beneficial immune response against the tumour, perhaps protecting against multi-drug resistance as well as leading to earlier presentation. Since the response can apparently begin when the tumours are very small, they must be remarkably immunogenic in high responder patients.

Interestingly, there is very little overlap between the SCLC - and the thymoma-associated syndromes (see Fig 5). While atypical carcinoids may resemble SCLCs histologically, MG and NMT are common in patients with thymoma and do not associate with SCLC. The associations with thymic tumours pose greater conceptual challenges partly because both the autoantibodies and the tumour pathology are so diverse, and partly be-

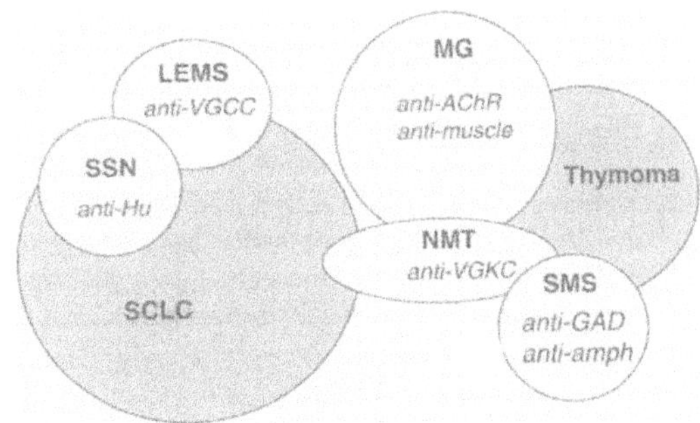

Figure 5. Venn diagram to illustrate some of the overlapping paraneoplastic syndromes and their associated autoantibodies.

cause none of the target autoantigens has been found in its complete form in the tumours. Moreover, few of these syndromes remit after surgery.

Since some of the thymic carcinoids and carcinomas contain few or no developing T cells, a general failure in self tolerance induction within thymomas appears improbable (see above). It seems far more likely that certain epitopes actively immunise specific helper or cytotoxic T cells in the tumours, and that these only induce B cell responses and antibody production after re-encountering antigen and MHC in the periphery; possibly myoid cells in the adjacent thymic remnant could play this role in MG (especialy in younger patients). The long delays inevitable in such a multi-step process could easily explain the poor clinical response to tumour resection as well as the late presentation of MG so often seen after surgery.

Remembering the epitope sharing between various muscle and neurofilament antigens, and the expression of some of them within thymomas, one could imagine that T cell responses to a very few shared determinants might easily induce antibodies to a variety of proteins. Further determinant spreading, both within and between molecules, might result from subsequent muscle damage and so broaden the range of autoantibodies yet further. To evaluate these speculations, we clearly need to know much more about the variety of epitopes/autoantigens expressed in the tumours. At present, we suspect that the 153kd polypeptide with its several B cell epitopes is not a sufficent explanation. Shared T cell epitopes are less easily identified, but it is clearly a high priority to study the repertoire of T cells recognising them in these tumours. That, in turn, may help to explain why they are so much more immunogenic than the generality of tumours elsewhere and why different tumours associate with different syndromes. For this reason, it is essential to look for the expression of muscle antigens in thymoma tissue, to demonstrate T cell responses against them, and to correlate these findings with antibody responses to a range of muscle antigens including AChR subunits. In addition, any putative thymoma epitopes should be tested for their ability to induce anti-AChR or anti-muscle antibodies in experimental animals.

REFERENCES

1. Souadjian, JV, Enriquez, P, Silverstein, MN, Pepin, J-M. The spectrum of diseases associated with thymoma. Arch Intern Med 134:374–379, 1974.
2. Drachman DB. Myasthenia gravis. 1994. *New England J Med* 330:1797–1810.
3. Vincent A, Whiting PJ, Schluep M et al. 1987. Antibody heterogeneity and specificity in myasthenia gravis. *Ann NY Acad Sci* 505:326–332.
4. Karlin A, Akabas MH. 1995. Toward a structural basis for the function of nicotinic acetylcholine receptors and their cousins. *Neuron* 15: 1231–1244.
5. Tzartos SJ, Lindstrom JM. 1980. Monoclonal antibodies used to probe acetylcholine receptor structure: localization of the main immunogenic region and detection of similarities between subunits. *Proc Natl Acad Sci USA* 77:755–759.
6. Tzartos SJ, Seybold ME, Lindstrom JM. 1982. Specificities of antibodies to acetylcholine receptors in sera from myasthenia gravis patients measured by monoclonal antibodies. *Proc Natl Acad Sci USA* 79:188–192.
7. Tzartos SJ, Barkas T, Cung MT, et al. 1991. The main immunogenic region of the acetylcholine receptor: structure and role in myasthenia gravis. *Autoimmunity* 8:259–270.
8. Compston DAS, Vincent A, Newsom-Davis J, Batchelor JR. 1980. Clinical, pathological, HLA antigen and immunological evidence for disease heterogeneity in myasthenia gravis. *Brain*, 103, 579–601.
9. Schluep M, Willcox N, Vincent A, Dhoot GK, Newsom-Davis J. 1987. Acetylcholine receptors in human thymic myoid cells in situ: an immunohistological study. *Ann Neurol* 22:212–222.
10. Scadding GK, Vincent A, Newsom-Davis J, Henry K. 1981. Acetylcholine receptor antibody synthesis by thymic lymphocytes: correlation with thymic histology. *Neurology* 31:935–943.

11. Heidenreich, F., A.Vincent, N.Willcox and J.Newsom-Davis. 1988. Anti-acetylcholine receptor antibody specificities in serum and in thymic culture supernatants from myasthenia gravis patients. *Neurology* 38:1784–1788.
12. Vincent A, Newsom-Davis J, Newton P, Beck N. 1983. Acetylcholine receptor antibody and clinical response to thymectomy in myasthenia gravis. *Neurology* 33:1276–1282.
13. Fujii Y, Monden Y, Nakahara K, Hashimoto J, Kawashima Y. 1984. Antibody to acetylcholine receptor in myasthenia gravis: production by lymphocytes from thymus or thymoma. Neurology 34; 1182–116.
14. Willcox N, Schluep M, Ritter MA, Schurman HJ, Newsom-Davis J, Christensson B. Myasthenic and non-myasthenic thymoma. An expansion of a minor cortical epithelial cell subset? Am J Pathol 1987; 127:447–460.
15. Somnier FE. Exacerbation of myasthenia gravis after removal of thymoma. Acta Neurol Scand 1994; 90:56–66.
16. Gilhus N-E, Aarli JA, Christensson B, Matre R. Rabbit Antiserum to a Citric Acid Extract of Human Skeletal Muscle Staining Thymomas from Myasthenia Gravis Patients. J Neuroimmunol 1984, 7: 55—64.
17. Kirchner T, Hoppe F, Schalke B, Muller-Hermelink HK. 1988. Microenvironment of thymic myoid cells in myasthenia gravis. *Virch Archiv B Cell Pathol* 54:295–302.
18. Marx A, Willisch A, Schultz A, Greiner A, Magi B, Pallini Vi, Schalke B et al. Expression of neurofilaments and of a titin epitope in thymic epithelial tumours. Implications for the pathogenesis of myasthenia gravis. Am J Pathol 1996; 148:1839–1850.
19. Gilhus NE, Willcox N, Harcourt G, Nagvekar N, Beeson D, Vincent A, Newsom Davis J. 1995. Antigen presentation by thymoma epithelial cells from myasthenia gravis patients to potentially pathogenic T cells. *J Neuroimmunol* 56:65–76.
20. Geuder KI, Marx A, Witzemann V, Schalke B, Kirchner T, Müller-Hermelink HK. 1992. Genomic Organization and Lack of Transcription of the Nicotinic Acetylcholine Receptor Subunit Genes in Myasthenia Gravis-Associated Thymoma. *Lab Invest* 66:452 -458.
21. Vincent A 1980. Immunology of acetylcholine receptors in relation to myasthenia gravis. *Physiol Rev* 60, 756–824.
22. Jacobson, L, Nagvekar, N, Vincent, A, Willcox, N, Newsom-Davis, J. Is the AChR α373–380 sequence a T or B cell epitope in thymoma associated-myasthenia gravis? Neuromusc Disord 4:S34, 1994.(Abstract)
23. Sommer N, Willcox N, Harcourt GC, Newsom Davis-J. 1990. Myasthenic thymus and thymoma are selectively enriched in acetylcholine receptor-reactive T cells. *Ann Neurol* 28:312–9.
24. Osborn M, Marx A, Kirchner T, Tzartos SJ, Plessman W, Weber K. 1992. A Shared Epitope in the Acetylcholine Receptor-α Subunit and Fast Troponin I of Skeletal Muscle. *Am J Pathol* 140:1215–1223.
25. Marx A; Kirchner T; Greiner A; Muller Hermelink HK; Schalke B; Osborn M. 1992. Neurofilament epitopes in thymoma and antiaxonal autoantibodies in myasthenia gravis. *Lancet* 339:707–8.
26. Williams CL, Lennon VA. 1986. Thymic B Lymphocyte Clones from Patients with Myasthenia Gravis Secrete Monoclonal Striational Autoantibodies Reacting with Myosin, α Actinin, or Actin. *J Exp Med* 164:1043–1059.
27. Kaminski HJ, Fenstermaker RA, Abdul Karim FW, Clayman J, Ruff RL. 1993. Acetylcholine receptor subunit gene expression in thymic tissue. *Muscle Nerve* 16:1332–7
28. Vincent A, Newsom-Davis J. 1982. Acetylcholine receptor antibody characteristics in myasthenia gravis. I. Patients with generalised myasthenia or disease restricted to ocular muscles. *Clin Exp Immunol* 49:257–265.
29. Lehmann PV, Sercarz EE, Forsthuber T, Dayan CM, Gammon G. Determinant Spreading and the Dynamics of the Autoimmune T-Cell Repertoire. *Immunology Today*, 1993, 14: 203 -208.
30. Vincent A, Jacobson L, Shillito P. 1994. Response to human acetylcholine receptor α138–199: determinant spreading initiates autoimmunity to self-antigen in rabbits. *Immunol Lett* 39:269–275.
31. Newsom-Davis J, Mills KR. 1993. Immunological associations of acquired neuromyotonia (Isaacs' syndrome). Report of five cases and literature review. *Brain* 116: 453–469.
32. Shillito P, Molenaar PC, Vincent A, et al 1995. Acquired neuromyotonia: evidence for autoantibodies against K+ channels of peripheral nerves. *Ann Neurol.* 38; 714–722.
33. Solimena, M, Folli, F, Denis-Donini, S, Comi, GC, Pozza, G, De Camilli, P, Vicari, AM. Autoantibodies to glutamic acid decarboxylase in a patient with stiff-man syndrome, epilepsy, and Type 1 diabetes mellitus. N Engl J Med 318:1012–1020, 1988.
34. O'Neill JH, Murray NM, Newsom-Davis J. 1988. The Lambert-Eaton myasthenic syndrome. A review of 50 cases. *Brain* 111:577–596.
35. Roberts A, Perera S, Lang B, Vincent A, Newsom-Davis J. 1985. Paraneoplastic myasthenic syndrome IgG inhibits $^{45}Ca^{2+}$ flux in a human small cell carcinoma line. *Nature* 317:737–739.

36. Motomura M, Johnston I, Lang B, Vincent A, Newsom-Davis J. 1995. An improved diagnostic assay for Lambert-Eaton myasthenic syndrome. *J Neurol Neurosurg Psychiatry* 58:85–87.
37. Lennon VA, Kryzer TJ, Griesmann GE, O'Suilleabhain PE, Windebank AJ, Woppmann A, Miljanich GP, Lambert EH. 1995. Calcium channel antibodies in the Lambert Eaton myasthenic syndrome and other paraneoplastic syndromes. *New Eng J Med* 332: 1467–1474.
38. Chalk CH, Murray NM, Newsom-Davis J, O'Neill JH, Spiro SG. 1990. Response of the Lambert-Eaton myasthenic syndrome to treatment of associated small-cell lung carcinoma. *Neurology* 40:1552–1556.
39. Antoine JC, Honnorat J, Thomas Angerion C, Aguera M, Absi L, Fournel P, Michel D. Limbic encephalitis and immunological perturbations in two patients with thymoma. J Neurol Neursurg Psychiatry 1995 58; 706–710.
40. Morris CS, Esiri MM, Marx A, Newsom-Davis J. 1992. Immunocytochemical characteristics of small cell lung carcinoma associated with the Lambert-Eaton myasthenic syndrome. *Am J Pathol* 140:839–845.

27

T-CELL DERIVED MECHANISMS IN THE PATHOGENESIS OF MYASTHENIA GRAVIS

Ann Kari Lefvert*

Department of Medicine and Immunological Research Laboratory
Karolinska Institute
S-171 76 Stockholm, Sweden

1. INTRODUCTION

Myasthenia gravis (MG) is often described as the prototype of an auto antibody-mediated autoimmune disease. The autoantibodies are directed against the nicotinic acetylcholine receptor on the skeletal muscle endplate, the disease is transmitted from mother to child and from humans to animals, and immunisation with acetylcholine receptor induces experimental myasthenia gravis in animals.[1] The disease-specific autoantibodies are, however, found in conditions not accompanied by neuromuscular symptoms, as in healthy first-degree relatives to patients, in monoclonal gammopathies, in primary biliary cirrhosis and in thymomas. Despite extensive efforts to try to distinguish the disease-causing antibodies found in myasthenia with those found in other conditions, no clear difference between these antibodies has been found. These observations together with the rather bad correlation between the concentration of autoantibodies in serum and the clinical symptoms suggest that mechanisms other than these antibodies may contribute by modulating the effects of autoantibodies on the neuromuscular junction.

This review will concentrate on the role of T cells and T cell products in the possible contribution of the pathophysiology in MG.

2. PROPERTIES OF PERIPHERAL BLOOD MONONUCLEAR CELLS (PBMC)

The phenotypic distribution of PBMC in patients is usually not different from that found in healthy persons.

The *in vitro* functional properties of peripheral blood mononuclear cells differ in some cases from that of healthy individuals.[2,3,4,5] The spontaneous proliferation measured

* Phone: 46-8-7293084; fax: 46-8-317058.

Epithelial Tumors of the Thymus, edited by Marx and Müller-Hermelink.
Plenum Press, New York, 1997

as increased DNA-synthesis, incorporation of ^{3}H-thymidine, tend to be higher in patients, especially in those with active disease. Patients with severe disease also have a higher percentage of cells bearing the IL- 2 receptor and a higher spontaneous production of TNF-α in cell culture than patients with mild disease. The response to mitogens was reduced, especially in cells from non-thymectomized patients as compared to cells from thymectomized patients and healthy individuals. These results indicate a partially altered T-cell function in myasthenia gravis which is most pronounced in patients before thymectomy.[2] Most of these changes might be secondary to an activation of the immune system *in vivo*, caused by the disease itself.

3. T-CELL STIMULATION BY AUTOANTIGENS

3.1. T-Cell Epitopes on the Acetylcholine Receptor α–Chain

The synthesis of acetylcholine receptor antibodies in myasthenia is regulated by acetylcholine receptor specific T-helper cells. These T-cells react predominantly with the α-subunit in one of the four different transmembranous subunits that form the penthameric acetylcholine receptor.[6,7] The amino terminal part of this subunit has a high degree of amphipaticity which is reported to be an important feature of T-cell epitopes and there are indeed several such epitopes located at this part of the receptor.[8] We examined the T-cell epitopes on the amino terminal part of the α-chain using T-cell stimulation measured as the number of IFN-γ secreting T-cells in response to 70 hexa-peptides overlapping with one amino acid and representing residues 10 to 84.[9] Twenty-one of the hexapeptides induced a higher number of IFN-γ producing cells in patients as compared with healthy individuals. A lack of T-cell stimulation in response to all the tested peptides was found only in 4% of the patients. Ninety-six % of the peptides induced T-cell stimulation in at least one of the patients as compared with 51% in the healthy individuals. One single hexa-peptide induce T-cell stimulation in a maximum of 37% of the patients. These results indicate that different epitopes and/or multiple T-cell-clones are involved in a T-cell-recognition of that special part of the acetylcholine receptor.

3.2. T-Cell Stimulation by Affinity-Purified Human Acetylcholine Receptor

T-cell stimulation induced by human acetylcholine receptor that had been affinity purified on α-bungarotoxin was measured as the induction of IL-2 and IFN-γ secretion from single cells using the ELISPOT-method.[10] The spontaneous production of both IFN-γ and IL-2 was lower from cells from patients than from cells from healthy individuals. Eighty-eight % of the patients responded with IFN-γ and 81% with IL 2-secretion when stimulated with the receptor. Corresponding values for healthy individuals was 7 and 8%. This T-cell stimulation was also dependent on HLA-DR and on the presence of monocytes/macrophages, indicating a conventional antigenic type of stimulation.

In a second investigation the number of cells secreting IL-4 was enumerated in patients and compared with the number of IFN-γ and IL-2 secreting cells. [11] IL-4 is typically secreted by Th2-type of cells that have a poor cytolytic activity but provide help to antibody-producing cells. IL-2 and IFN-γ are secreted in higher concentration by Th1-type of cells that have a higher cytolytic activity.[12,13,14] Forty % of the patients had a Th1 response with IL-2 and IFN-γ secretion, 46 % a Th0 or mixed response and only 9% an exclusive Th2 response.[15] Thus, these figures indicates a dominant Th1 response in most patients.

3.3. T-Cell Stimulation with Human Monoclonal Idiotypic and Anti-Idiotypic Antibodies

The specific auto antibody repertoire in MG contains not only antibodies binding directly to the acetylcholine receptor but also antibodies bearing receptor-antibody related idiotypes and anti-idiotypic antibodies against the receptor antibodies.[16,17] Interactions between idiotypic and anti-idiotypic antibodies are probably important in the regulation of the disease. Before the start of disease and in early disease there is a relatively higher concentration of anti-idiotypic antibodies than idiotypic immunoglobulins.[18] A shift from idiotype to anti-idiotype dominance is seen in patients who are recovering from MG precipitated by penicillamine treatment and in healthy children to MG mothers.[17,18,19] We therefore proceeded to examine also the T-cell recognition of idiotypes.[20,21,22] In these studies we analysed the IFN-γ, IL-2 and IL-4 secretion induced by two human monoclonal antibodies, one idiotypic and one anti-idiotypic. These monoclonal antibodies had been prepared by Epstein-Barr virus transformation and subsequent cloning of peripheral blood B-cells from patients with MG, and recognised recurrent idiotypes.[23] T-cell-stimulated to secrete one or more of the cytokines were found in 33/34 patients. These T-cell responses were MHC class 2 restricted.

According to the cytokine secretion pattern, the idiotype-reactive cells corresponded to Th1, Th2 and/or Th0-cells. The anti-idiotypic antibody, on the other hand, induced most frequently a Th1-type response. On the basis of the functional properties of T-cell subsets an interesting hypothesis can be made. Anti-idiotype reactive T-cells might regulate B cells secreting anti-idiotypic antibodies. As these anti-idiotype-reactive T-cells are predominantly of Th1 type, the interaction between these T-cells and B-cells should thus be a down regulation of, or a cytotoxic effect on the B-cells. This down regulation or killing of the B-cells that secrete anti-idiotypic antibodies will result in up regulation of the anti-acetylcholine receptor antibody secreting B-cells and consequently to a more active disease. As mentioned above, there is indirect evidence that regulatory mechanisms such as anti-idiotypic antibodies have an effect of the expression of acetylcholine receptor antibodies. These data show that a change in the clinical condition of the patient in some situations is reflected by the balance between the idiotypic and anti-idiotypic antibodies. According to our present result, T-cells with different functional properties stimulated by idiotypic and anti-idiotypic antibodies, respectively, might be an additional way by which a network is regulated.

3.4. Immune Reactivity against the β2-Adrenergic Receptor

Antibodies against the β2-adrenergic receptor are present in 18% of MG patients.[24] In a recent investigation, it was found by us that auto reactive T and B cells to β2-adrenergic receptor were present in 67% and 50%, respectively, of MG patients.[25] The β2-adrenergic receptor is present on a number of cell types, including lymphocytes and skeletal muscle cells and regulates both immune and muscle functions. Agonist stimulation increases muscle glycogenolysis [26] and decreases the concentration of plasma potassium.[27] Agonists thus increase muscle contractility [28] while antagonists may lead to muscle fatigue by decreasing the availability of energy stores, or by decreasing the uptake of K^+.[29]

The β2-adrenergic receptor on human lymphocytes represents a link between the sympathetic nervous system and the immune system. The role of the sympathetic nervous system in the modulation of immune responses is incompletely known. Some data suggest that it may be involved in antibody synthesis [30] and suppressor T-cell functions.[31] Two ways in which the immune reactivity against the β2-adrenergic receptor may influence the disease MG may thus be envisioned: affection of muscle and/ or immune functions.

To investigate the possible functional effects of this immune reactivity we have recently made an evaluation of the density and affinity of the receptors in MG. In a preliminary study we investigated the density and affinity of the β2-adrenergic receptor on peripheral blood mononuclear cells in patients with MG. Our results show that cells from these patients have a lower density of the receptor than cells from healthy individuals and from patients with other neurological disorders. The affinity of the receptor and the concentration of cAMP in the cells did not differ between the groups.

3.5. Immune Reactivity against the Pre-Synaptic Membrane Receptor

The β-bungarotoxin-binding protein, pre synaptic membrane receptor, has been suggested to be one of the auto antigens in MG along with other muscle antigens.[32] In our own study, the majority of patients had T and B-cells specific for the affinity-purified β-bungarotoxin binding protein. IFN-γ secretion was induced in 60% and IL-4 secretion in 48% of MG patients.[33] There was, moreover, a positive correlation between the numbers of T-cells stimulated by the pre synaptic membrane receptor and those stimulated by the acetylcholine receptor. If this immune reactivity can influence the course or severity of disease remains to be determined.

4. T-CELL RECEPTOR Vα/β GENE USAGE

Patients with myasthenia gravis have a bias in their usage of TCR Vα/β gene products. In order to determine the extent of V-gene heterogeneity of blood T lymphocytes in patients, we used 8 and in a later preliminary study, 12 available monoclonal antibodies against different Vα and Vβ gene products. [34] Using two-and three colour immunofluorescence methods, we could calculate the expression of α/β V segments within the CD4+ and CD8+ subsets. In the first study, 25% of the patients had T cells showing signs of abnormal expansions. In our second, preliminary study, 18% patients had CD4+ expansions, and 38% had CD8+ expansion. There was no clear restriction to certain Vα/Vβ. The phenotype of the expanded cells were mainly CD45RA and there was often an increased HLA-DR and IL-expression, indicating the activated stage of the cells. Functional studies have until now not shown any preferential auto reactivity restricted to the expanded cells.

5. EFFECTS OF IMMUNOMODULATORY TREATMENT

5.1. Thymectomy

Several lines of evidence indicate a crucial rule of the thymus in the pathogenesis of myasthenia gravis. The patients have a high prevalence of thymic abnormalities,[35] the autoantigen, the acetylcholine receptor, is expressed by thymic myoid cells and an acetylcholine receptor-like protein is expressed by thymic epithelial cells.[36,37] B-cells secreting antibodies against the receptor and T-cells that are reactive with a receptor are present in thymic tissue.[38,39] Thymectomy leads to improvement of muscle function and increases the remission rate, especially in patients with thymic hyperplasia.[40] The mechanism responsible for this improvement is unclear.

In a prospective study by my group we followed 11 patients for 3 years after thymectomy.[41] Five of them had thymus hyperplasia, 3 had thymomas and 3 had normal thymus histology. A marked improvement of muscle-function was evident in 7 of the patients one year after thymectomy and in 10 patients after 3 years. All 3 patients with thymomas deteriorated after the operation but improved after initiation of immunosupressive treatment. Only one patient with hyperplasia and 7 years duration of disease did not improve.

The numbers of PBMC cells that spontaneously secreted IFN-γ and IL-2 decreased after thymectomy. The T-cell response to disease-specific auto-antigens were investigated using affinity-purified human acetylcholine receptor and a human monoclonal anti-receptor antibody as antigens.[20,21] Before thymectomy, 73% of the patients had T-cells that responded with cytokine secretion and/or proliferation to the acetylcholine receptor. Three years after thymectomy, the corresponding figure was 18%. Also the numbers of cells secreting IFN-γ in response to acetylcholine receptor decreased after thymectomy while the frequency of T-cells reactive with the monoclonal antibody was not affected. Reactivity against this monoclonal anti-receptor antibody could thus reflect a beneficial immune response counteracting anti-receptor antibody reactivity.

Auto-reactive lymphocytes were present in thymus in eight patients. Such cells were preferentially localised to the thymus in a few patients with short duration of disease. This could explain the clinical observation that the highest remission-rate is found in patients with duration of MG less than one year, and further emphasises the importance of early thymectomy in MG.

5.2. Treatment with Anti CD4 Monoclonal Antibodies

Monoclonal antibodies against the CD4 antigen on T-cells have been effective in treatment of experimental autoimmune diseases including experimental myasthenia gravis and some human autoimmune disorders.[42,43,44] We treated a patient with myasthenia with a one-week course of a chimaeric anti-CD4 monoclonal antibody.[42] A marked clinical and electrophysiological improvement was evident on the forth day of treatment. This improvement was most pronounced during the second to eight week and was still present at the five month follow-up. A progressive deterioration started three months after initiation of treatment. There was a rapid decrease in percentage of both CD4+ and CD8+ cells. The CD4+ cells recovered very slowly and were still about 50% of pre-treatment value at the five months follow-up.

The IL-2 production from single cells and T-cell proliferation was abolished during the anti-CD4 treatment, both spontaneously and in response to the acetylcholine receptor, and the human monoclonal anti-receptor and anti-idiotypic antibodies, all of which induced T-cell-stimulation prior to treatment. During several months after completion of therapy, T-cells were spontaneously more activated than before therapy. The treatment did not induce any changes in the level of receptor antibodies in serum. Thus, this treatment induced a striking immunomodulation. These findings support that CD4+ lymphocytes play an important role in the pathogenesis of myasthenia and suggests that chimaeric anti-CD4 monoclonal antibodies could be helpful in the treatment of severe myasthenia resistant to conventional therapy.

6. T-CELL SUBTYPES IN EARLY MYASTHENIA GRAVIS

The autoantibody pattern in early myasthenia is consistently characterized by a switch from dominance of anti-idiotypic antibodies to that of idiotypic, including antibodies that bind to the receptor. In the few cases in whom it has been possible to examine serum samples taken long before the start of overt disease, there were high concentrations of anti-idiotypic and low of receptor antibodies. We therefore made a study to examine the cellular components of the idiotypic network.

The T-cell cytokine pattern was studied in six patients with myasthenia of less than four months duration. The cytokine secreting cells were enumerated in response to the auto antigens, the acetylcholine receptor, the idiotypic and anti-idiotypic antibodies. There were no differences in the number of IL-4 secreting cells, induced by either antigen. There was, however, a significant increase of the number of IFN-γ secreting cells induced by the monoclonal idiotypic antibody. These idiotype-reactive, "anti-idiotypic T cells" might presumably have the effect of down-regulating idiotypic and autoantibody-producing B cells and also T-cells reactive with the anti-idiotypic antibody. Such a down-regulation might have a beneficial effect on the disease process. Thus, also studies of the cellular arm of the idiotypic network suggests that idiotypic regulation plays a role in the development of disease.

REFERENCES

1. Lefvert AK. Human and experimental myasthenia gravis. In: Coutinho A, Kazatchine M, Wiley-Liss, Inc. Eds. Autoimmunity: Physiology and Disease. New York 1994; 267–305.
2. Åhlberg RE, Pirkanen R, Lefvert AK. Defective T lymphocyte function in nonthymectomized patients with myasthenia gravis. *Clin. Immunol. Immunopathol.* 1991; **60:** 93–105.
3. Dropcho EJ, Richman DP, Antel J, Arnason BGW. Defective mitogenic responses in myasthenia gravis and multiple sclerosis. *Ann. Neurol.* 1982; **11:** 456–462.
4. Zilko PJ, Dawkins RL, Holmes K, Witt C. Genetic control of suppressor lymphocyte function in myasthenia gravis: Relationship of impaired suppressor function to HLA-B8/DRW3 and cold reactive lymphocytotoxic antibodies. *Clin. Immunol. Immunopathol.* 1979; **14:** 222–230.
5. Mischak RP, Dau PC, Gonzales RL, Spitler LE. In vitro testing of suppressor cell activity in myasthenia gravis. In: Dau PC, Ed. Plasmapheresis and the Immunobiology of myasthenia gravis. Houghton, Boston,1979.
6. Hohlfeld R, Kalies I, Kohleisen B, Heininger K, Conti-Tronconi BM, Toyka KV. Myasthenia gravis: Stimulation of antireceptor autoantibodies by autoreactive T cell lines. *Neurology* 1986; **36:** 618–621.
7. Hohlfeld R, Toyka KV, Tzartos SJ, Carson W, Conti-Tronconi BM. Human T-helper lymphocytes in myasthenia gravis recognize the nicotinic receptor α subunit. *Proc. Natl. Acad. Sci. USA* 1987; **84:** 5379–5383.
8. Hohlfeld R, Toyka KV, Miner LL, Walgrave SL, Conti-Tronconi BM. Amphipatic segment of the nicotinic receptor alpha subunit contains epitopes recognized by T lymphocytes in myasthenia gravis. *J. Clin. Invest.* 1988; **81:** 657–660.
9. Åhlberg R, Yi Q, Eng H, Pirskanen R, Lefvert AK. T-cell epitopes on the human acetylcholine receptor α-subunit residues 10–84 in myasthenia gravis. *Scand. J. Immunol.* 1992; **36:** 435–442.
10. Yi Q, Pirskanen R, Lefvert AK. Human muscle acetylcholine receptor reactive T and B lymphocytes in the peripheral blood of patients with myasthenia gravis. *J. Neuroimmunol.* 1993; **42:** 215- 222.
11. Yi Q, Åhlberg R, Pirskanen R, Lefvert AK. Acetylcholine receptor-reactive T cells in myasthenia gravis: Evidence for the involvement of different subpopulations of T helper cells. *J. Neuroimmunol.* 1994; **50:** 177–186.
12. Romagnani S. Human T_H1 and T_H2 subsets: doubt no more. *Immunol. Today* 1991; **12:** 256–257.
13. Del Prete GF, De Carli M, Mastromauro C, *et als.*. Purified protein derivative of *Mycobacterium tuberculosis* and excretory-secretory antigen(s) of *Toxocara canis* expand in vitro human T cells with stable and opposite (type 1 T helper or type 2 T helper) profile of cytokine production. *J. Clin. Invest.* 1991; **88:** 346–350.

14. Del Prete GF, De Carli M, Ricci M, Romagnani S. Helper activity for immunoglobulin synthesis of T helper type 1 (Th1) and Th2 human T cell clones: the help of Th1 clones is limited by their cytolytic capacity. *J. Exp. Med.* 1991; **174:** 809–813.
15. Yi Q, Åhlberg R, Pirskanen R, Lefvert AK. Acetylcholine receptor-reactive T cells in myasthenia gravis: Evidence for the involvement of different subpopulations of T helper cells. *J. Neuroimmunol.* 1994; **50:** 177–186.
16. Lefvert Ak, Sundén H, Holm G. Acetylcholine receptor antibodies and anti-idiotypic antibodies produced in blood lymphocyte cultures from patients with myasthenia gravis. *Scand. J. Immunol.* 1986; **23:** 655–662.
17. Lefvert AK. Idiotypes and anti-idiotypes of human autoantibodies to the acetylcholine receptor. In: Karger S, Ed. Monographs in allergy. Basel 1987; **22:** 57–70.
18. Lefvert AK. The start of an autoimmune process: idiotypic networks during the development of myasthenia gravis. *Ann. Inst. Pasteur* 1988; **139:** 633–643.
19. Lefvert AK. Anti-idiotype antibodies in myasthenia gravis. In: Bona C, Ed. Biological applications of anti-idiotypes. CRC Press Inc, Boca Raton, Fl. 1988; **Vol IIC:** 69–91.
20. Yi Q, Åhlberg R, Lefvert AK. T cells with specificity for idiotypic determinants on human monoclonal autoantibodies in myasthenia gravis. *Res. immunol.* 1992; **143:** 149–156.
21. Yi Q, Lefvert AK. Idiotypic and anti-idiotypic T and B lymphocytes in myasthenia gravis. *J. Immunol.* 1992; **149:** 3423- 3426.
22. Yi Q, Lefvert AK. Idiotype- and anti-idiotype-reactive T lymphocytes in myasthenia gravis: Evidence for the involvement of different subpopulations of T helper lymphocytes. *J. Immunol.* 1994; **153:** 3353–3359.
23. Lefvert AK, Holm G. Idiotypic network in myasthenia gravis demonstrated by human monoclonal B-cell lines. *Scand. J. Immunol.* 1987; **26:**573.
24. Eng H, Magnusson Y, Matell G, Lefvert AK, Saponja R, Hoebeke J. β2-adrenergic receptor antibodies in myasthenia gravis. *J. Autoimmunity* 1992; **5:** 213–227.
25. Yi Q, He W, Matell G, Pirskanen R, Magnusson Y, Eng H, Lefvert AK. T and B lymphocytes reacting with the extracellular loop of the β2-adrenergic receptor (β2AR) are present in the peripheral blood of patients with myasthenia gravis. *Clin. Exp. Immunol.* 1996; **103:** 133–140.
26. Meyer SE, Stull JT. Cyclic AMP in skeletal muscle. *Ann. NY Acad.Sci.* 1971; **185:** 433–448.
27. Elfellah MS, Reid JL. The role of skeletal muscle β- adrenoreceptors in the regulation of plasma potassium. *J. Auton. Pharmac.* 1987; **7:** 175–184.
28. Marooned CD, Meadow JC. The effect of adrenaline on the contraction of human muscle. *J. Physiol.* 1970; **207:** 429–448.
29. Sjogaard G. Water and electrolyte fluxes during exercise and their relation to muscle fatigue. *Acta Physiol. Scand.* 1986; **128:** 129- 136.
30. Cross RJ, Jackson JC, Brooks WH, Sparks DL, Markesbery WR, Roszman TL. Neuroimmunomodulation: impairment of humoral immune responsiveness by 6-hydroxydopamine treatment. *Immunology* 1986; **57:** 145–152.
31. Depelchin A, Letesson JJ. Adrenaline influence on the immune response II. its effects through action on the suppressor T cells. *Immunol. Lett.* 1981; **3:** 207–213.
32. Lu C-Z, Link H, Mo X-A, *et al.*Anti-presynaptic membrane receptor antibodies in myasthenia gravis. *J. Neurol. Sci.* 1991; **102:** 39–45.
33. Yi Q, Pirskanen R, Lefvert AK. Presynaptic membrane receptor- reactive T lymphocytes in myasthenia gravis. *Scand J Immunol.* 1996; **43**: 81–87.
34. Grunewald J, Åhlberg R, Lefvert AK, DerSimonian H, Wigzell H, Jansson CH. Abnormal T cell expansion and V gene usage in myasthenia gravis patients. *Scand.J.Immunol.* 1991; **34**:161–168.
35. Castleman B. The pathology of the thymus gland in myasthenia gravis. *Ann. NY Acad. Sci.* 1966; **135:** 496–503.
36. Engel WK, Trotter JL, McFarlin DE, Mc Intosh CL. Thymic epithelial cell contains acetylcholine receptor. *Lancet* 1977; **1:** 1310–1311.
37. Kirchner T, Tzartos S, Hoppe F, Schalke B, Wekerle H, Müller- Hermelink HK. Pathogenesis of myasthenia gravis: Acetylcholine receptor-related antigenic determinants in tumor-free thymuses and thymic epithelial tumors. *Am. J. Pathol.* 1988; **130:** 268–280.
38. Vincent A, Scadding GK, Thomas HC, Newsom-Davis J. In-vitro synthesis of anti-acetylcholine-receptor antibody by thymic lymphocytes in myasthenia gravis. *Lancet* 1978; **1:** 305–307.
39. Melms A, Schalke BCG, Kirchner T, Müller-Hermelink HK, Albert E, Wekerle H. Thymus in myasthenia gravis: Isolation of T- lymphocyte lines specific for the nicotinic acetylcholine receptor from thymuses of myasthenic patients. *J. Clin. Invest.* 1988; **81**:902–908.

40. Papatestas AE, Genkins G, Kornfeld P, *et al*. Effects of thymectomy in myasthenia gravis. *Ann. Surg.* 1987; **206:** 79–88.
41. Åhlberg R, Yi Q, Pirskanen R, *et al.* The effect of thymectomy on autoreactiv T- and B- lymphocytes in myasthenia gravis. Submitted
42. Åhlberg R, Yi Q, Pirskanen R, *et al.* Treatment of myasthenia gravis with anti-CD4 antibody: Improvement correlates to decreased T-cell autoreactivity. *Neurology* 1994; **44:** 1732–1737.
43. Herzog C, Walker C, Müller W, *et al.* Anti-CD4 antibody treatment of patients with rheumatoid arthritis: 1. Effect on clinical course and circulating T cells. *J. Autoimmun.* 1989; **2:** 627–642.
44. Hiepe F, Volk H-D, Apostoloff E, von Baehr R, Emmrich F. Treatment of severe systemic lupus erythematosus with anti-CD4 monoclonal antibody. *Lancet* 1991; **338:** 1529–1530.

28

THYMOMAS EXPRESS RYANODINE RECEPTOR EPITOPES

Åse Mygland,[1] Goro Kuwajima,[2] Katsuhiko Mikoshiba,[3] Johan A. Aarli,[4] and Nils Erik Gilhus[4]

[1]Department of Neurology
Vest-Agder Central Hospital, Kristiansand, Norway
[2]Shinogi Institute for Medical Science
Osaka, Japan
[3]Tokyo University
Tokyo, Japan
[4]Department of Neurology
University of Bergen, Bergen, Norway

1. ABSTRACT

Myasthenia gravis (MG) patients with thymoma have antibodies against the Ca^{2+}release channel of striated muscle, the ryanodine receptor (RyR). Thymomas were examined for immunoreactivity with a panel of polyclonal antibodies against RyR peptides. An antibody raised against a peptide in the transmembrane segment of cardiac and skeletal muscle RyR immunostained thymoma epitehlial cells in sections of 17/23 thymomas, and detected a 40 kDa peptide in membrane fractions of thymoma. The RyR peptide was not detected in normal thymus, tonsil or carcinoma of colon. The results indicate that neoplastic thymoma cells express epitopes shared by skeletal and cardiac muscle RyR.

2. INTRODUCTION

About 50% of all thymoma patients develop myasthenia gravis (MG)[1], an autoimmune disease with fluctuating weakness of skeletal muscle. The symptoms in thymoma-associated MG as well as in non-paraneoplastic MG are mainly caused by autoantibodies to acetylcholine receptors (AChR) in the postsynaptic membrane of the neuromuscular junction. In non-paraneoplastic MG the autoimmune response is restricted to the AChR, whereas MG patients with thymoma have antibodies against various proteins in the striated muscle cell[2–5].

Epithelial Tumors of the Thymus, edited by Marx and Müller-Hermelink.
Plenum Press, New York, 1997

Among the striated muscle antibodies, those against ryanodine receptor (RyR) have the most specific relation to thymoma. RyR antibodies are restricted to about 50% of MG patients with thymoma. They have not been detected in patients with other muscular disorders or in MG patients without thymoma[2,6]. RyR is a Ca^{2+} release channel located in the region of the sarcoplasmic reticulum membrane (SR) that is in contact with T-tubular invaginations of the muscle cell surface membrane[7]. The RyR molecule consists of four homologous 564 kDa subunits around a central pore. Each subunit has a C-terminal transmembrane region and a large cytoplasmic N-terminal domain that provides contact with the T-tubule[7]. RyR plays a key role in the excitation-contraction coupling by releasing Ca^{2+} from SR as a response to depolarization of the surface membrane[8]. MG thymoma patients with RyR antibodies have a more severe course and a higher mortality than MG thymoma patients without RyR antibodies[9]. This may be due to functional effects of RyR antibodies on calcium fluxes in the striated muscle cell, or the presence of RyR antibodies may just be an innocent marker of an especially aggressive autoimmune response to muscle.

The association between striated muscle antibodies and the presence of a thymoma indicates that the autoimmmune response is related to events in the thymoma. Production of autoantibodies against protein antigens is dependent on autoreactive $CD4^+$ T lymphocytes with similar antigen specificity. In the thymus T lymphocytes are educated to be immunocompetent against foreign antigens but tolerant to self-antigens. Developing T lymphocyte clones that can recognize foreign antigens presented by thymic epithelial cells are selected for survival and expansion («positive selection»). Potentially self-reactive T lymphocyte clones that can recognize self antigens presented by other thymic stroma cells are subjected to elimination or functionally silencing («negative selection»)[10]. Thymomas consist of neoplastic epithelial cells surrounded by maturing T lymphocytes. Neoplastic epithelial cells express various muscle epitopes[11–13] that are not detected in epithelial cells of normal thymus. It is possible that developing T lymphocytes in thymoma recognize muscle epitopes presented by neoplastic epithelial cells[14] and thus are subjected to abberant positive selection resulting in survival and expansion of potentially muscle-autoreactive T lymphocytes.

In the present study we investigated the origin of RyR antibodies by examining whether neoplastic thymoma cells express RyR epitopes and thus could sensitize developing T lymphocytes.

2. MATERIALS AND METHODS

2.1. Materials

Twenty-three thymomas (lymphoepitheliomas) were analyzed. Twenty thymomas were from MG patients, and three where from patients without MG. Four of the thymomas showed local invasive growth. The neoplastic epithelial cells were classified as polygonal-cell in nine thymomas, spindle-cell in three, and mixed-cell in 11. Sera from four of the thymoma patients were availible.Two of them were anti-RyR antibody positive (MG patients) and two were anti-RyR antibody negative (non-MG patients).

Normal thymus tissue obtained during elective cardiac surgery on children aged 2–3 years, tonsillar tissue, and tissue from carcinoma of colon served as control tissues.

Table 1. Reactivity of anti-RyR peptide antibodies in Western blot with skeletal muscle RyR, cardiac muscle RyR and brain RyR

	Anti-C2[16]	Anti-C4[16]	Anti-S4[16]	Anti-S5[a]	Anti-B4[a]
RyR skeletal	+	–	+	+	–
RyR cardiac	+	+	–	–	–
RyR brain	+	+	–	–	+

[a]Data not shown

2.2. Panel of Anti-RyR Antibodies

There are three isoforms of RyR; skeletal muscle, cardiac muscle and brain RyR. The isoforms have amino acid sequence differencies in their N-terminal cytoplasmic domain, whereas the C-terminal transmembrane segment has a high degree of similarity[7,15]. The C-terminal transmembrane segment of RyR also shows extensive homolgy across species. Human and rabbit RyR exhibit complete identity in the transmembrane segment.

We prepared polyclonal antibodies against the following short peptides with amino acid sequences of rabbit RyR[7,15]: C2 (Asn4929-Arg4949) and C4 (Glu2791-Gln2810) of cardiac RyR, S4 (Ala2826-Gln2844) and S5 (Glu1367-Lys1386) of skeletal RyR and B4 (Lys2692-Gln2711) of brain RyR. The peptides were synthesized, conjugated to keyhole limpet hemocyanin and injected into rabbit as previously described[16]. The antibodies were purified by ammonium-sulphate precipitation and affinity chromatography with agarose gel conjugated with the peptides. The reactivity of the five different antibody preparations is shown in Table 1.

2.3. Immunohistochemistry

Immunostaining (ABC technique) were performed on air-dried, acetone-fixed cryostat sections (5µ) at room temperature and involved 1) blocking procedure for endogenous biotin; 2) incubation for 15 minutes with 10% normal swine serum; 3) incubation over night at 4°C with anti-RyR peptide antibody diluted to 2 µg/ml; 4) incubation for 60 minutes with biotinylated swine-antibodies against rabbit; 5) incubation for 30 minutes with peroxidase-conjugated biotin-avidin complex; 6) colour development with 3-amino-9-etyl-carbazole benzidine.

Immunofluorescence double-staining involved 1) incubation for 120 minutes with anti-C2 RyR antibody (2 µg/ml); 2) incubation for 120 minutes with a mixture of the two monoclonal anti-cytokeratin antibodies MNF116 and LP34 (Dako); 3) incubation for 30 minutes with FITC-conjugated swine antibodies to rabbit IgG; 4) incubation for 30 minutes TRITC-conjugated rabbit antibodies to mouse IgG.

2.4. Western Blots

Membrane fractions from thymoma, normal thymus and tonsil were prepared by a differential centrifugation technique[17]. The membrane fractions were electrophoresed on 4–20% SDS-polyacrylamide gradient gels and transblotted onto nitrocellulose[18]. The blots were 1) blocked for 60 minutes with 5% dry milk; 2) incubated for 120 minutes with anti-RyR peptide antibodies diluted to 0.5 µg/ml or MG serum diluted to 1:50; 3) incubated for 60 minutes with biotinylated swine antibodies to rabbit IgG; 4) incubated for 30 minutes with peroxidase-conjugated biotin-avidin complex; 5) colour developed with 4-chloro-1-naphtol or immunostained with patient serum as previously described[6].

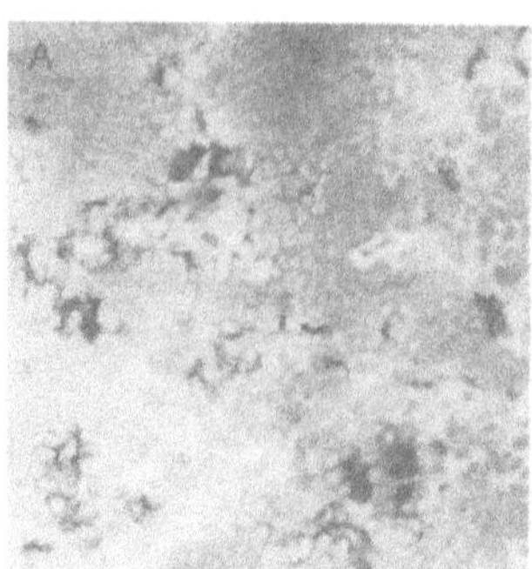

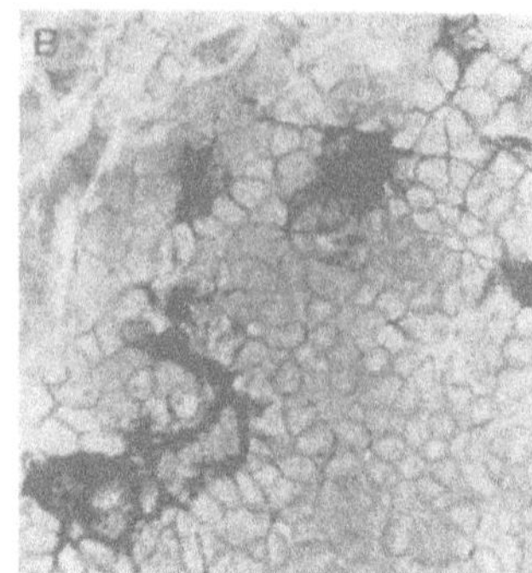

Figure 1. Immunoperoxidase staining of thymoma epitehlial cells by an antibody raised against a RyR peptide (C2) common to skeletal and cardiac muscle RyR. Magnifications: (A) x300; (B) x600.

3. RESULTS

3.1. Immunohistochemistry

The antibody against peptide C2 of RyR (anti-C2), stained sections from 17/23 thymomas (15 with MG, and 2 without MG). Anti-C2 stained scattered cells or groups of cells spread throughout the thymoma sections (Fig 1). The staining was cytoplasmic, often with an accentuation at the cell membrane. The pattern was similar with immunoperoxidase and immunofluorescence staining.

Cells stained by anti-C2 RyR antibody were also stained by anti-cytokeratin antibodies (not shown). Cells stained by anti-C2 comprised less than 25% of the anti-cytokeratin positive cells.

The staining of anti-C2 was not due to unspecific binding of IgG because control sections incubated with PBS without primary antibody were negative and no staining was seen on sections incubated with the anti-RyR peptide antibodies apart from the anti-C2 antibody.

Sections from 6/23 thymomas (5 with MG and 1 without MG) were not stained by anti-C2. Five of the anti-C2 negative thymomas were of the mixed epithelial cell type, one was polygonal cell thymoma. All the invasive thymomas were anti-C2 positive. Anti-C2 RyR antibody did not stain any cells in the sections from normal thymus, tonsils or carcinoma of colon.

The other anti-RyR peptide antibodies; anti-C4, anti-S4, anti-S5 and anti-B4, did not stain any cells in sections of the thymomas or the control tissues. Thymoma sections from the four patients with known RyR antibody status; two MG patients with circulating RyR antibodies and two non-MG patients without RyR antibodies, were all anti-C2 positive.

3.2. Western Blots

The anti-C2 RyR antibody stained a peptide in the thymoma membrane fraction. The anti-C2 reactive peptide had a molecular weight of about 40 kDa (Fig 2). Sections from the same thymoma were positive against anti-C2 in immunohistochemical studies. Anti-C2 did not stain any peptide in a similar membrane preparation from normal thymus and tonsil. The other anti-RyR peptide antibodies; anti-C4, anti-S4, anti-S5 and anti-B4,

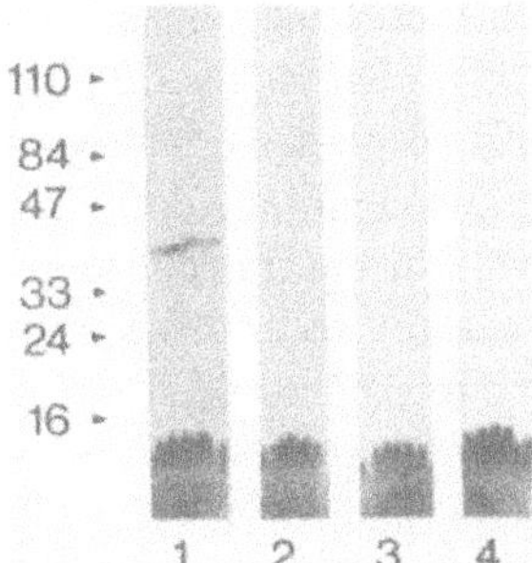

Figure 2. Western blots of membrane preparations from thymoma, normal thymus and tonsil electrophoresed on a 5–12% SDS/polyacrylamide gradient gel (100μg protein per lane). Lane 1: Anti-C2 RyR antibody raised against a peptide (C2) from the transmembrane region of RyR stains a 40kDa band in thymoma preparation. Lane 2: Thymoma preparation incubated with the anti-S5 RyR antibody. No staining. Lane 3: Normal thymus preparation incubated with anti-C2 RyR antibody. No staining. Lane 4: Tonsil preparation incubated with anti-C2 RyR antibody. No staining.

did not stain any peptide in the membrane preparation from the thymoma, nor from normal thymus or tonsil.

None of the anti-RyR antibodies stained any 564 kDa peptide in Western blots of the membrane preparations. MG patient sera containing anti-RyR antibodies did not stain the 40 kDa peptide or the 564 kDa native RyR in membrane preparations.

4. DISCUSSION

MG patients with thymoma have circulating antibodies against RyR of skeletal and cardiac muscle[2,19]. This study shows that thymomas from such patients express a RyR epitope. Anti-peptide antibodies raised against a short peptide (C2) from the C-terminal transmembrane region of RyR reacted with thymoma epithelial cells in tissue sections. The anti-C2 antibody similarly reacted with a 40 kDa protein in Western blot of thymoma membrane preparations. The 40 kDa protein is specific for neoplastic thymus, since it was not detected in normal thymus. Neither was it detected in tissue from tonsils or from carcinoma of colon. Thus, neoplastic epithelial thymoma cells seem to express a thymoma-specific protein with an epitope shared by the C-terminal transmembrane segment of RyR.

Thymoma specific RyR epitopes could be responsible for sensitization of developing T lymphocytes against RyR and subsequent stimulation of RyR specific B lymphocytes to anti-RyR antibody production. The 40 kDa thymoma specific RyR epitope was not detected by anti-RyR antibodies in sera from MG patients, but this does not exclude the possibility for cross-reactivity between thymoma and skeletal muscle RyR at T lymphocyte level.

C2 is the only one of the peptides used in this study that is common to cardiac and skeletal muscle RyR. Cardiac and skeletal muscle RyR show a high degree of sequence similarity in the C-terminal transmembrane region, where C2 is located, whereas there are more sequence differences in the N-terminal cytoplasmic domain. RyR antibodies raised by immunizing an animal with purified native RyR of one isotype does not usually cross-react with the other isotype[19,20], probably because antigen-presenting cells tend to present N-terminal cytoplasmic RyR epitopes to T lymphocytes. The RyR antibodies occurring in MG patients, however, cross-react with cardiac and skeletal muscle RyR[19]. This indicates that immunization to

RyR in MG involves special antigen-presenting cells expressing shared C-terminal epitopes, for example neoplastic thymoma cells presenting the C2 peptide.

The RyR resembles the AChR. Both are ligand-gated ion-channel proteins consisting of subunits with a C-terminal transmembrane domain and a N-terminal extra-membranous domain. AChR plays a key role in the transmission of signal from nerve to muscle cell surface membrane. RyR plays a key role in the transmission of signal from muscle cell surface membrane to cytoplasmic contractile filaments. There are limited sequence-homology between the transmembrane segments of AChR and RyR, especially between amino acid residue 4628–4861 of RyR and residue 231–301 of the AChR alpha-subunit[15]. Marx et al.[12] previously showed that thymoma epithelial cells express a 153 kDa protein with an epitope (residue 371–378) mapped to the transmembrane region of the AChR alpha-subunit. Neoplastic thymoma cells may have a specific tendency to express transmembrane epitopes of ligand-gated ion-channels.

The classification of thymomas into cortical, medullary or mixed-cell types is based on predominant phenotypical features of the neoplastic epithelial cells. However, most thymomas are heterogenous with a mixture of epithelial cells of different phenotype[21]. This may reflect that all thymoma epithelial cells are derived from a common tumor pluripotent stem cell, and that the epithelial cells are arrested at various stages of maturation. The restriction of RyR epitope expression to a small fraction of thymoma epithelial cells, may reflect that it is limited to certain stages of epithelial cell maturation.

The RyR epitope was detected in thymomas from MG patients as well as in thymomas from asymptomatic patients, and it was detected in thymomas from patients without circulating RyR antibodies. This is in agreement with previously observed similarities between mysthenic and non-myasthenic thymomas[21], and probably reflects that most thymoma patients are at risk of developing autoimmunity against striated muscle.

In conclusion, this study shows that neoplastic thymoma epithelial cells express an epitope shared by skeletal and cardiac muscle RyR. This thymoma specific epitope may be important in the development of autoimmunity against RyR in thymoma-associated MG.

REFERENCES

1. Lewis JE, Wick MR, Scheithauer BW, Bernatz PE, Taylor WF. Thymoma. A clinicopathologic review. Cancer 1987:60:2727–2743.
2. Mygland Å, Tysnes O-B, Matre R, Volpe P, Aarli JA, Gilhus NE. Ryanodine receptor autoantibodies in myasthenia gravis patients with a thymoma. Ann Neurol 1992:32:589–591.
3. Aarli JA, Stefansson K, Marton LSG, Wollmann RL. Patients with myasthenia gravis and thymoma have in their sera IgG autoantibodies against titin. Clin Exp Immunol 1990:82:284–288.
4. Gautel M, Lakey A, Barlow DP, Holmes Z, Scales S, Leonard K, Labeit S, Mygland Å, Gilhus NE, Aarli JA. Titin antibodies in myasthenia gravis; identification of a major immunogenic region of titin. Neurology 1993:43: 1581–1585.
5. Williams CL, Lennon VA. Thymic B lymphocyte clones from patients with myosin, alpha-actinin, or actin. J Exp Med 1986:164:1043–1059.
6. Mygland Å, Tysnes O-B, Aarli JA, Flood PR, Gilhus NE. Myasthenia gravis patients with a thymoma have antibodies against a high molecular weight protein in sarcoplasmic reticulum. J Neuroimmunol 1992:37:1–7.
7. Otsu K, Willard HF, Khanna VK, Zorzato F, Green NM, MacLennan DH. Molecular cloning of cDNA encoding the Ca2+ release channel (ryanodine receptor) of rabbit cardiac muscle sarcoplasmic reticulum. J Biol Chem 1990:265:13472–13483.
8. Mc Pherson PS, Campbell KP. The ryanodine receptor/Ca2+ release channel. J Biol Chem 1993:268:13765–13768.

9. Mygland Å, Aarli JA., Matre R, Gilhus NE. Ryanodine receptor antibodies related to severity of thymoma-associated myasthenia gravis. J Neurol Neurosurg Psychiat 1994:57:843–846.
10. Boyd RL, Tucek TL, Godfrey DI, Izon DJ, Wilson TJ, Davidson NJ, Bean AGD, Ladyman HM, Ritter MA, Hugo P. The thymic microenvironment. Immunol Today. 1993:14:445–459.
11. Gilhus NE, Aarli JA, Christensson B, Matre R. Rabbit antiserum to a citric acid extract of human skeletal muscle staining thymomas from myasthenia gravis patients. J Neuroimmunol 1984/85:7:55–64.
12. Marx A, O'Connor R, Geuder KI, Hoppe F, Schalke B, Tzartos S, Kalies I, Kirchner T, Müller-Hermelink, H.K. Characterization of a protein with an acetylcholine receptor epitope from myasthenia gravis-associated thymomas. Lab Invest 1990:62:279–286.
13. Dardenne M, Savino W and Bach J-F. Thymomatous epithelial cells and skeletal muscle share a common epitope defined by a monoclonal antibody. Am J Pathol 1987:126:194–198.
14. Gilhus NE, Willcox N, Harcourt G, Nagvekar N, Beeson D, Vincent A, Newsom-Davis J. Antigen presentation by thymoma epithelial cells from myasthenia gravis patients to potentially pathogenic T cells. J Neuroimmunol 1995:56:65–76.
15. Takeshima H, Nishimura S, Matsumoto T, Ishida H, Kangawa K, Minamino N, Matsuo H, Ueda M, Hanaoka M, Hirose T, Numa S. Primary structure and expression from complementary DNA of skeletal muscle ryanodine receptor. Nature 1989:339:439–445.
16. Kuwajima G, Futatsugi A, Niinobe M, Nakanishi N, Mikoshiba K. Two types of ryanodine receptors in mouse brain: skeletal muscle type exclusively in Purkinje cells and cardiac muscle type in various neurons. Neuron 1992:9:1133–1142.
17. Jones LR, Besch HR Jr, Fleming JW, McConnaughey MM, Watanabe AM. Separation of vesicles of cardiac sarcolemma from vesicles of cardiac sarcoplasmic reticulum: comparative biochemical analysis of component activities. J Biol Chem 1979 254:530–539.
18. Towbin H, Stahelin T, Gordon J. Electrophoretic transfer of proteins from polyacrylamide gels to nitrocellulose sheets: procedure and some applications. Proc Natl Acad Sci. USA 1979:76:4350–4354.
19. Mygland Å, Tysnes O-B, Matre R, Aarli JA, Gilhus NE. Anti-cardiac ryanodine receptor antibodies in thymoma-associated mysthenia gravis. Autoimmunity 1994:17:327–331.
20. Imagawa T, Takasago T, Shigekawa M. Cardiac ryanodine receptor is absent in type 1 slow skeletal muscle fibers: immunochemical and ryanodine binding studies. J Biochem 1989:342–348.
21. Willcox N, Schluep M, Ritter MA, Schuurman HJ, Newsom-Davis J, Christensson B. Myasthenic and non-myasthenic thymoma: an expansion of a minor cortical epithelial cell subset? Am J Pathol 1987:127:447–460.

29

TITIN EPITOPE IN THYMOMA

A. Wilisch,[1] A. Schultz,[1] A. Jung,[2] T. Kirchner,[2] B. Schalke,[3] K. V. Toyka,[3] V. Pallini,[4] S. Tzartos,[5] H. K. Müller-Hermelink,[1] and A. Marx[1]

[1]Institute of Pathology
University of Würzburg
[2]Institute of Pathology
University of Erlangen
[3]Department of Neurology
University of Würzburg
[4]Department of Molecular Biology
University of Siena
[5]Helenic Pasteur Institute, Athens

1. ABSTRACT

Autoantibodies against striated muscle proteins (particularly against titin), neuronal structures and the acetylcholine receptor are a hallmark of paraneoplastic Myasthenia gravis (MG). The stimulus for this autoimmunity remains enigmatic, because complete titin or nicotinic acetylcholine receptors are not found in these tumors. This study reports, that a monoclonal antibody (mAb 155) directed against the "Very Immunogenic Cytoplasmic Region" (VICE-α) of the acetylcholine receptor (α373 - 380) crossreacts with a 153 kD molecule only in cortical type thymomas. We could show by immunostaining and westernblotting that this molecule might be the medium molecular weight neurofilament NF-M. Since NF-M and titin share a common epitope, we observed that a crossreactive anti-titin antibody showed a similar staining pattern in cortical type thymomas as antibodies against NF-M and mAb 155. We suggest that one molecule, NF-M, which does contain titin and AChR epitopes and which is expressed in an inappropriate cortical environment in thymoma, might autosensitize maturing T-cells and initiate autoimmunity in patients with paraneoplastic MG against the three main autoantigen targets: AChR, titin and neuronal structures.

2. INTRODUCTION

Myasthenia gravis is an autoimmune disease which is caused by autoantibodies against the acetylcholine receptor (AChR) located at the neuromuscular junction (Oos-

Epithelial Tumors of the Thymus, edited by Marx and Müller-Hermelink.
Plenum Press, New York, 1997

terhuis, 1992). In 10 to 15 % of MG cases there is an association with a thymoma or a well-differentiated thymic carcinoma (Müller-Hermelink, 1986; Kirchner, 1992). Typical for this paraneoplastic MG is the existence of other autoantibodies. In 90% of thymoma-associated MG patients antibodies against striated muscle proteins like titin (van der Geld, 1966; Aarli, 1990; Gautel, 1993) and against neuronal structures (Marx, 1993) are found. This is not the case in non-neoplastic MG patients with thymitis.

Thymomas and well-differentiated thymic carcinomas are epithelial tumors that share morphological features with the normal thymus (Müller-Hermelink, 1986; Kirchner, 1992). They usually retain their unique thymic functions of attracting T-cells and promoting their maturation. However, it may be that in the course of these processes autoreactivity is induced (Kirchner,1992; Marx,1992).

One of the main unresolved questions is how the antigen specificity of this autoimmune reaction is induced, because neither complete AChR (Kirchner, 1988; Geuder, 1992) nor titin molecules (Marx, 1992) are expressed in these thymic epithelial tumors (TETs). A loss of self tolerance is notable in these tumors, but the responsible antigen is not yet identified.

In this study we identified a titin epitope which is aberrantly expressed in cortical-type TETs. We suggest that this abnormal expression in thymoma might trigger autoimmunity against titin.

3. MATERIALS AND METHODS

3.1. Materials

Thymic epithelial tumors (TETs) obtained on ice within 0.5 to 4 h after surgery, were studied using cryostat sections from snap frozen tissue. TETs were classified according to Müller-Hermelink and co-workers (Müller-Hermelink,1986; Kirchner,1992). Non-neoplastic thymuses were obtained from patients undergoing thoracic surgery.

Antibodies against the medium molecular weight neurofilament (NN18 and BF10) were bought from Boehringer Mannheim and the guinea pig anti-keratin antiserum was bought from Sigma. mAb 155 was kindly provided by S. Tzartos, Athens, (Tzartos, 1992) and mAb 63/15 was kindly provided by V. Pallini, Siena (Mencarelli, 1991).

3.2. Immunohistochemistry

The three step immuno-peroxidase labelling for single antigens in air-dried, acetone fixed sections was described previously (Marx, 1989)

3.3. Affinity Chromatography

A triton X-100 extract from tissue sections was prepared as described by Marx (1989). Affinity chromatography was performed using Tresyl-activated sepharose (Pharmacia) with bound monoclonal antibody 155.

3.4. Protein Extraction and Western Blotting

Detergent Triton X-100 insoluble fractions of thymoma and of control tissues were prepared from 0.5 g of snap frozen tissue or 10^7 cells following the method of Bennett (1988). Western blots were prepared as described previously (Marx,1996).

3.5. Protein Expression

pNF-M (36), a clone encoding base pairs 1374 to 2211 of the medium molecular weight neurofilament was kindly provided by I. Screpanti (Screpanti, 1989) and cloned into an expression vector (Pharmacia). Protein expression was carried out with the GST-Protein expression kit from Pharmacia according to the manufacturers instruction.

4. RESULTS AND DISCUSSION

Normal thymus and thymic epithelial tumors were analyzed using different antibodies against the AChR. While most autoantibodies react with the MIR (= *m*ain *i*mmunogenic *r*egion) of AChR, respective monoclonal antibodies label only myoid cells in the normal thymus, but not epithelial cells of thymoma. Instead mAb 155 which is directed against the VICE-alpha epitope of AChR (VICE = *v*ery *i*mmunogenic *c*ytoplasmic *e*pitope, α373 - 380), stains myoid cells and a few epithelial cells in the vicinity of Hassall's corpuscles in normal thymus and neoplastic cells in almost all cortical type thymic epithelial tumors (fig.1a,b).

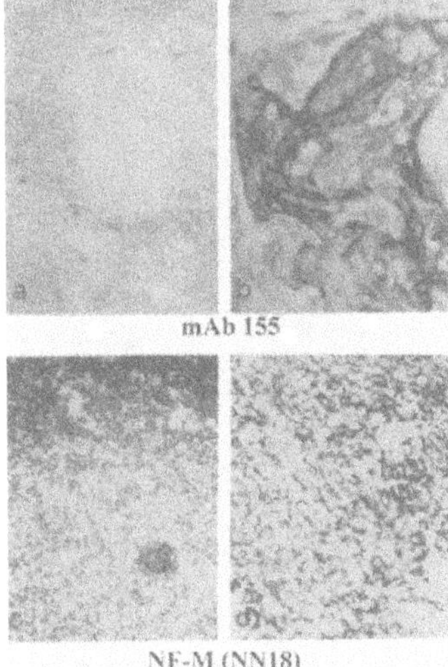

Figure 1. Expression of an AChR epitope (labeled by mAb 155) and an NF-M epitope (labeled by mAb NN18) in normal thymus and cortical thymoma.**(a.)** Faint immunoreactivity for AChR epitopes in the normal thymus in myoid cells and in single epithelial cells in the vicinity of a Hassall's corpuscle. **(b.)** Strong immunoreactivity for AChR epitopes in almost all epithelial cells in a cortical thymoma. **(c.)** weak expression of a NF-M epitope in normal thymus only around a Hassall's corpuscle. **(d)** Again strong immunoreactivity for an NF-M epitope in almost all epithelial cells in a cortical thymoma. (Immunoperoxidase, a. - b.: x 400; c. - d.: x 160).

Kirchner and co-workers found a highly significant correlation between the staining of thymic epithelial cells with mAb 155 and MG (Kirchner, 1987).

The antigen with the epitope against which mAb 155 is directed, was isolated from normal thymus and thymoma using affinity chromatography. In normal thymus a reaction of mAb 155 with the AChR alpha-subunit of myoid cells and a crossreaction with a protein of about 153 kD was detected. In thymoma, where no myoid cells can be found, we could only detect the 153 kD band representing the crossreacting antigen (fig.2).

It is known (Kirchner, 1988) from earlier observations that mAb 155 also recognizes neurons in nerve tissue. Therefore we had the idea that the 153 kD protein might be identical with the medium molecular weight neurofilament (NF-M), which has a molecular weight of about 160 kD. The fact that NF epitopes have been identified in thymomas and that antiaxonal antibodies have been found in the sera of most patients with paraneoplastic MG supported this idea (Marx, 1993).

To check this hypothesis, phosphorylation dependent (P-D, mAb BF10) and phosphorylation independent (P-I, mAb NN18) antibodies against NF-M were used for immunostaining. Using these antibodies a focal expression in single cells scattered throughout the medulla, especially around Hassall's corpuscles was observed in most normal thymuses (fig.1c). Expression was mainly detectable with P-I antibodies. Epitopes recognized by P-D antibodies were very rare and only detected in some medullary cells. The cortex was always negative for staining. It was shown by double immunostaining with an anti-keratin antibody that NF-M epitopes could only be detected in epithelial cells.

In contrast, cortical type thymomas showed much stronger expression of P-I and P-D epitopes of NF-M (fig.1d). The signal intensity was comparable for P-I and P-D antibodies. Medullary and mixed thymomas exhibited no reactivity with anti-NF-M antibodies.

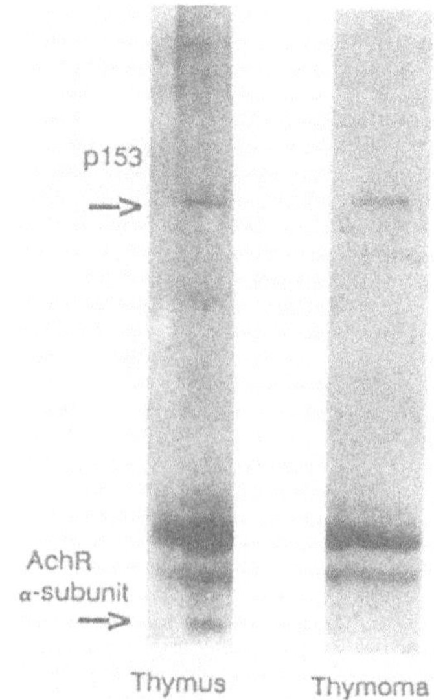

Figure 2. Identification of p153, bearing an AChR epitope, in normal thymus and thymoma using mAb 155 affinity chromatography. Westernblot with mAb 155 reveals a 153 kD band in both, normal thymus (lane 1) and thymoma (lane 2), whereas the AChR α-subunit (43 kD) is only detected in normal thymus (lane 1).

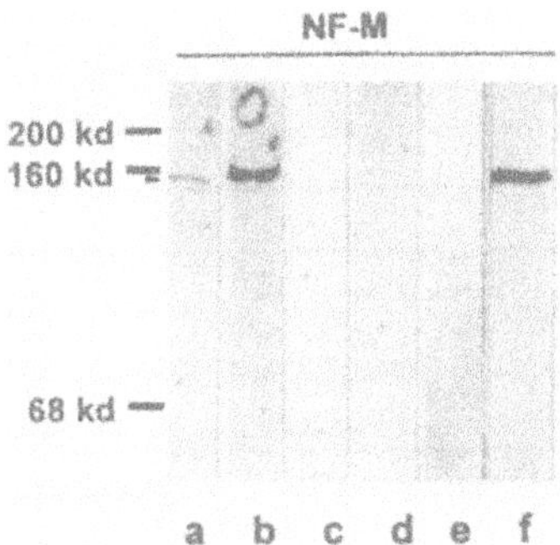

Figure 3. Detection of neurofilament NF-M in a TET by immunoblotting. Blots of cytoskeleton extracts of a well-differentiated thymic carcinoma (lane a), a mature ganglioneuroma (lane b), a squamous cell carcinoma of the lung (lane c), the cervical carcinoma cell line A 431 (lane d), normal human thymus (lane e) and a commercial preparation of bovine NF-M (lane f) were developed with anti-NF-M mAb NN18. The band in the TET extract that represents NF-M is marked with an arrowhead. The faint band at about 130 kD may represent degradation products or lymphophosphorylated NF-M.

To test whether the epitopes were expressed on authentic NF polypeptides, we checked their size and antigenicity by immunoblotting. We compared an epithelial thymoma with a mature ganglioneuroma and a commercial bovine NF preparation.

With the anti-NF-M mAb NN18 the expected 160 kD band was detected in the ganglioneuroma extract and the bovine NF, and a 153 kD band was detected in the thymoma (fig.3). This 153 kD band is typical of hypophosphorylated NF-M specifically detected by this P-I antibody. Taken together, these data demonstrate that the expression of NF-M is very similar to the expression of p153, bearing the AChR epitope, which is recognized by mAb 155. Furthermore, p153 is, like NF-M, restricted to cortical TETs.

A hallmark of thymoma-associated MG is the existence of autoantibodies against striated muscle proteins (van der Geld, 1966), particularly and most specifically against titin (Aarli, 1990, Gautel, 1993). However, titin molecules, like AChR molecules, are not expressed in cortical type epithelial tumors (Marx, 1992). Given the known occurence of epitopes shared between titin and NF-M (Shimizu, 1988), we also tested mAb 63/15 that was raised against fish titin and crossreacts with a titin epitope in neurofilament of fish (Mencarelli, 1991). This antibody also crossreacts with human skeletal muscle, thymic myoid cells and ganglion cells and binds to NF-M of human spinal cord in Western blots. Interestingly it also reacted with thymomas mainly of cortical types (fig.4a/b). Expression

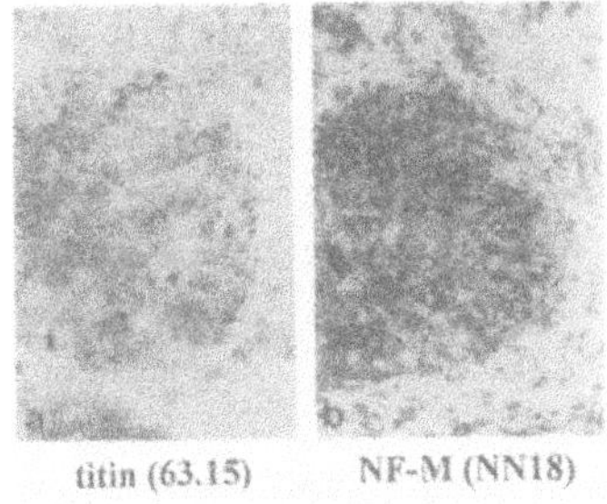

Figure 4. An epitope shared by NF-M and titin (labeled by mAb 63/15) is expressed **(a.)** in a cortical thymoma that **(b.)** stains more intensely with the anti-NF-M mAb NN18 (Immunoperoxidase, x 160).

Table 1. Expression of the medium molecular weight neurofilament NF-M (mAb NN18) and of a titin epitope (mAb 63/15) in thymic epithelial tumors of various histological subtypes

Tumor type	NF-M	Titin epitope
Medullary thymoma	none out of 3	none out of 3
Mixed thymoma	none out of 7	3 (focal) out of 7*
Cortical thymoma	7 out of 8	5 out of 8
WDTC**	7 out of 7	4 out of 7

* The detection of the titin epitope in NF-M negative thymomas is probably caused by the reaction of mAb 63/15 with high molecular neurofilament NF-H that is focally present in thymomas (Marx, 1996)
** WDTC = well differentiated thymic carcinoma

correlated well with that of NF-M epitopes and - again - with the staining pattern of mAb 155 (table 1).

To further test the hypothesis that NF-M expresses a titin and AChR epitope we performed a western blot with recombinant human NF-M that was synthesized in bacteria. In this immunoblot the antibody NN18 (directed against NF-M), mAb 155 (directed against AChR) and mAb 63/15 (directed against against titin) all recognized the recombinant human NF-M.

5. CONCLUSION

In patients with paraneoplastic MG autoantibodies against AChR, against titin and against neuronal structures are identified. However, complete AChR and titin molecules are not found in thymic epithelial tumors of these patients. Instead a neuronal protein, the medium molecular weight neurofilament NF-M, which is expressed particularly in cortical type TETs and which combines epitopes of AChR and titin in one molecule can be detected.

In cortical type thymomas but not in the normal thymus, the expression of NF-M occurs close to immature $CD1^+$ thymocytes. Therefore, there is an 'aberrant hyperexpression' of NF-M in an inappropriate microenvironment in cortical TETs that is not seen in normal thymus. We suggest that this abnormal environment and the crossreacting epitopes in NF-M trigger the autoreactivity to AChR, titin and neuronal structures.

ACKNOWLEDGMENT

We thank E. Oswald, C. Kohaut and E. Schmitt for technical support and M. Neumann for critically reading of the manuscript. This work was supported by grant Ki 370/ 1 - 3 and Ma 1484/ 2 - 1 of the DFG and by the project "Autoimmunitäts-forschung" of the BMBF to Alexander Marx and Thomas Kirchner.

REFERENCES

Aarli,JA., Stefansson,K., Marton,LSG., Wollmann,RL. (1990); Patients with Myasthenia gravis have in their sera IgG autoantibodies against titin; Clin.Exp.Immunol. 82, 284 - 288

Bennett,GS., Hollander,BA., Laskowska,D. (1988); Expression and phosphorylation of the mid-sized neurofilament protein NF-M during chick spinal chord neurogenesis; J.Neurosci.Res 21, 376 - 390

Gautel,M., Lakey,A., Barlow,DP., Holmes,Z., Scales,S., Leonard,K., Labeit,S., Mygland,A., Gilhus,NE., Aarli,JA. (1993); Titin antibodies in myasthenia gravis: identification of a major immunogenic region of titin; Neurology 43, 1581 - 1585

Geuder,KI., Marx,A., Witzemann,V., Schalke,B., Kirchner,Th., Müller-Hermelink,HK. (1992); Genomic organisation and lack of transcription of the nicotinic acetylcholine receptor subunit genes in myasthenia gravis-associated thymoma; Lab.Invest. 66, 452 - 458

Kirchner,Th., Hoppe,F., Müller-Hermelink,HK. Schalke,B., Tzartos,S. (1987); Acetylcholine receptor epitopes on epithelial cells of thymoma in myasthenia gravis; Lancet I, 218

Kirchner,Th., Tzartos,S., Hoppe,F., Schalke,B., Wekerle,H., Müller-Hermelink,HK. (1988); Acetylcholine receptor related antigenic determinants in tumor-free thymuses and thymic epithelial tumors; Am.J.Pathol. 130, 268 - 280

Kirchner,Th., Schalke,B., Buchwald,J., Ritter,M., Marx,A., Müller-Hermelink,HK.(1992); Well-differentiated thymic carcinoma; Am.J.Surg.Pathol. 16, 1153 - 1169

Marx,A., Kirchner,Th., Hoppe,F., O'Connor,R., Schalke,B., Tzartos,S., Müller-Hermelink,HK. (1989); Proteins with epitopes of the acetylcholine receptor in epithelial cell cultures of thymomas in myasthenia gravis; Am.J.Pathol. 134, 865 - 877

Marx,A., Osborn,M., Tzartos,S., Geuder,KI., Schalke,B., Nix,W., Kirchner,Th., Müller-Hermelink,HK. (1992); A striational muscle antigen and myasthenia gravis associated thymomas share an acetylcholine receptor epitope; Dev.Immunol. 2, 77 - 84

Marx,A., Kirchner,Th., Greiner,A., Schalke,B., Müller-Hermelink,HK. (1993); Myasthenia gravis-associated thymic epithelial tumors express neurofilaments and are associated with antiaxonal autoimmunity; Ann.N.Y.Acad:Sci. 681, 107 - 109

Marx,A., Wilisch,A., Schultz,A., Greiner,A., Magi,B., Pallini,V., Schalke,B., Toyka, KV., Nix,W., Kirchner,Th., Müller-Hermelink,HK. (1996); Expression of neurofilaments and of a titin-epitope in thymic epithelial tumors: Implications for the pathogenesis of myasthenia gravis; Am.J.Pathol. (148:1839–1850)

Mencarelli,C., Magi,B., Marzocchi,B., Armellini,D., Pallini,V. (1991); Evolution of the titin epitope in neurofilament proteins; Comp.Biochem.Physiol.B. 100, 741 - 744

Müller-Hermelink,HK., Marino,M., Palestro,G. (1986); Pathology of thymic epithelial tumors. The Human Thymus: Histopathology and Pathology; Current topics in Pathology Vol 75; editor HK. Müller-Hermelink, Springer Berlin, 207 - 268

Oosterhuis,HJGH., Kuks,JBM. (1992); Myasthenia gravis and myasthenic syndromes; Current Opinions Neurology Neurosurgery 5, 638–644

Screpanti,I., Meco,D., Scarpa,S., Morrone,S., Frati,L., Gulino,A., Modesti,A. (1992); Neuromedullary loop mediated by nerve growth factor and interleukin 6 in thymic stromal cell cultures; Proc.Natl.Acad.Sci. 89, 3209 - 3212

Shimizu,T., Matsumara,K., Itoh,Y., Mannen,T., Maruyama,K. (1988); An immunological homology between neurofilament and muscle elastic filament. A monoclonal antibody cross-reacts with neurofilament subunits and connectin; Biomed.Res. 9, 227 - 233

Tzartos,S., Remoundos,MS. (1992); Precise epitope mapping of monoclonal antibodoes to the cytoplasmic side of the acetylcholine receptor alpha subunit. Dissecting a potentially myasthenogenic epitope; Eur.J.Biochem. 207, 915 - 922

Van der Geld,HWR., Strauss,AJL. (1966); Immunological relationship between striated muscle and thymus; Lancet I, 57 - 60

30

ACCESSORY MOLECULE EXPRESSION IN HUMAN THYMOMAS AND THYMUS

S. Appiah-Boadu, J. A. Aarli, G. O. Skeie, and N. E. Gilhus

Department of Neurology
University of Bergen
Bergen, Norway

1. ABSTRACT

Paraneoplastic MG is probably caused by sensitisation of T-cells to muscle-like epitopes presented on the neoplastic epithelial cells. Accessory molecules on antigen-presenting cells and T-cells are important for the outcome of the immunisation process. In this study, cryostat sections from 13 thymomas (11 with MG, 2 without; 10 non-invasive, 3 invasive; 3 spindle-cell, 10 polygonal-cell thymomas) and 6 normal thymuses from children were examined for the accessory molecules ICAM-1, VCAM-1, LFA-3 and CD28 using commercially available mouse monoclonal antibodies and immunoperoxidase staining.

In the normal thymus, ICAM-1, LFA-3 and CD28 all stained the medulla stronger than the cortex. VCAM-1 was expressed sparsely but equally in both cortex and medulla.

ICAM-1 was expressed more in non-invasive than in invasive thymomas. ICAM-1 expression was independent of thymoma histology and of the presence of MG. VCAM-1 expression was strongest in our invasive polygonal-cell thymomas and weak in the non-invasive spindle-cell thymomas, as was LFA-3 expression. CD28 expression did not vary to the same extent as VCAM-1 and LFA-3 and was independent of histology and invasiveness of the thymoma and the presence of MG.

The presence of these accessory molecules in thymomas supports the idea that sensitisation against muscle-like epitopes can take place within the tumour itself.

2. INTRODUCTION

Thymomas consist of neoplastic epithelial cells mixed with non-neoplastic maturing T-cells. 10–15% of all myasthenia gravis (MG) patients have a thymoma. The incidence of MG in patients with a thymoma is 30–50% (Monden et al., 1988). MG is therefore viewed as a classical paraneoplastic disease. Paraneoplastic MG is probably caused by sensitisation of T-cells to muscle epitopes presented on the neoplastic epithelial cells. The

Epithelial Tumors of the Thymus, edited by Marx and Müller-Hermelink.
Plenum Press, New York, 1997

neoplastic epithelium maintains its capacity to induce T-cells (Gilhus et al., 1995). Striated muscle epitopes including acetylcholine receptor (AChR) epitopes have been detected in thymomas (Gilhus et al., 1984; Marx et al., 1989). Thymoma patients with MG have circulating autoantibodies against serveral muscle antigens (Mygland et al., 1992; Gautel et al., 1993; Willcox, 1995).

Normally T-cell clones that are able to react to these self antigens are eliminated or functionally depressed by clonal deletion or clonal anergy (Boyd and Hugo, 1991). In the MG thymoma, these processes are changed, and specifically so for muscle antigens.

The outcome of immune sensitisation depends on the antigen as well as the accessory or adhesion molecules present. Accessory molecules orient antigen receptors for optimal recognition. Activation, proliferation, costimulation, anergy or deletion are all accessory-molecule dependent as are cell migration, invasion, spread and recirculation (Hemler, 1992; Pignatelli and Vessey, 1994). Accesory molecules may thus be important for the outcome of the immunisation against self muscle epitopes within a thymoma, determining MG or no MG.

We have examined human thymomas for the presence of the accessory molecules ICAM-1, VCAM-1, LFA-3 and CD28, looking for patterns related to presence of MG, tumour invasiveness and histology.

3. MATERIAL AND METHOD

Fresh thymomas were obtained during surgery, immediately divided into pieces, mounted on blocks and frozen in liquid nitrogen. They were then stored at -80°. 5um sections were made from the mounted blocks, acetone-fixed for 10 minutes, air dried for 24 hours, acetone-fixed for another 10 minutes and air-dried for 24 hours. They were then wrapped up in aluminium foil and kept at -80°C until staining.

Sections from 13 thymomas were examined, 6 of them kindly provided by Dr. Nick Willcox, Oxford. Patient age range at the time of thymectomy was 17–78 years. 11 of the thymomas were associated with MG, 2 were not. 3 thymomas were macro- and microscopically invasive and 10 non-invasive. 3 thymomas were histologically of the spindle-cell type and 10 of the polygonal-cell type. 6 fresh-frozen normal thymus samples were obtained as controls, from heart patients at age range 1–5 years.

Frozen sections were defrosted at room temperature and then rinsed in phosphate-buffered saline pH 7.4 (PBS) for 5 minutes. Sections were then washed in a solution of 0.3% H_2O_2 in PBS for 5 minutes and rinsed in PBS for 10 minutes.

To prevent endogenous biotin from binding to avidin-biotin system reagents, the sections were incubated for 15 minutes at room temperature with avidin D solution (Blocking Kit: Vector Lab.; Burlingame, CA, USA), rinsed in PBS for 15 minutes, incubated in biotin-blocking solution (Blocking Kit: Vector Lab.) for 15 minutes and rinsed in PBS for another 15 minutes.

The sections were incubated for 15 minutes at room temperature with normal rabbit serum and washed to avoid non-specific binding of the biotinylated rabbit anti-mouse IgG secondary antibody.

The sections were then incubated with the primary mouse monoclonal IgG antibodies listed in table 1, at 4°C over night and then rinsed in PBS for 5 minutes. Sections were then incubated with biotinylated anti-mouse IgG (E354; DAKO, Glostrup, Denmark) for 30 minutes and rinsed in PBS for 5 minutes.

Table 1. Antibodies used for antigen examination of thymus and thymomas

Antibody	Antigen	Source
6.5B5; M7063	ICAM-1	DAKO; Glostrup, Denmark
1G11B1	VCAM-1	Monosan; Uden, The Netherlands
AICD58.9	LFA-3	Boehringer Mannheim; Mannheim, Germany
antileu 28	CD28	Becton Dickinson; San Jose, CA
LP34; M717	cytokeratin	DAKO
B2-TP3b	CD3	Monosan

Avidin-biotinyl peroxidase complex solution was made by mixing avidin (DAKO), biotinylated horseradish peroxidase (DAKO), and PBS in the volume ratio 1:1:125. The sections were incubated with the complex for 45 minutes and then washed.

Colour was developed in a solution of 10 mg 3-amino-9-etyl-carbaxol in 6 ml dimethyl sulphoxide mixed with 50 ml 0.02 M NaAc pH 5.5 and 4 ul 30% H_2O_2 for 15 minutes, washed and counter-stained with hematoxyline before mounting.

4. RESULTS

4.1. Normal Thymus

Thymus epithelial cells were stained along the cell surface by the anti-cytokeratin antibody, especially in the medulla and subcapsular region, forming a network in the medulla. Hassall's corpuscles were stained.

Anti-CD3 strongly stained the membrane of many medullary thymocytes and fewer cortical thymocytes. Hassall's corpuscles were not stained.

Anti-ICAM-1 stained many cells in the medulla, few in the cortex. The intensity of the staining was also greater in the medulla. Anti-ICAM-1 stained Hassall's corpuscles and peri vascular cells in the medulla. The anti-ICAM-1 and anti-cytokeratin antibodies stained the same cells.

Anti-VCAM-1 staining was sparse both in the cortex and the medulla. Very few cells were stained, and neither intensity nor proportion of positive cells differed in cortex and medulla. Anti-VCAM-1 positive cells varied in morphology. The cells were neither typical epithelial nor T cells according to the morphology and to the distribution of the cytokeratin and CD3 stained cells.

Anti-LFA-3 intensely stained many cells in the medulla whereas staining was almost undetectable in the cortex. LFA-3 stained the cell surface. The anti-LFA-3 staining did not form any network. Hassall's corpuscles were negative or faintly stained. The stained cells were epithelial in morphology and distribution.

Anti-CD28 strongly stained many cells in the medulla. Few cells were weakly stained in the cortex. Anti-CD28 did not stain Hassall's corpuscles. Staining was seen along the cell surface of rounded cells without strands, identical to CD-3 positive lymphoid cells.

4.2. Thymomas

4.2.1. Anti-Cytokeratin and Anti-CD3. Anti-cytokeratin stained as intensely in the thymomas as in the normal thymic medulla. The stained cells were often big, some with

Table 2. Expression of accessory molecules in thymomas and normal thymus

	ICAM-1	VCAM-1	LFA-3	CD28
Thymomas	++(+)	0 – +++	0 – +++	+ – +++
Normal thymus	+	+	++(+)	+++

stellate-like cytoplasm forming a network. Anti-cytokeratin did not stain one polygonal, non-invasive thymoma from a MG patient thymectomised 17 years old. Otherwise cytokeratin staining showed little variation in intensity and distribution among the thymomas.

Anti-CD3 staining intensity and number of stained cells varied much more among the thymomas than among the normal thymuses. The anti-CD3 staining pattern was not related to the presence of MG, thymoma invasiveness and histology.

4.2.2. Anti-Icam-1. Anti-ICAM-1 stained the thymomas similarly to the normal thymus medulla, both regarding proportion of positive cells and staining intensity (table 2). The cells were stained along the surface forming a network. Many of the positive cells in the polygonal-cell thymomas had strands. Anti-ICAM-1 staining was found in all thymomas but on more cells and was more intense in the non-invasive ones (table 3). The expression of ICAM-1 did not differ in patients with or without MG nor according to histology.

4.2.3. Anti-VCAM-1. Anti-VCAM-1 staining of the thymomas varied from intense to undetectable (table 2). It was detected in only 1 of the 3 spindle-cell thymomas but in all polygonal-cell thymomas. Anti-VCAM-1 stained more intensely and also many more cells in sections of the 2 invasive polygonal-cell thymomas than in the non-invasive polygonal-cell thymomas and also more than in the normal thymus cortex and medulla (tables 2 and 3). Where expressed, VCAM-1 was seen on scattered cells not forming any network and with varied morphology. Mainly membrane but also weak cytoplasmic staining was seen. Anti-VCAM-1 staining did not differ in thymomas from patients with or without MG.

4.2.4. Anti-LFA-3. Anti-LFA-3 staining varied greatly among the thymomas both in intensity and in proportion of stained cells (table 2). Anti-LFA-3 staining occurred mainly on the surface of the epithelial cells. The 2 spindle-cell thymomas that did not stain for anti-VCAM-1 did not stain for anti-LFA-3 either (table 3). The staining intensity and distribution was not related to the presence of MG or thymoma invasiveness.

Table 3. Expression of ICAM-1, VCAM-1, and LFA-3 in thymomas according to invasiveness and histology respectively

Molecule	Non-invasive	Invasive	Polygonal-cell	Spindle-cell
ICAM-1	+++	+	++(+)	++(+)
VCAM-1	+(+)*	+++*	++(+)	0 – ++
LFA-3	+	+	+	0 – ++

*Only in polygonal-cell thymomas

4.2.5. Anti-CD28. Anti-CD28 staining intensity and number of stained cells varied among the thymomas but not as much as for LFA-3 and VCAM-1 staining (table 2). Most thymomas stained weaker than normal thymus medulla. Weak anti-CD28 staining tended to correspond to weak staining of anti-CD3. Most of the stained cells had big nuclei with scant cytoplasm, uniform size and shape. Anti-CD28 staining occurred mainly on the cell surface. The anti-CD28 staining was independent of MG, invasiveness and histology.

5. DISCUSSION

This study shows the presence of the accessory molecules ICAM-1 and LFA-3 on thymoma epithelial cells, VCAM-1 on accessory cells and CD28 on lymphoid cells within the tumours. ICAM-1 was expressed strongly in all thymomas. Only 1 of the 3 spindle-cell thymomas expressed VCAM-1 and LFA-3 whereas all the polygonal-cell thymomas did so. Spindle-cell thymomas are much more rarely associated with MG (Monden et al., 1988) and also seldom grow invasively (Kuo and Lo, 1993; Quintanilla-Martinez et al., 1993). These differences may be due to differences in the expression of accessory molecules as shown here.

ICAM-1, LFA-3 and CD28 were all expressed to a greater extent in the normal thymus medulla than in the cortex whereas VCAM-1 was equally expressed in both cortex and medulla as has also been previosly reported (Marx et al., 1994). ICAM-1/LFA-1 has been implicated in clonal deletion or negative selection (Pircher et al., 1992) whilst CD28/B7(BB1) has been linked to clonal selection, deletion (Turka et al., 1991) and anergy (Harding et al., 1992). The functional importance of LFA-3/CD2 and VCAM-1/VLA-4 in the normal thymus has still not been clearly defined. All these accessory molecules that are present in the normal thymus are also present in the thymomas. From this, it is tempting to assume that normal thymus functions, such as selection and deletion of T-cell clones also take place in the thymomas.

There was no obvious differences in expression of the accessory molecules between thymomas from patients with MG and the two thymomas from patients without MG. Two spindle-cell thymomas did not stain for VCAM-1 and LFA-3 and one of the two was from a non-MG patient. However low numbers prohibit general conclusions.

The initiating autoimmunisation is believed to take place in the thymoma. MG thymomas contain a higher number of AChR-specific T-cells than hyperplastic and normal thymus (Sommer et al., 1990). AChR and other striated muscle antigens are present in the thymomas (Gilhus et al., 1984; Marx et al., 1989). Cultured thymic epithelial cells are able to present antigens to specific T-cells (Gilhus et al., 1995). This interaction between neoplastic epithelial cells and T-cells is accessory molecule dependent as the T-cell proliferation was blocked almost completely by anti-LFA-3, but marginally increased by anti-ICAM-1 and anti-CD28. Therefore the presence of these accessory molecules in the thymomas, and especially the presence of LFA-3, may be crucial for the interaction between the neoplastic epithelial cells and T-cells. We do not know why one MG associated thymoma did not express LFA-3 (and VCAM-1). Maybe the expression in some thymomas differs markedly in various areas. It is also possible that accessory molecule expression can fluctuate over years. The primary sensitisation in MG can occur many years before the debut of overt clinical symptoms which in our patient lead to the thymectomy (Namba et al., 1978).

Invasive thymomas expressed less ICAM-1 but more VCAM-1 than non-invasive ones. Such differences in adhesion molecule expression may be a causative factor for tumour invasiveness and spread (Weiss, 1994; Tang and Honn, 1994).

In conclusion, this study supports the idea of the thymoma as the focus for the primary autoimmune sensitisation in MG, and it also points to a possible role for accessory cell surface molecules in the invasive growth of thymic epithelial tumours.

6. ACKNOWLEDGMENT

Samuel Appiah-Boadu receives a student research scholarship from the Norwegian Cancer Society.

7. REFERENCES

Boyd RL, Hugo P. Towards an integrated view of thymopoiesis. Immunol Today. 1991;12(2):71–9.

Gautel M, Lakey A, Barlow DP, Holmes Z, Scales S, Leonard K, Labeit S, Mygland A, Gilhus NE, Aarli JA. Titin antibodies in myasthenia gravis: identification of a major immunogenic region of titin. Neurology. 1993;43(8):1581–5.

Gilhus NE, Aarli JA, Christensson B, Matre R. Rabbit antiserum to a citric acid extract of human skeletal muscle staining thymomas from myasthenia gravis patients. J Neuroimmunol. 1984;7(1):55–64.

Gilhus NE, Willcox N, Harcourt G, Nagvekar N, Beeson D, Vincent A, Newsom-Davis J. Antigen presentation by thymoma epithelial cells from myasthenia gravis patients to potentially pathogenic T cells. J Neuroimmunol. 1995;56(1):65–76.

Harding FA, McArthur JG, Gross JA, Raulet DH, Allison JP. CD28-mediated signalling co-stimulates murine T cells and prevents induction of anergy in T-cell clones. Nature. 1992;356(6370):607–9.

Hemler ME. Adhesion molecules. In; Encyclopedia of Immunology Ivan M. Roitt (ed.) London: Academic Press, 1992. Vol.1, 22–26

Kuo TT, Lo SK. Thymoma: a study of the pathologic classification of 71 cases with evaluation of the Muller-Hermelink system [published erratum appears in Hum Pathol 1993 Oct;24(10):1152] Hum Pathol. 1993;24(7):766–71.

Marx A, Kirchner T, Hoppe F, O'Connor R, Schalke B, Tzartos S, Muller-Hermelink HK. Proteins with epitopes of the acetylcholine receptor in epithelial cell cultures of thymomas in myasthenia gravis. Am J Pathol. 1989;134(4):865–77.

Marx A, Schomig D, Schultz A, Gattenlohner S, Jung A, Kirchner T, Melms A, Muller-Hermelink HK. Distribution of molecules mediating thymocyte-stroma-interactions in human thymus, thymitis and thymic epithelial tumors. Thymus. 1994;23(2):83–93.

Monden Y, Uyama T, Taniki T, Hashimoto J, Fujii Y, Nakahara K, Kawashima Y, Masaoka A. The characteristics of thymoma with myasthenia gravis: a 28-year experience. J Surg Oncol. 1988;38(3):151–4.

Mygland A, Tysnes OB, Matre R, Volpe P, Aarli JA, Gilhus NE. Ryanodine receptor autoantibodies in myasthenia gravis patients with a thymoma. Ann Neurol. 1992;32(4):589–91.

Namba T, Brunner NG, Grob D. Myasthenia gravis in patients with thymoma, with particular reference to onset after thymectomy. Medicine. 1978;57(5):411–33.

Pignatelli M, Vessey CJ. Adhesion molecules: novel molecular tools in tumor pathology. Hum Pathol. 1994;25(9):849–56

Pircher H, Muller KP, Kyewski BA, Hengartner H. Thymocytes can tolerize thymocytes by clonal deletion in vitro. Int Immunol. 1992;4(9):1065–9.

Quintanilla-Martinez L, Wilkins EW Jr, Ferry JA, Harris NL. Thymoma—morphologic subclassification correlates with invasiveness and immunohistologic features: a study of 122 cases. Hum Pathol. 1993;24(9):958–69.

Sommer N, Willcox N, Harcourt GC, Newsom Davis J. Myasthenic thymus and thymoma are selectively enriched in acetylcholine receptor-reactive T cells. Ann Neurol. 1990;28(3):312–9.

Tang DG, Honn KV. Adhesion molecules and tumor metastasis: an update. Invasion Metastasis. 1994–95;14(1–6):109–22.

Turka LA, Linsley PS, Paine R 3d, Schieven GL, Thompson GB, Ledbetter JA. Signal transduction via CD4, CD8, and CD28 in mature and immature thymocytes. Implications for thymic selection. J Immunol. 1991;146(5):1428–36.

Weiss L. Cell adhesion molecules: a critical examination of their role in metastasis. Invasion Metastasis. 1994–95;14(1–6):192–7.

Willcox-N. Myasthenia gravis. Curr Opin Immunol. 1993;5(6): 910–7.

31

CD40-EXPRESSION IN THYMOMA

A. Schultz,[1] A. Greiner,[1] R. Nenninger,[1] D. Schömig,[1] A. Wilisch,[1] E. Oswald,[1] R. A. Kroczek,[2] B. Schalke,[3] H. K. Müller-Hermelink,[1] and A. Marx[1]

[1]Institute of Pathology
University of Würzburg
[2]Robert-Koch-Institute, Berlin
[3]Department of Neurology
University of Würzburg

1. ABSTRACT

Overexpression of CD40 on neoplastic epithelium has been found in most Myasthenia gravis (MG) associated thymoma. Whether CD40 is functionally expressed in thymoma and is involved in the generation of autoimmunity, has not been elucidated. To check the function of CD40, the proliferation of thymic epithelial cells (TEC) was induced by triggering the cells with soluble CD40 ligand. No difference between normal and neoplastic TEC was detected. IFN-γ could not modulate the CD40-dependent proliferation. In contrast IL-4 blocked the proliferative response of epithelial cells from normal thymus and cortical thymoma, but not from medullary thymoma. Since CD40/CD40 ligand interaction has been implicated in negative selection of immature T-cells, we compared the number of positively selected (immature) double positive $CD69^+$ thymocytes with the number of (mature) single positive $CD69^+$ cells, which are thought to have escaped negative selection. The ratio of mature to immature thymocytes was markedly reduced in thymoma. One explanation might be an enhanced deletion of positively selected thymocytes. Our results demonstrated, that CD40 is functionally expressed on normal and neoplastic epithelial cells *in vitro*. The data suggest, that maturation of autoaggressive T-cells in paraneoplastic MG is probably not caused by an unspecific inefficiency of negative selection.

2. INTRODUCTION

The thymic microenviroment is essential for T-cell development and maturation. On the one hand thymocytes are dependent on signals provided by the stroma, on the other hand signals from the lymphocytes are necessary for the survival of the stroma cells (Rit-

Epithelial Tumors of the Thymus, edited by Marx and Müller-Hermelink.
Plenum Press, New York, 1997

ter M.A. et al., 1993). Thymocytes and stroma cells interact via direct cell-cell-contact or soluble molecules. Recently, CD40/CD40 ligand interaction was found to be a candidate to guide such a cross-talk. CD40 is expressed on B-cells, monocytes, dendritic cells, T-cells and thymic epithelial cells. CD40L is mainly expressed on T-cell subsets. Functionally, CD40 was described as B-cell proliferation and maturation factor in conjunction with IL-4 (Clark E.A. et al., 1986). Stimulation of TEC with anti-CD40 antibody in addition to IL-1 and IFN-γ leads to enhanced GM-CSF secretion (Galy A.M. 1992). CD40 as well as CD40 ligand can provide a T-cell costimulatory signal: when triggering T-cells with anti-CD3 antibodies or suboptimal concentrations of Phytohemagglutinin (PHA) the proliferation, interleukine production and expression of activation markers could be enhanced by additional CD40 or CD40 ligand stimulation (Armitage R.J. et al., 1993, I; Cayabya M. et al., 1994).

The essential role of CD40/CD40 ligand in negative selection of thymocytes was analysed by Foy et al. (1995). They demonstrated the dependence of negative selection on CD40 ligand costimulation. So far it has not been elucidated, whether CD40L is involved in the generation of autoimmunity. As we report here, overexpression of CD40 on neoplastic epithelium is found in most Myasthenia gravis-associated thymoma. The aim of our studies was first to investigate whether CD40 is functional on normal and neoplastic TEC and second to analyse whether negative selection might be different in thymoma compared to normal thymus.

3. MATERIAL AND METHODS

3.1. Patients and Tumors

The clinical data of the patients are given in table 1. Tumors were classified according to Müller-Hermelink et al. (1994).

Normal thymuses (n = 5) were obtained from patients undergoing cardiothoracic surgery (age 0 - 58).

3.2. Immunohistochemistry

Cryostat sections of normal thymuses, cortical and medullary thymoma were immunohistochemically investigated by applying a standard immunoperoxidase technique (Marx A. et al. 1996). The monoclonal antibody anti-CD40 (mAb 89) was kindly provided by J. Banchereau, Dardilly, France and the anti-CD40 ligand (TRAP) by R. H. Kroczek, Berlin, Germany.

3.3. Cell Preparation and Culture

Thymocytes were prepared from thymus or thymoma by passing minced tissue through a stainless steel sieve. The lymphocytes were isolated by Ficoll-hypaque density gradient centrifugation. Lymphocytes form tonsils were prepared in the same way. The B-cells were isolated by depletion using directly conjugated anti-CD3 and anti-CD14 magnetic beads (Dynal). The cells were analysed by FACS to guaranted more than 97 % $CD19^+$ B-cells.

TEC and fibroblasts were isolated from five normal thymuses, two cortical and one medullary thymoma as described previously (Marx A. et al. 1989). For the cultivation of

Table 1. Clinical data of patients and tumors investigated in this study

Case	Age (years)	Sex	MG*	Histologial diagnosis
3028/93	83	m	–	MDT
1006/95	73	f	NA	MDT
14839/95	56	m	–	MXT
17821/94	37	f	NA	MXT
24864/95	75	f	+	MXT
2306/91	42	m	+	MXT
11688/89	69	f	+	MXT
29117/86	64	f	+	MXT
5697/88	53	f	+	CT
2516/95	48	m	NA	CT
3792/95	59	m	NA	CT
15173/94	58	m	+	CT
4858/95	61	m	+	CT
6942/88	50	m	+	CT
15977/87	76	f	+	CT
16204/95	61	f	NA	WDTC
13562/95	30	m	+	WDTC
H1942/91	78	f	NA	WDTC
22401/88	63	f	+	WDTC
2080/92	71	m	+	WDTC
12830/92	63	m	+	WDTC

NA, not available
MDT, medullary thymoma; MXT, mixed thymoma; CT, cortical thymoma
WDTC, well differentiated thymic carcinoma
m, male; f, female
* Absence (–) or presence (+) of MG

epithelial cells DMEM/HAM's F12 (3 parts DMEM plus 1 part HAM's F12) supplemented with 10% (v/v) FCS, 2 mM Glutamine, 100 IU/ml Penicillin and 100 IU/ml Streptomycin, 5 μg/ml Transferrin, 5 μg/ml Insulin, 2 x 10^{-9} M Triiodothyronine, 10^{-10} M Choleratoxin, 0,4 μg/ml Hydrocortisone and 20 ng/ml EGF (Sigma) was used. Fibroblasts were grown in DMEM supplemented with 10% (v/v) FCS, 2 mM Glutamine, 100 IU/ml Penicillin and 100 IU/ml Streptomycin. The cell cultures were analysed by FACS using a monoclonal antibody anti-cytokeratin. More than 95% of the epithelial cell lines and less than 3% of the fibroblast cell lines express cytokeratin.

3.4. Proliferation Assay

The thymic stroma cells were transferred into 96-well flat bottom plates. Cell numbers (5 x 10^3 – 2 x 10^4/well) were chosen to achieve near confluence of cells. 12 hours after plating, the standard medium was removed and replaced by fresh medium without serum. 3 hours later the medium was again removed and the cells received serum-free medium supplemented with the reagents to be tested.

Purified B-cells (5 x 10^4/well) were cultured in RPMI 1640 supplemented with 1% gentamycin, 10% FCS and 50μg/ml transferrin (Sigma, St.Louis, MO). For activation, B-cells were cultured in the presence of reagents which should to be analysed. The soluble

CD40 ligand, the vector control and the anti-CD40 ligand antibody (TRAP) were a gift from R.A. Kroczek. INF-γ was ordered by Sigma and recombinant human IL-4 was kindly provided by W. Sebald, Würzburg, Germany. After 3 days cells were pulsed with 5 μCi ^{3}H-thymidin/ml for 5 hours, harvested and counted. During the whole assay the cells were cultivated at 37°C and 5% CO_2 .

3.5. FACS Analysis

For three colour FACS analysis a direct immunofluorescence staining of cell surfaces and a single colour FACS analysis of intracellular markers was performed as described by Becton Dickinson. For each staining 2 x 10^5 cells were used. The following antibodies were obtained from Becton Dickinson: anti-CD69 (clone Leu-23, FITC-labeled), anti-CD8 (clone Leu-2b, PE-labeled), anti-CD54 (clone Leu-54, FITC-labeled) and anti-cytokeratin (clone cam 5.2, FITC-labeled). Isotype controls and anti-CD4 (clone Q4120, Quantum-Red-labeled) were supplied by Sigma. The antibody anti-CD8 (clone B9.11, FITC-labeled) was obtained from Dianova and anti- CD25 (clone ACT-1, PE-labeled) and anti-CD19 (clone HD37, FITC-labeled) were ordered from Dako. Data sampling and analysis were performed on a Becton Dickinson FACScan flow cytometer equiped with a 15-mW air-colled 488 nm Argon-ion laser. Data were analysed and histogramms generated using the Lysis II software (Becton Dickinson)

3.6. Semiquantitative RT-PCR

The snap frozen tissue of two normal thymuses, three cortical, two mixed and two medullary thymoma were analysed by RT-PCR as described previously (Marx A. et al. 1996). The sequences of the used oligonucleotide primers were:

CD40 ligand-oligonucleotides	forward: cag tgg gct gaa aaa gga tac reverse: gac aaa cac cga agc acc tgg
GAPDH-oligonucleotides	forward: tga agg tcg gag tca acg gat ttg gt reverse: cat gtg ggc cat gag gtc cac cac

Amplification were carried out at 60°C, 30 cycles for CD40 ligand primer and 60°C, 25 cycles for GAPDH primers. The amplification of the "house keeping gene" GAPDH was used to quantify the amounts of mRNA as described by Huettner et al. (1995)

4. RESULTS

4.1. Expression of CD40 and CD40 Ligand in Normal Thymus and Thymoma

In the normal thymus CD40 was strongly expressed in the medulla but only low expression was detected in the cortex. In contrast, the CD40 expression in medullary and cortical thymoma was much higher than expression in the normal thymic cortex and resembled the expression in the normal medulla. (Tab. 2, Fig. 1). By cytological criteria CD40 seems to be mainly expressed on epithelial cells in thymoma. CD40 ligand could not be detected in thymus or thymoma by immunohistochemistry or FACS analyses (Data

Table 2. Expression of CD40 in thymic epithelial tumors

Case	Histological diagnosis*	CD40 expression**
3028/93	MDT	+++
1006/95	MDT	++++
24864/95	MXT	+++
2306/91	MXT	+++
11688/89	MXT	+++
29117/86	MXT	+++
6942/88	CT	++
15977/87	CT	+++
H1942/91	WDTC	+++
22401/88	WDTC	++
2080/92	WDTC	++
12830/92	WDTC	+++

*MDT, medullary thymoma; MXT, mixed thymoma; CT cortical thymoma; WDTC, well differentiated thymic carcinoma

**CD40 expression in thymoma was estimated according to the expression of CD40 in the medulla (+++) and cortex (+) of normal thymus (n=5)

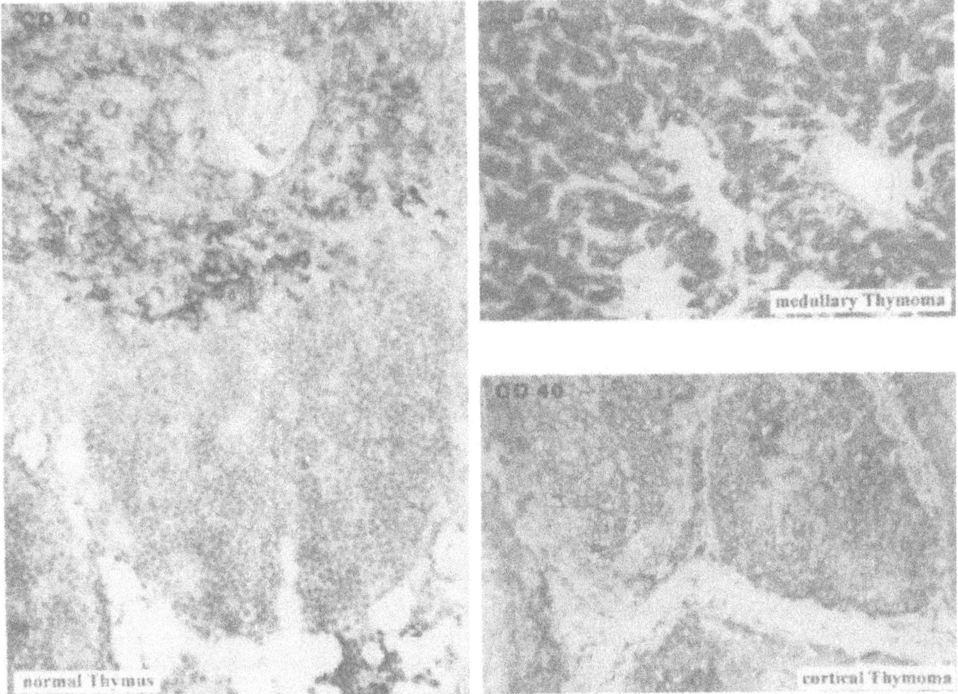

Figure 1. Immunohistochemistry of normal thymus, cortical and medullary thymoma. Expression of CD40 in the normal thymus is strong in the medulla, but faint in the cortex. In cortical and medullary thymoma CD40 is over-expressed. (Immunoperoxidase, X125.)

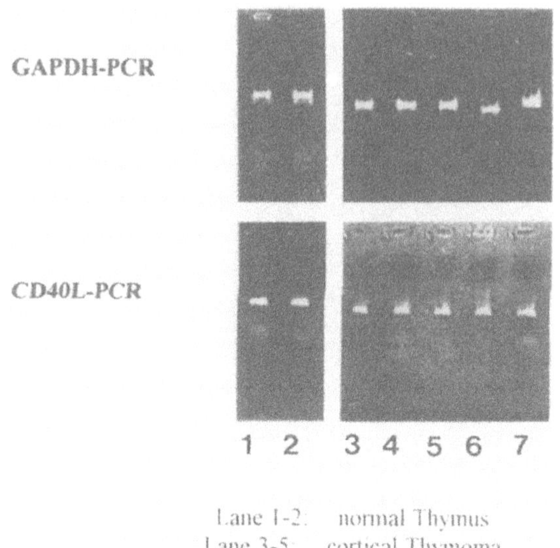

Figure 2. Detection of CD40 ligand specific mRNA in normal thymus and thymoma by RT-PCR. Expression of CD40 ligand gene and GAPDH gene as a control in normal thymus (lane 1–2), cortical thymoma (lane 3–5).

not shown). To investigate whether the CD40 ligand expression might be too low in thymus and thymoma to be detected, a semiquantitative RT-PCR was performed. RNA from two normal thymuses, three cortical and two medullary thymoma were isolated and the expression of CD40 ligand specific mRNA was analysed. In all samples CD40 ligand specific mRNA could be detected (Fig. 2). By this approach expression was reduced in thymoma compared to normal thymus, but cortical and medullary thymoma exhibited similar quantities of CD40 ligand mRNA.

4.2. The CD40-Specific Proliferation of TEC and Modulation by IFN-γ and IL-4

The CD40-dependent proliferation of TEC was tested and compared with fibroblasts and B-cells as negative and positive control, respectively. Thymic epithelial cells and B-cells proliferated after stimulation with soluble CD40 ligand. There was no difference between epithelial cells from normal thymus and from cortical and medullary thymoma. Fibroblast proliferation could not be achieved by solube CD40 ligand (Fig. 3). The proliferation of TEC and B-cells could be blocked by the CD40 ligand specific antibody TRAP (Data not shown).

To check the influence of cytokines on the CD40-dependent proliferation we tested IFN-γ and IL-4 in conjunction with soluble CD40 ligand. IFN-γ did not modulate the proliferation of epithelial cells neither in combination with CD40 ligand nor without (data not shown). B-cell proliferation could be stimulated by IL-4 or by CD40 ligand alone and could be enhanced by stimulation with soluble CD40 ligand in conjunction with IL-4. By contrast IL-4 alone could not stimulate normal or neoplastic TEC. Interestingly the CD40-specific proliferation of epithelial cells from normal thymus and cortical thymoma was reduced by IL-4 (Fig. 4). The proliferation of medullary thymoma epithelial cells was not modulated by IL-4.

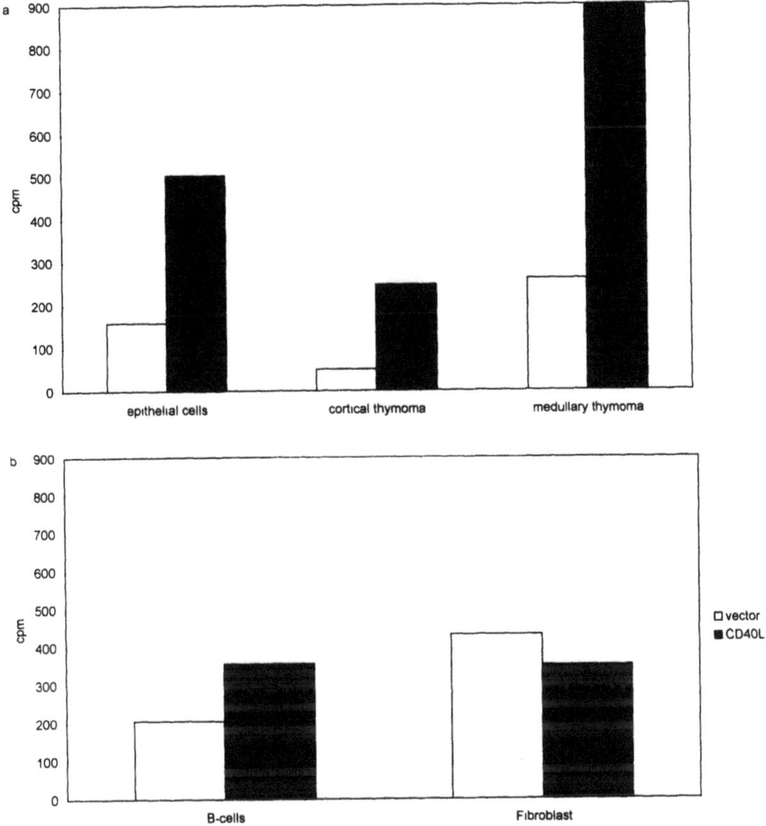

Figure 3. The proliferative response of epithelial cells from normal thymus, cortical and medullary thymoma stimulated with soluble CD40 ligand (500 U/ml) (a). Fibroblasts and B-cells were used as negative and positive control respectively (b).

4.3. Expression of CD69 and Activation Markers by DP and SP Thymocytes from Normal Thymus and Thymoma

We performed three-colour FACS analyses with freshley isolated thymocytes of thymoma and normal thymus using monoclonal antibodies against CD4, CD8 and CD69. The number of immature DP $CD69^+$ cells was nearly equal in normal thymus compared to cortical and mixed thymoma. In contrast, only some DP $CD69^+$ thymocytes were detected in medullary thymoma. The number of mature SP $CD4^+CD69^+$ was markedly reduced in thymoma (Tab. 3). The expression of CD54 and CD25 is low in normal thymus, but it is even lower in thymoma. Exceptions were one medullary Thymoma (1006/95) and one mixed thymoma (17821/94). An increased number of CD54- and CD25-positive cells were detected in these two cases.

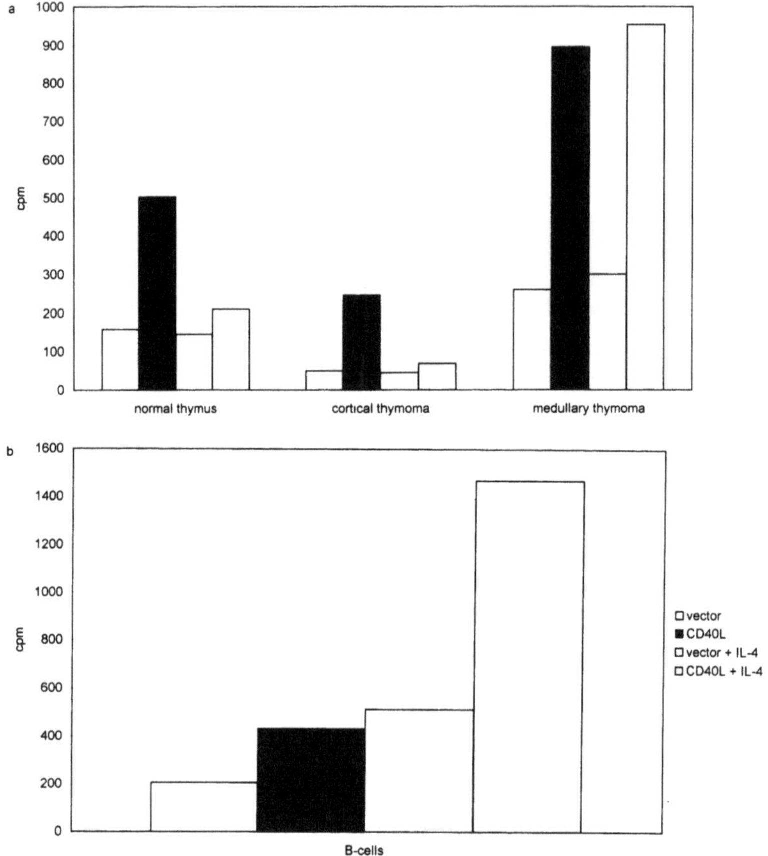

Figure 4. The proliferation evoked by soluble CD40 ligand (500 U/ml) is modulated by IL-4 (50 U/ml). IL-4 enhanced the CD40 specific proliferation of B-cells (b) but reduced the proliferation of epithelial cells from normal thymus and cortical thymoma (a).

5. DISCUSSION

CD40 ligand is known to be essential for negative selection in the normal murine thymus (Foy et al. 1995). As we show here, overexpression of CD40 was a feature of thymoma associated with paraneoplastic Myasthenia gravis. However, it has not been elucidated whether CD40/CD40 ligand interaction is involved in the generation of autoimmunity in thymic epithelial tumors, which are highly associated with Myasthenia gravis (Kirchner et al. 1992; Müller-Hermelink et al. 1993). Surprisingly we could not detect CD40 ligand protein on tissue sections by immunohistochemistry or on unstimulated thymocytes by FACS analyses. Foy et al. (1995) could show, that CD40 ligand is expressed on DP and SP $CD4^+$ thymocytes after activation with PHA/ionomycin or Concanavalin A (Con A). In addition, we could detect CD40 ligand specific mRNA by semiquantitative RT-PCR (Fig. 2). The different results of immunohistochemistry, FACS analyses and RT-PCR could be caused by a low level of CD40 ligand expression. In addition, it is possible that the CD40 ligand is not translated after the transcription of the gene. Although the importance of CD40/CD40 ligand for the response of peripheral T-cells to

Table 3. Three-colour-FACS analysis. Expression of CD69, CD54 and CD25 on SP and DP thymocytes from thymoma of various histological subtypes and normal thymus. Numbers represent the number of immunoreactive cells per 20.000 cells investigate were analysed per staining

	CD69+				CD54+			CD25+		
Case	SP CD4+	DP CD4+8+	SP CD8+	DP CD4+8+/ SP CD4+	SP CD4+	DP CD4+8+	SP CD8+	SP CD4+	DP CD4+8+	SP CD8+
MDT										
1006/95	85	52	411	0,6	90	179	450	308	9	350
MXT										
14839/95	183	1430	668	7,8	3	191	13	0	62	0
24864/94	136	1196	183	8,8	52	371	66	0	41	0
17821/94	365	1527	1582	4,2	N.A.	N.A.	N.A.	967	962	35
CT										
2516/95	327	1383	51	4,2	38	49	3	11	82	0
3792/95	303	2234	1234	7,3	4	126	12	0	16	4
15173/94	300	1445	677	4,8	N.A.	N.A.	N.A.	60	10	0
4858/95	676	1410	1256	2,1	N.A.	N.A.	N.A.	59	15	0
NT										
1	1624	1688	1183	1,0	127	284	129	209	94	17
2	2783	1013	1048	0,4	139	567	149	219	85	17
3	1491	2341	871	1,6	191	565	49	207	33	0
4	2291	2378	254	1,0	50	188	18	78	158	0
5	2972	5332	1514	1,8	200	238	162	174	558	74

MDT, medullary thymoma; MXT, mixed thymoma; CT, cortical thymoma; NT, normal thymus.
SP, single positive; DP, double positive; NA, not available.

thymus dependent antigens was shown by Renshaw et al. (1994) and the essential role of CD40 ligand in the thymic selection in the mouse (Foy et al. 1995), we do not know the function of the CD40/CD40 ligand interaction in the human thymus.

It is the main finding of the present investigation that the CD40 receptor is functionally expressed on neoplastic TEC. A CD40 dependent proliferation of TEC could be induced by soluble CD40 ligand. In agreement with the results of Galy and Spits (1992) we did not find proliferation after triggering with anti-CD40 antibody (data not shown). Therefore the signals induced by soluble CD40 ligand and anti-CD40 antibody seem to be different. In addition, the opposing effect of IL-4 on CD40-triggered proliferation of epithelial cells and B-cells is a novel observation. While IL-4 stimulates CD40-dependent proliferation in B-cells, it blocks proliferation of epithelial cells from normal thymus and cortical thymoma. The proliferation of TEC from medullary thymoma is not modulated. The reason for the different effects of IL-4 on B-cells and TEC is unclear so far. In contrast, the different influence of IL-4 on epithelial cells from normal thymus and cortical thymoma and from medullary thymoma might be explained by the data of Mat et al. (1991) and Kirchner et al. (1992), who described a low expression of IL-4 receptor in the thymic medulla but a high expression in the normal thymic cortex and cortical-type thymic epithelial tumors. As a consequence IL-4 may modulate the proliferation only of cortical but not of medullary epithelium. Interestingly Mat et al. found a downregulation of IL-4 receptor in high grade breast tumors and hypothesized IL-4 to be involved in the tumorigenesis.

Whether the overexpression of CD40 in thymoma may influence the maturation of thymocytes by interaction with CD40 ligand is unknown. In contrast to positive selection (Takahama Y. et al. 1994) negative selection seems to require a secondary signal. Beside LFA-1/ICAM-1 (Carol D. A. 1992) and B7/CD28 (Punt J.A. 1994) also CD40/CD40 ligand (Foy T.M. et al. 1995) is discussed to be important. To get a hint whether CD40 may have an influence on negative selection in thymoma, we compared the number of double positive $CD69^+$ and single positive $CD69^+$ thymocytes from normal thymus and thymoma. During positive selection the thymocytes express CD69 after the first TCR/MHC contact (Swat W. et al. 1992) and thereafter the phentotype switchs from CD4/CD8 double positive $CD69^-$ to CD4/CD8 double positive $CD69^+$. During maturation cells pass through negative selection and downregulate CD4 or CD8 and become single positive $CD69^+$. Consequently the high ratio of double positive $CD69^+$ to single positive $CD69^+$ cells (Tab.3) suggests no inefficient negative selection after the first step of positive selection. Alternatively, the reduced number on mature thymocytes in thymoma could be explained by an inefficient multistep positive selection process (Pircher H. et al. 1994). However, using FACS analyses we can not distinguish between these two possibilities.

Beside the effects on thymocyte maturation CD40 is also known to costimulate the activation of mature CD4+ T-cells (Cayabyab M. et al. 1994). Therefore CD40 overexpression by thymoma epithelial cells could potentially cause an increased number of activated mature T-cells. In conjunction with the overexpression of proteins with acetylcholine receptor- and striational muscle epitopes in thymoma epithelial cells (Kirchner et al. 1992; Marx et al. 1996) the overexpression of CD40 could be expected to specificly induce the activation and proliferation of autoaggressive T-cells. However this seems not to be the case as shown by our FACS analyses (Tab. 3): with few exceptions the expression of CD54 - an early activation marker - and CD25 - a late activation marker- seems to be reduced in thymoma compared to normal thymus.

6. CONCLUSION

CD40 is functionally expressed on normal and neoplastic TEC. The overexpression of CD40 on neoplastic epithelial cells does not lead to an inappropriate activation of potentially autoaggresive T-cells *in situ*. Negative selection inside the tumors seems more rather than less effective than in the normal thymus. Therefore, we suggest that the generation of autoreactive T-cells in paraneoplastic Myasthenia gravis may be caused by an abnormal intratumorous positive selection.

We thank A. Homburger and M. Reichert for assistance with FACS analysis and cell culture, Prof. Kirchner for normal thymus sampels and J. Banchereau and W. Sebald for gift of antibodies and cytokines.

This work was supported by the grants Ma 1484/2–1 (DFG) and 94025.1 (Sander Stiftung) .

REFERENCES

Armitage R. J.; Tough T. W.; Macduff B. M. (1993, I) CD40 ligand is a T cell growth factor. Eur. J. Immunol. 23: 2326

Armitage R. J.; Macduff B. M.; Spriggs M. K.; Fanslow W. C. (1993, II) Human B cell proliferation and Ig secretion induced by recombinant CD40 ligand are modulated by soluble cytokines. J. Immunol. 150 (9): 3671

Carlow D. A.; van Oers N. S. C.; Teh S.-J.; The H.-S. (1992) Deletion of antigen-specific immature thymocytes by dendritic cells requires LFA-1/ICAM interations. J. Immunol. 148: 1595

Cayabyab M.; Phillips J. H. Lanier L. L. (1994) CD40 preferentially costimulates activation of $CD4^+$ T Lymphocytes. J. Immunol. 152: 1523

Clark E. A.; Ledbetter J. A. (1986) Activation of human B cells mediated through two distinc cell surface differentiation antigens, Bp35 and Bp50. Proc. Natl. Acad. Sci. USA 83: 4494

Foy T. M.; Page D. M.; Waldschmidt T. J.; Schoneveld A.; Laman J. D.; Masters S. R.; Tygrett L.; Ledbetter J. A.; Aruffo A.; Claassen E.; Xu J. C.; Flavell R. A.; Oehen S.; Hedrichk S. M.; Noelle R. J. (1995) An essential role for gp 39, the ligand for CD40, in thymic selection. J. Exp. Med. 182: 1377

Galy A. H. M.; Spits H. (1992) CD40 is functionally expressed on human thymic epithelial cells. J. Immunol. 149: 775

Huettner C.; Paulus W.; Roggendorf W. (1995) Messenger RNA expression of the immunosuppressive cytokine IL-10 in human gliomas. Am. J. Pathol. 146: 317

Marx A.; Kirchner T.; Hoppe F.; O'Connor R.; Schalke B.; Tzartos S.; Müller-Hermelink H. K. (1989) Protein with epitopes of the acetylcholine receptor in epithelial cell cultur of thymomas in myastenia gravis. Am. J. Pathol. 134: 865

Marx A.; Wilisch A.; Schultz A.; Greiner A.; Magi B.; Pallini V.; Schalke B.; Toyka K.; Nix W.; Kirchner T.; Müller-Hermelink H.K. (1996) Expression of neurofilaments and of titin-epitope in thymic epithelial tumors: implications for the pathogenesis of Myasthenia gravis. Am. J. Pathol. 148: 1839–1850

Mat I.; Melcher D.; Ritter M.A. (1991) Epithelial cell expression of Interleukin-4 receptor complex. Lymphatic tissues and in vivo immune responses. Edited by Imhof B. A.; Berrih-Aknin S.; Ezine S. Marcel Dekker, Inc. 27

Müller-Hermelink H. K.; Marx A.; Geuder K. I.; Kirchner T. (1993) The pathological basis of thymoma-associated Myasthenia gravis. Ann N. Y. Acad. Sci: 681: 56

Müller-Hermelink H.K.; Marx A.; Kirchner T. (1994) Advances in the diagnosis and classification of thymic epithelial tumors. Rec Adv Histopathol 1994, 16: 49

Pircher H.; Ohashi P. S.; Boyd R. L.; Hengartner H.; Brduscha K. (1994) Evidence for a selective and multi-step model of T-cell differentiation: $CD4^+CD8^{low}$ thymocytes selected by a transgenic T-cell receptor on major histocompatibility complex class I molecules. Eur. J. Immunol. 24: 1982

Punt J. A.; Osborne B. A.; Takahama Y.; Sharrow S.; Singer A. (1994) Negative Selection of $CD4^+$ and $CD8^+$ thymocytes by T cell receptor-induced apoptosis requires a costimulatory signal that can be provided by CD28. J. Exp. Med. 179: 709

Renshaw B. R.; Fanslow III; Armitage R. J.; Campbell K. A.; Liggitt D.; Wright B.; Davison B. L.; Maliszewski C. R. (1994) Humoral immune response in CD40 ligand-deficient mice. J. Exp. Med. 180: 1889

Ritter M.A.; Boyd R.L; (1993): Development in the thymus: it takes two to tango. Immmunol. today 51: 462

Swat W.; Dessing M.; Boehmer H.; Kisielow P. (1992) CD69 expression during selection and maturation of $CD4^+$ $CD8^+$ thymocytes. Eur. J. Immunol. 23: 739

Takahama Y.; Suzuki H.; Katz K. S.; Grusby M. J.; Singer A. (1994) Positive selection of $CD4^+$ T cells by TCR ligation without aggregation even in the absence of MHC. Nature 371: 67

32

MYASTHENIA GRAVIS WITH THYMOMA AND FAS ANTIGEN

S. Kawanami,[1] S. Mori,[1] S. Yoneda,[2] T. Shirakusa,[2] K. Nishimaru,[1] and M. Kikuchi[3]

[1]First Department of Internal Medicine
[2]Second Department of Surgery
[3]First Department of Pathology
Fukuoka University, Fukuoka

Fas is a 45 kD transmembrane protein which is able to induce apoptosis, belongs to the tumor necrosis factor-receptor (TNF-R) super family[1] and was expressed in a variety of epithelial cells[2]. Fas ligand (FasL) is a 40 kD membrane protein and one of the TNF family[3]. Fas-L induces apoptosis to the cell having Fas antigen after binding to Fas. In the thymus, Fas is present and known to work on negative selection by deletion of autoreactive T-cell clones[4]. In patients with myasthenia gravis (MG) and thymoma, the value of anti-acetylcholine receptor (AChR) antibody is often found high[5]. The pathogenesis of the anti-AChR-antibody has not been fully elucidated. The messenger RNA of AChR-αsubunit was reported in cultured thymoma cells[6]. In the mechanism producing anti-AChR autoantibody, abnormal Fas-FasL system may have a role. The purpose of the present study is to find the localization and to detect function of Fas in thymomas of patients with MG.

PATIENTS AND METHODS

Nineteen patients with both MG and thymomas presented at Fukuoka University Hospital during the 19-year period from 1977 to 1996 (Table 1). These patients comprised 18.4 % of all MG patients admitted to the hospital. Eighteen of them underwent a thymomectomy. The mean post operative follow-up duration was 99.4 months. Five normal thymuses obtained at cardiac surgery were examined as controls. To determine the presence of Fas antigen in the thymomas, we used immunohistochemistry, by means of the labeled streptoavidin-biotin-alkaline phosphatase method (LSAB). Antibodies against Fas (CH11, MBL, 50x), keratin (Dako, 400x), S-100 (Dako, 200x), desmin (Dako, 40x), and

Epithelial Tumors of the Thymus, edited by Marx and Müller-Hermelink.
Plenum Press, New York, 1997

Table 1. Patients with thymoma and myasthenia gravis

No.	age	sex	preop duration (m)	post op duration (m)	TA (1)	TA (2)	anti-AChR Ab, nM	pred.
1	26	F	3	170	M	B	308.0	+
2	63	F	20	162	MED	B	NE	+
3	59	F	18	154	M	B	21.5	-
4	25	M	10	150	Mc	M	NE	+
5	31	M	4	138	C	B	105	+
6	60	F	4	92	Mc	M	5.5	+
7	66	F	3	78	MED	B	81.0	+
8	32	M	0	68	C	B	1.40	-
9	59	F	40	37	Mc	B	4.77	-
10	73	M	4	8	Mm	B	163	+
11	57	F	1	6	Mc	M	13.4	+
12	23	F	6	245	M	M	NE	+
13*	47	M	13	227	Mc	M	0.97	+
14*	62	M	5	119	Mc	B	1.36	-
15*	25	F	1	67	C	M	NE	+
16*	47	M	22	52	C	M	NE	-
17*	58	F	12	11	Mc	M	NE	-
18*	34	F	5	3	C	B	4.94	-
19	47	F	120	0	NE	M	1.1	+

polyclonal antibody against acetylcholine receptor-like protein isolated from the thymus, made by us (250x) were used. To determine the degree of apoptosis induced by Fas antigen, in situ cell death detection was performed using a kit from Boehringer Mannheim.

The acetylcholine receptor-like protein (AChR-LP) was isolated from the fetal calf thymus after performing both solubilization with Triton-X-100 and affinity chromatography with cobrotoxin-Sepharose[7]. Japanese white rabbits were immunized with this protein emulsified in complete Freund's adjuvant. Anti-sera were obtained from rabbits induced with experimental autoimmune myasthenia gravis (EAMG)[8].

Apoptosis was detected by terminal deoxynucleotidyl transferase (TdT) mediated fluorescein d-UTP nick end labeling (TUNEL) methods[9]. Anti-fluorescein antibody conjugated with alkaline phosphatase was used and the positive reaction was found by staining with Fuchsin.

RESULTS AND DISCUSSION

Table 1 shows the clinico-pathological findings of all 19 patients. The five patients with asterisks all died, four due to metastasis of the thymoma, and one because of myasthenic crisis. Ten patients had benign thymomas, while nine were malignant. According to the European histological classification[10], five cases were cortical type, eleven cases were mixed, and two were medullary type. Anti-AChR-antibody was measured by the immunoprecipitation method.

The survival of patients with MG was compared according to the histological type of thymoma. No significant differences were observed between the non-invasive, benign type and malignant type thymoma. According to the European histological classification of thymomas cortical type had a shorter survival than either mixed or medullary type by means of Kaplan-Meier method (Fig.1). These findings are in accordance with those reported from Italy[11].

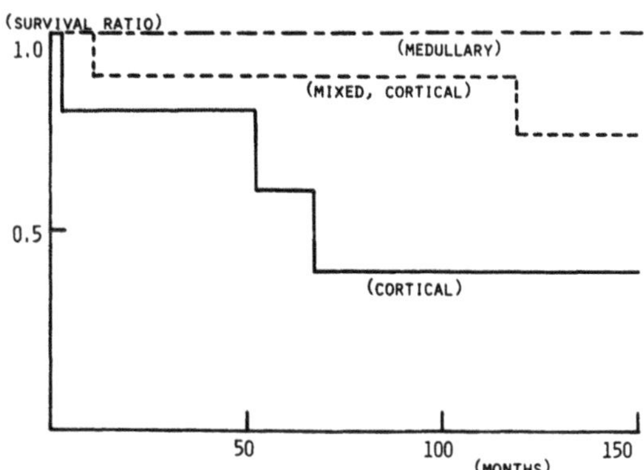

Figure 1. Survival of patients with thymoma and mysthenia gravis according to the European classification of thymoma.

In normal control thymus, Fas was found in the subcapsular, cortical and medullary epithelial cells. In a frozen mixed cortical predominant type thymoma section, the neoplastic epithelial cells were diffusely stained with anti-Fas antibody. By double-staining of keratin and Fas in a paraffin embedded section, the keratin was stained LSAB-horse radish peroxidase (HRP) and Fas with on alkaline phosphatase. The cortical type thymoma showed positive reactions in the neoplastic cortical epithelial cells (Fig.2). In mixed, predominantly cortical type thymoma, the subcapsular epithelial cells had positive staining (Fig. 3). The mixed cortical predominant type thymoma was immunostained with anti-AChR-LP antibody, while some of the epithelial cells were also positively stained.

By the TUNEL method using an in situ cell death detection kit, the apoptosis positive nuclei stained red (Fig.4). The positive cells were identified in some neoplastic epithelial cells, lymphocytes and subcapsular epithelial cells. In the subcapsular region, 500 cells were counted to calculate the percentage of positive cells at the three different views. The post operative survival and the results of TUNEL were then compared for both mixed type and cortical type thymomas. No correlation was found between the survival, based on post operative duration, and apoptosis by the TUNEL method. A correlation between the results of TUNEL and the anti-AChR antibody by the immunoprecipitation method was detected, and a negative correlation existed between them, r=-0.795(Fig. 5). These results show that in patients with a high value of anti-AChR antibody, the ratio of apoptosis in the thymoma is low, which thus suggests the blockage of the Fas antigen by anti-AChR antibody probably due to the presence of co-antigen between the AChR and the Fas antigen. In paraffin embedded section of mixed, cortical predominant type thymoma, double stain-

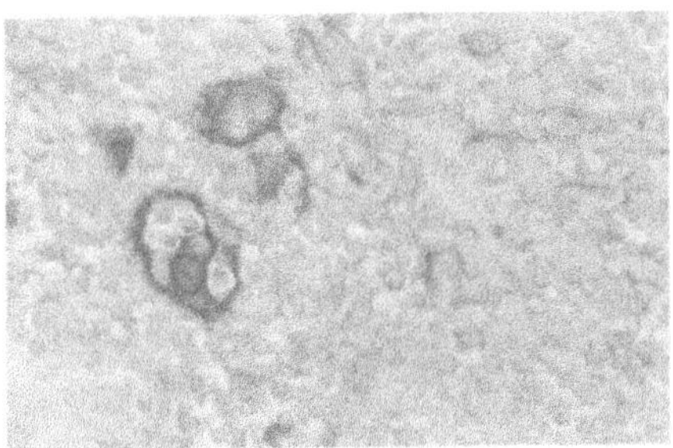

Figure 2. Double staining of keratin and Fas in paraffin embedded section of cortical type thymoma (400x).

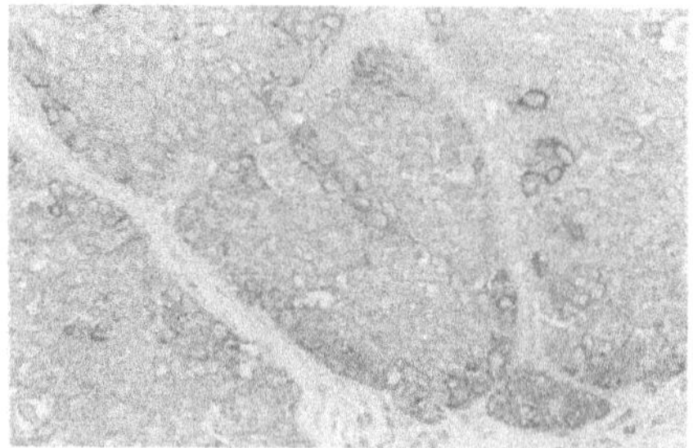

Figure 3. Double labeling of Fas and keratin in paraffin embedded section of mixed, predominantly cortical type (200x).

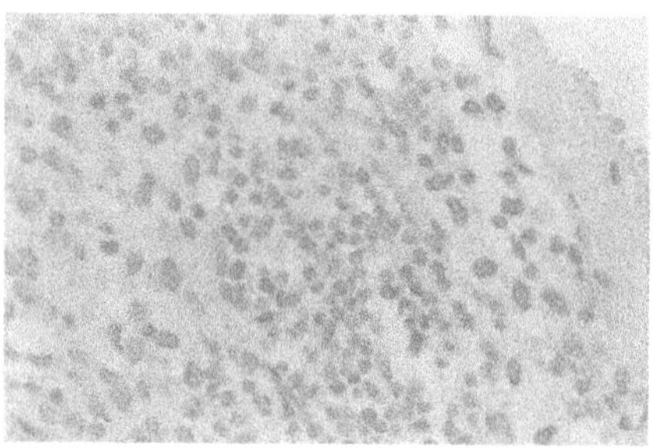

Figure 4. In situ cell death detection by TUNEL method using a kit (Boehringer Manheim)

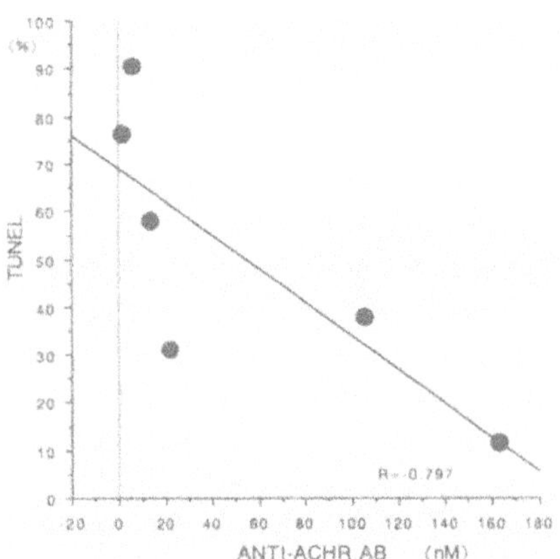

Figure 5. Correlation between apoptosis in the thymoma and anti-acetylcholine receptor antibody.

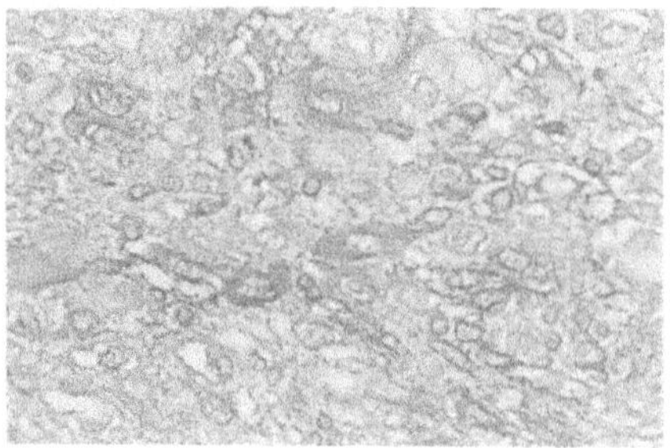

Figure 6. Double labeling of Fas and AChR-LP in paraffin embedded section of mixed, predominantly cortical type (400x).

ing with AChR-LP and Fas revealed positive reactions in some of the epithelial cells (Fig. 6).

In conclusion, 1. Based on the above findings, Fas antigen was found to be present in a part of the neoplastic subcapsular, cortical and medullary epithelial cells of thymomas with MG. 2. A negative correlation was observed between anti-AChR antibody and apoptosis as detected using the TUNEL method. When the antibody titer was high, the rate of apoptosis was low, thus suggesting that anti-AChR antibody masked Fas antigen in the thymus. The presence of co-antigen between the Fas and AChR-LP in the thymus is therefore suggested.

ACKNOWLEDGMENTS

We would like to express our gratitude to Drs. Michio Kimura, Yukito Ichinose, Syousaku Noda, Kazuhiko Muta and colleagues of The First Dept. of Internal Medicine. We would appreciate excellent technical assistance by Ms. Hiromi Wada, Mariko Kishimomto and Midori Sugihara. This work was supported in part by grants-in aids from the Ministry of Public Welfare.

REFERENCES

1. Yonehara S, Ishii A, Yonehara M (1989) A cell-killing monoclonal antibody (Anti-Fas) to a cell surface antigen codownregulated with the receptor of tmornecrosis factor. J Exp Med 169:1747–1756.
2. Leithauser F, Dhein J, Mechtersheimer G et al. (1993) Constitutite and induced expression of APO-1, a new member of the nerve growth factor/tumor necrosis factor receptor superfamily, in normal and neoplastic cells. Lab invest 69:415–429.
3. Suda T, Takahashi T, Goldstein P et al. (1993) Molecular cloning and expression of the Fas ligand, a novel member of tumor necrosis factor family. Cell 75:1169–1178.
4. Yonehara S, Nishimura Y, Kishi S et al. (1994) Involvement of apoptosis antigen Fas in clonal deletion of human thymocytes. Int Immunol 6:1849–1856.
5. Kawanami S, Tsuji R, Oda K (1984) Enzyme-linked immunosorbent assay for antibody against the nicotinic acetylcholine receptor in human myasthenia gravis. Ann Neurol 5:195–200.
6. Hara Y, Ueno S, Uemichi T et al. (1991) Neoplastic epithelial cells express α-subunit of muscel nicotinic acetylcholine receptor in thymomas from patients with myathenia gravis. FEBS Lett 279:137–140.
7. Kawanami S, Conti-Tronconi B, Racs J et al. (1988) Isolation and characterization of nicotinic acetylcholine receptor-like protein from fetal calf thymus. J Neurol Sci 87:195–209.
8. Kawanami S, Mori S (1994) Experimental autoimmune myasthenia gravis induced by thymic acetylcholine receptor-like protein. Fukuoka Acta Med 85: 120–127.
9. Gavrieli Y, Sherman Y, Ben-Sasson SA (1992) Identification of programmed cell death in situ via specific labeling of nuclear DNA fragmentation. J cell Biol 119:493–501.
10. Marino M, Muller-Hermelink HK (1985) Thymoma and thymic carcinoma-Relation of thymoma epithelial cells to the cortical and medullary differentiation of thymus. Virchow Arch [Pathol Anat] 407:119–149.
11. Pescarmona E, Rendina EA, Venuta F et al. (1990) The prognostic implication of thymoma histologic subtyping- A study of 80 consecutive cases. Am J Clin Pathol 93:190–195.

MYASTHENIA GRAVIS PATIENTS HAVE A CELLULAR IMMUNE RESPONSE AGAINST TITIN

Geir Olve Skeie,[1] Johan A. Aarli,[1] Roald Matre,[2] Alexandra Freiburg,[3] and Nils Erik Gilhus[1]

[1]Department of Neurology
[2]Department of Immunology
University of Bergen
Bergen, Norway
[3]European Molecular Biology Laboratory
Heidelberg, Germany

1. ABSTRACT

Myasthenia gravis (MG) is caused by antibodies against the acetylcholine receptor (AChR). However, some MG patients have antibodies against non-AChR epitopes of skeletal muscle including titin. In this study, we tested peripheral blood lymphocytes from 11 MG patients and 13 blood donors in a lymphocyte transformation test using the antigen MGT-30, a titin epitope that represents the main immunogenic region. Stimulation index (SI) was defined as counts per minute (cpm) in stimulated culture minus background divided by cpm in unstimulated culture minus background. MGT-30 caused a significant stimulation of T-cells from titin-antibody positive MG patients; SI=1.84±0.77, compared with titin-antibody negative patients; SI=0.67±0.28 (p=0.01), and blood-donors; SI=0.65±0.21 (p=0.0005). SI after PHA stimulation was similar in MG patients with and without titin-antibodies and blood-donors. After MGT-30 stimulation, IL-4 concentrations in the supernatant were 84–150pg/mL in all 4 titin-positive patients examined. IL-4 levels were below the detection limit for the ELISA used (60pm/ml) in the cultures from the 8 blood-donors and the 1 titin-negative MG patient that were tested. Thus, MG patients with anti-titin antibodies also have a T-cell mediated immune reactivity against titin.

2. INTRODUCTION

Myasthenia gravis (MG) is characterized by fatiguability of skeletal mucle caused by antibodies against the acetylcholine receptor (AChR) at the muscle endplate (Lind-

Epithelial Tumors of the Thymus, edited by Marx and Müller-Hermelink.
Plenum Press, New York, 1997

strom et al.,1988). The production of AChR-antibodies is regulated by AChR-spesific $CD4^+$ T helper (Th) cells (Willcox 1993). Some patients with MG have antibodies to non-AChR skeletal muscle antigens including titin (Aarli et al., 1990). Titin is a myofibrillar protein unique to striated muscle and it comprises about 10% of the myofibril mass (Trinick et al., 1984). It is the largest protein identified to date, molecular mass about 3000kD (Labeit and Kolmerer 1995). Its function is to hold the sarcomere together, to keep the thick filaments centred within the sarcomere during force generation, and it plays an important role in the elastic recoil of striated muscle (Wang 1984, Horowitz et al., 1986).

Titin-antibodies are related to thymus pathology in MG as 90% of thymoma patients and about half of the patients with late-onset MG and thymic atrophy have titin-antibodies. Titin antibodies do not occur in MG patients with thymic hyperplasia nor in patients with other autoimmune diseases (Gautel et al., 1992). There is a relationship between the severity of MG and the presence of titin antibodies in late-onset MG patients (Skeie et al., 1995) but whether the antibodies are directly pathogenic is not known.

The mechanisms that initiate and regulate titin-antibody production have not been studied, but the relationship to thymus pathology makes a T-cell response likely. The aim of this study was to look for such a T-cell mediated immunity against titin in order to see if the production of titin-antibodies could be T-cell dependent.

3. MATERIALS AND METHODS

3.1. Patients

The study included 11 MG patients, age range 17–85 years. The diagnosis of MG was based on conventional clinical criteria, edrophonium (Tensilon) test, neurophysiological investigations and the presence of anti-AChR antibodies in all the patients. Seven of the MG patients had antibodies against the titin antigen MGT-30 in ELISA (Gautel et al., 1992). Of the patients with titin-antibodies 4 had a thymoma and 3 were non-thymoma late-onset MG patients. Among the 4 patients with no titin-antibodies 2 had late-onset MG and 2 had early-onset MG and thymic hyperplasia. Four of 7 titin-positive and 2 of the 4 titin-negative patients used immunosuppressive drugs; prednisone, azathioprine or both. Three of 7 titin-positive and 2 of 4 titin-negative patients had autoimmune diseases in addition to MG; rheumatoid arthritis (2), thyroiditis (2), aplastic anemia(1).

Thirteen healthy blood-donors were used as controls. None of them had titin antibodies.

3.2. Lymphocyte Transformation Test

Venous blood (10ml) was drawn into a sodium-heparinised tube (Vacutainer®, Becton Dickinson, Meylan, France) and experiments started immediately. Mononuclear cells were separated by density gradient centrifugation using Lymphoprep ™ (Nycomed Pharma AS, Oslo, Norway). The cells were washed 2 times by centrifugation at 1200rpm(400G) for 10 minutes in phosphatebuffered saline pH 7.4(PBS) and then in culture medium RPMI 1640 (Flow Laboratories, Irvine, Scotland) containing 10% (200mM, 29.23mg/ml) heat-inactivated foetal calf serum (Flow Laboratories), supplemented with 1% L-glutamin (Flow Laboratories), 2% solution of 5000IU/ml benzylpenicillin and 5000IU/ml streptomycin (Flow Laboratories). The cells were resuspended in the culture

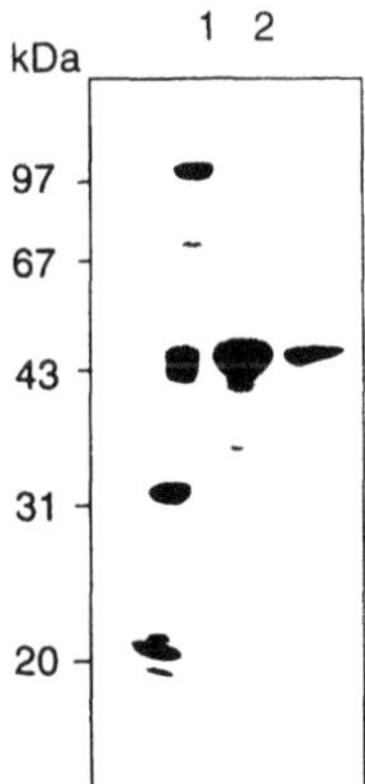

Figure 1. Purity of the MGT-30 peptide. There is only 1 visible band in the gel after the second step of purification.

medium and the concentration was adjusted to 3.3 x 10^5 cells/ml. 150µl of this cell suspension were seeded into each well of a 96-well round-bottom microtiter plate (Nunclon, Roskilde, Denmark).

The recombinant titin peptide MGT-30 was used as antigen (Gautel et al.,1993). This 30kD peptide represents the main immunogenic region of the titin molecule. MGT-30 was expressed in BL21[DE3]plysS as previously described (Gautel et al.,1993) using the pET8c E.Coli expression vector (Studier et al., 1990). The His_6 -tagged protein was purified by metal-chelate affinity chromatography on Ni^{2+} -nitrilo-tetraacetic acid agarose (Quiagen, Chatsworth, CA) (LeGrice and Grununger-Leitch, 1990). Further purification was performed by anion-exchange chromatography on a MonoQ column (Pharmacia, Uppsala, Sweden) at pH 8 and pH 9.5 (Figure 1).

MGT-30 diluted in PBS to final concentrations 70µg/ml, 7.0µg/ml, 0.7µg/ml and 0.07µg/ml was added to the wells containing the mononuclear cells.

PHA (phytohaemagglutinin) (Wellcome Diagnostics, England) 2.5µg/ml was used as a positive control for mononuclear blood cell reactivity. A non-stimulated cell suspension was included as a control for spontaneous cell proliferation. Medium alone was cultured as background control. All cultures were run in 4 parallels.

After adding the antigen, the plates were kept at 37ºC in a humidified atmosphere with 5% CO_2 for 4 days before adding 1µCi ^{3}H-thymidine (Amersham International, Amersham, England) to each well. After another 18 hours the cultures were harvested (Skatron, Lierbyen, Norway). Incorporation of thymidine was measured in a liquid scintillator β-counter (Packard Tri-Carb 300, Packard Instruments, Zürich, Switzerland).

The lymphocyte response was expressed as SI (Stimulation Index). SI= (MS-BG):(MU-BG). In this equation, MS(mean of stimulated cultures) represents the median count of 4 parallel samples of the mononuclear blood cell cultures stimulated with MGT-30 or PHA and MU(mean of unstimulated cultures) represents the corresponding value of the mononuclear blood cell cultures without antigen added. BG (background) represents the median counts from the wells with medium only.

The statistical analyses were performed using SPSS. The Mann Whitney U test and Student's t-test were used to test for statistical difference between groups.

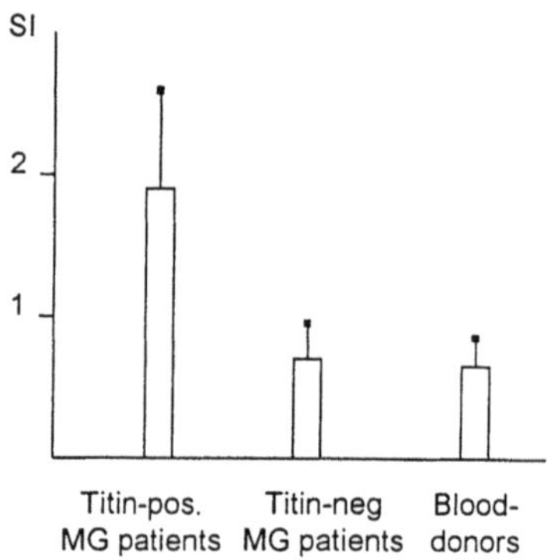

Figure 2. Stimulation index (mean + 1SD) for MG-patients with and without titin antibodies and for blood-donors after mononuclear blood cell cultures were stimulated with MGT-30 0.7µg/ml.

3.3. IL-4 Supernatant Detection

Supernatant (50µl) was collected from wells where cultured mononuclear blood cells from 5 MG patients and 8 blood-donors had been incubated with MGT-30 for 90 hours. This supernatant was immediately frozen at -20ºC. For the IL-4 detection, we used the protocol recommended for Duoset ELISA developmental system (Genzyme Diagnostics, Cambridge, USA) with minor modifications.

4. RESULTS

4.1. Lymphocyte Transformation Test

The stimulation index (SI) in the cell cultures from MG patients with titin-antibodies after incubation with MGT-30 0.7µg/ml was 1.84±0.77 (mean ±1SD). This was an increased SI compared with the MG patients without anti-titin antibodies; SI=0.67 ±0.28 (p=0.01) and also compared with the blood-donors; SI=0.65±0.21(p=0.0005)(Figure 2).

In addition to SI, the absolute lymphocyte proliferation was calculated. In MGT-30 stimulated cultures the mean absolute counts were higher in MG patients with titin-antibodies than in patients without titin-antibodies and blood-donors (Table 1). The counts for thymidin incorporation without antigen stimulation were similar in MG patients with titin-antibodies and in MG and non-MG controls. In cultures from MG patients with titin-antibodies cpm's tend to increase after MGT-30 stimulation. This contrasts with the decreased cpm's in MGT-30 stimulated cultures from MG patients without titin-antibodies and blood-donors (Figure 3).

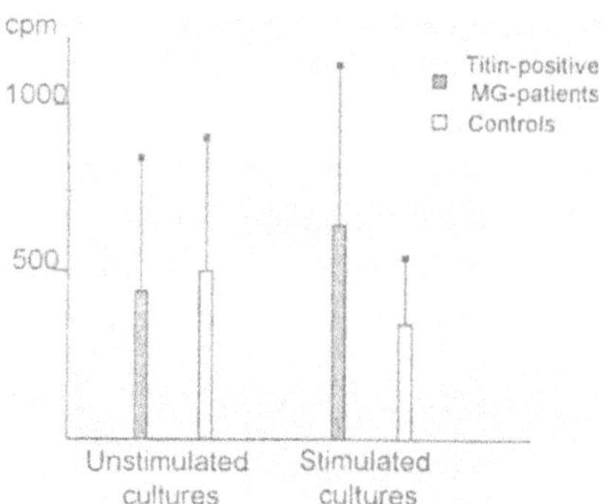

Figure 3. ^{3}H-thymidine uptake (Mean +1SD) in unstimulated cultures and cultures stimulated with MGT-30 in titin-positive MG-patients and controls (blood-donors and titin-negative MG-patients).

Table 1. β-counts and stimulation indexes from 5 titin-positive MG patients and 17 MG and non-MG controls in unstimulated lymphocyte cultures and in cultures stimulated with 0.7μg/ml MGT-30. Mean ±1SD

	MG-patients titin-pos	MG patients titin-neg and blood donors	p-value
Unstimulated cultures (cpm)	433±388	504±400	0.793
Cultures with MGT-30 (cpm)	617±490	326±221	0.01
Stimulation Index	1.84±0.77	0.66±0.21	0.0005

The optimal MGT-30 concentration for the stimulation experiments was 0.7μg /ml (Figure 4). This concentration gave the best discrimination between a positive and a negative response. MGT-30 at high concentrations had an inhibiting effect on T-cell proliferation in all cultures.

Two of the titin-positive patients were tested both during an MG relapse and when in clinical remission. SI was 1.50 and 2.26 during the exacerbation and 0.74 and 0.70 respectively in remission. MG patients on immunosuppressive treatment tended to have lower SI than patients without such treatment. For the 3 MG patients with titin-antibodies without immunosuppression, SI was 1.4, 1.6 and 3.4 compared with SI 1.4, 1.5 and 1.6 for the MG patients with titin-antibodies who used immunosuppressive treatment. For MG patients without titin-antibodies and no immunosupressive treatment SI was 0.6 and 1.06 compared with SI 0.44 and 0.5 for the MG patients without titin-antibodies who used immunosuppressive treatment. The response to PHA did not differ significantly between different groups of MG patients and blood-donors. Titin-positive MG patients had SI=52.9±32.4, titin-negative MG patients had SI=48.97±56.73 and blood-donors had SI=53.8±49.94.

SI's after stimulation with MGT-30 did not differ significantly between MG patients with or without additional autoimmune diseases.

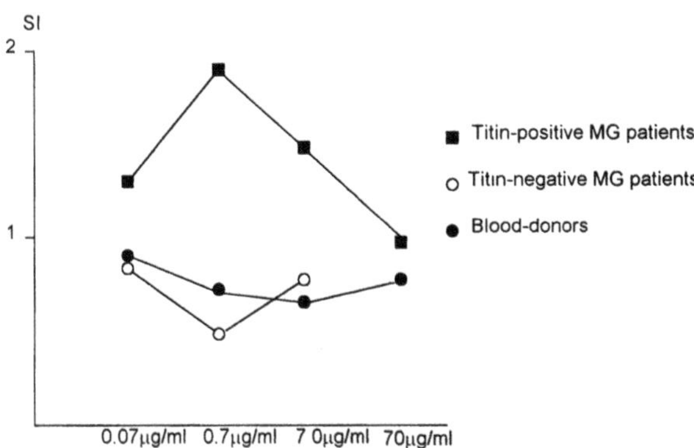

Figure 4. Stimulating indexes (SI)(mean) in cell cultures from MG patients and blood donors for 4 different MGT-30 concentrations.

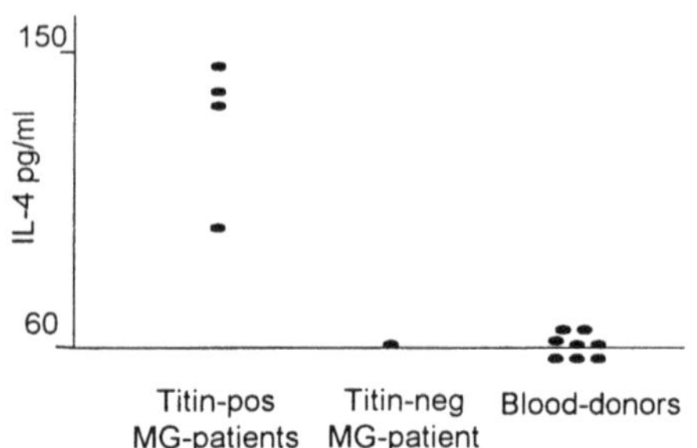

Figure 5. IL-4 supernatant concentrations in cultures stimulated with MGT-30 0.7 μg/ml. Four titin-positive MG-patients, one titin-negative MG-patient and 8 blood-donors were examined.

4.2. IL-4 ELISA

The IL-4 concentration was significantly increased in the culture supernatants from MG patients with titin-antibodies after MGT-30 stimulation. All 4 titin-positive MG patients tested had IL-4 concentrations 84–150pg/ml in cultures stimulated with 0.7μg/ml MGT-30 (Figure 5). In contrast, none of the 8 blood-donors or the titin-negative MG patient had levels of IL-4 above the detection limit of 60pg/ml. In unstimulated cultures and cultures stimulated with PHA, levels of IL-4 were below the detection limit both in all the titin-positive MG patients and controls.

5. DISCUSSION

This study shows that MG patients with circulating autoantibodies against titin also have T-cell reactivity against a titin epitope within the MGT-30 peptide. The recombinant peptide MGT-30 caused a significant stimulation of cultured mononuclear blood cells reflected by increased thymidine incorporation, a measure for cell proliferation, as well as by increased production of the cytokine IL-4. The T-cell reactions were not vigorous, probably due to most patient being in clinical remission and some even on immunosuppressive drugs. The fact that 2 of the titin-positive MG patients had an increased stimulation index during a clinical relapse indicates that the intensity of the T-cell titin reactivity fluctuates with disease severity.

MGT-30 is the main immunogenic region of titin for B-cells as most titin antibodies bind to this domain (Gautel et al. 1993). However, T-cell and B-cell epitopes are not identical (shown for AChR (Hohlfeld et al., 1987)). MG patients could well have additional autoreactive T-cells against titin epitopes outside the MGT-30 domain. Furthermore, MGT-30 is a large protein which requires processing by antigen-presenting cells. We do not know if the processing was optimal in our assay.

MG patients without titin-antibodies showed the same stimulation index as healthy blood donors. Thus, the stimulation is not unspecific and due to the MG itself, the presence of a thymoma or to AChR reactivity, but is related to a specific immunity against the titin epitope. As the patients have both T cell reactivity and autoantibodies against the same titin domain it is highly unlikely that this represents just cross-reactivity against another molecule with one similar antigen epitope.

We used a recombinant peptide as the antigen. In theory, contamination with E.Coli proteins could affect the result. However, MGT-30 is highly purified and there is no joining sequence. Proliferation assays with measurement of thymidine incorporation in cultured peripheral mononuclear blood cells reflect primarily the Th(1) cell response. IL-4 on the other hand is secreted by Th(2) cells. Thus, both Th(1) and Th(2) cells are involved in the immune reactivity against titin. Testing T-cell lines and clones specific for titin epitopes and a better characterization of the cytokine profile would further elucidate the immune response against titin in MG patients.

Some thymoma MG patients have a myositis with muscle lymphorhagias that is not related to the muscle endplate (Engel et al., 1966). The antigen specificity for this immune reaction are not known, but titin is one of several candidates. The mononuclear cell stimulation observed in our experiments could reflect activation of cytotoxic T-cells against titin.

SI was lower at high MGT-30 concentrations in all cultures. A paradoxical high dose suppression is reported for other antigens as well. Critchfield have shown that high antigen doses induce apoptosis in reactive T-cells, in a feed-back mechanism called propriocidal regulation, to protect the body from its own immune response (Critchfield et al., 1994).

Thymomas express AChR epitopes as well as RyR-epitopes (Marx et al., 1990, Mygland et al., 1995) and epithelial thymoma cells can present AChR antigens to T-cells in an immunogenic manner (Gilhus et al., 1995). Intrathymic immunization is thus suspected for AChR reactive T-cells at least in thymomas. Titin-antibodies are closely related to the presence of a thymoma and an intrathymic immunization is suspected for titin-reactive cells as well although titin epitopes have not been identified in thymomas so far (Marx et al., 1992).

In conclusion, we have found a titin specific T-cell response in titin-positive MG patients and therefore believe that the titin-antibody production seen in these MG patients is T-cell mediated.

REFERENCES

Aarli JA, Stefansson K, Marton LSG, Wollmann RL. (1990) Patients with myasthenia gravis and thymoma have in their sera IgG autoantibodies against titin. Clin Exp Immunol 82, 284–288

Critchfield JM, Racke MK, Zuniga-Pflucker JC, Cannella B, Raine CS, Goverman J, Lenardo MJ. (1994) T cell deletion in high antigen dose theraphy of autoimmune encephalomyelitis. Science 263,1139–1143

Engel WK, McFarlin DE. (1966) Muscle lesion in myasthenia gravis; discussion. Ann NY Acad Sci 135, 68–77

Gautel M, Lakey A, Barlow PD, Holmes Z, Scales S, Leonard K, Labeit S, Mygland Å, Gilhus NE, Aarli JA. (1993) Titin antibodies in myasthenia gravis: identification of a major immunogenic region of titin. Neurology 43, 1581–1585

Gilhus NE, Willcox N, Harcourt G, Nagvekar N, Beeson D, Vincent A, Newsom-Davis J. (1995) Antigen presentation by thymoma epithelial cells from myasthenia gravis patients to potentially pathogenic T cells. J Neuroimmunol 56, 65–76

Hohlfeld R, Toyka KV, Tzartos SJ, Carson W, Conti-Tronconi BM. (1987) Human T-helper lymphocytes in myasthenia gravis recognize the nicotinic receptor alpha subunit. Proc Natl Acad Sci 84, 5379-

Horowitz R, Kempner ES, Bisher ME, Podolsky RJ. (1986) A physiological role for titin and nebulin in skeletal muscle. Nature 323, 160–164

Kurzban GP, Wang K. (1988) Giant polypeptides of skeletal muscle titin: sedimentation equilibrium in guanidine hydrochloride. Biochem Biophys Res Comm 150, 1155–1161

Labeit S, Kolmerer B. (1995) Titins: giant protins in charge of muscle ultrastructure and elasticity. Science 270, 293–296.

LeGrice SFJ, Gruninger-Leitch F. (1990) Rapid purification of homodimer and heterodimer HIV-1 reverse transcriptase by metal chelate affinity chromatograpgy. Eur J Biochem 187, 307–314.

Lindstrom J, Schelton D Fujii Y. (1988) Myasthenia gravis. Adv. Immunol 42, 233–284.

Marx A, Osborn M, Tzartos S, Geuder KI, Schalke B, Nix W, Kirchner T, Müller-Hermelink HK. (1992) A striatonal muscle antigen and myasthenia gravis associated thymomas share an acetylcholine-receptor epitope. Dev Immunol 2, 77–84.

Marx A, O'Connor R, Geuder KI, Hoppe F, Schalke B, Tzartos S, Kalies I, Kirchner T, Müller-Hermelink HK. (1990) Characterisation of a protein with an acetylcholine receptor epitope from myasthenia gravis associated thymomas. Lab Invest 62, 279–286.

Mygland Å, Kuwajima G, Mikoshiba K, Tysnes OB, Aarli JA, Gilhus NE. (1995)Thymomas express epitopes shared by the ryanodine receptor. J Neuroimmunol 62, 79–83.

Skeie GO, Mygland Å, Aarli JA, Gilhus NE. (1995) Titin antibodies in patients with late-onset myasthenia gravis: clinical correlations. Autoimmunity 20, 99–105.

Studier FW, Rosenberg AH, Dunn JJ, Dubendorff JW. (1990) Use of T7 RNA polymerase to direct expression of cloned genes. Methods Enzymol 185, 60–89.

Trinick J, Knight P, Whiting A. (1984) Purification and properties of native titin. J Mol Biol 180, 331–356.

Wang K. (1984) Cytoskeletal matrix in striational muscle: the role of titin, nebulin and intermediate filaments. Adv Exp Med Biol 170, 285–305.

Willcox N. (1993) Myasthenia gravis. Curr Opin Immunol 5, 910–917.

34

TUMOR NECROSIS FACTOR GENE POLYMORPHISMS IN THYMOMA AND NON-THYMOMA MYASTHENIA GRAVIS

M. M. Lino,[1] G. Zelano,[2] A. P. Batocchi,[1] A. Evoli,[1] and P. Tonali[1]

[1]Institute of Neurology
Catholic University of Rome
[2]Institute of Anatomy
Catholic University of Rome
00168 Roma -Largo Francesco Vito 1

INTRODUCTION

Myasthenia Gravis (MG) is an autoimmune disease. Clinical symptons include muscle weakness after repeated exercise and diurnal fluctuations of the symptoms. Laboratory examinations generally reveal frequent occurrence of thymic hyperplasia or thymoma, precence of antiacetylcholine receptor antibodies and waning phenomenon on electromyographic examination.

Genetic analyses indicate that genes whithin the major histocompatibility complex (MHC) can be involved in autoimmune diseases susceptibility.[1]

TNFβ is a lymphokine, produced by T-lymphocytes, which plays an important role in the regulation of the immune response as part of the cytokine network.[2]

The gene encoding tumor necrosis factor beta (TNF) is tandemly arranged with TNT α gene within the MHC, centromeric to HLA-B and telomeric to class II genes.

The fact that TNF is so closely linked to HLA raises the possibility that it might be involved in the susceptibility to autoimmune diseases.

Some MHC linked autoimmune diseases,[3] such as Insulin-dependent diabetes mellitus (IDDM),[4,5] Systemic Lupus erythematosus (SLE)[6] and Graves disease[7] are associated with TNFB polymorphism and are characterized by abnormal levels of its expression.

Early-onset MG with thymic hyperplasia has been found to be associated with HLA A1, B8 and DR3, antigens,[8] while no clear HLA association has been observed in patients with thymoma.[9] The purpose of this study is to verify if TNT β play a role in the susceptibility to MG.

Epithelial Tumors of the Thymus, edited by Marx and Müller-Hermelink.
Plenum Press, New York, 1997

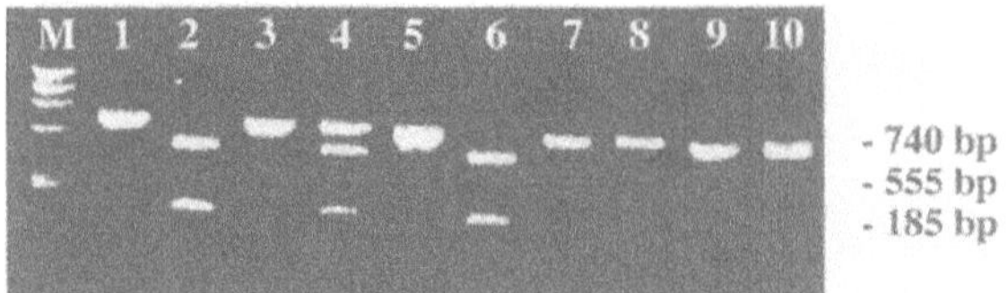

Figure 1. Lanes 1-3-5-7-9 are PCR amplification; lanes 2-4-6-8-10 are the digestion of the amplified fragments shown in the preceding lanes. Homozygotes TNB1 show two bands: 555 bp and 185 bp (lanes 2–6); homozygotes TNFB2 show one band of 740 bp (lanes 8–10, heterozygotes TNFB 1/2 show all the three bands (lane 4). M is the molecular weight marker.

MATERIAL AND METHODS

We analyzed an NcoI restriction fragment polymorphism, located within the first intron of TNFβ locus, in MG patients and controls.

In our study we included 63 MG patients and 93 healthy individuals.

Patients were sub-divided in 3 groups according to thymic pathology. We analyzed: 26 MG patients with thymic hyperplasia,17 MG patients with thymoma, 6 MG patients with involuted thymus and 14 unthymectomized patients.

Genomic DNA was purified from peripheral blood mononuclear cells (PBMC). The typing was achieved by appling a PCR/RFLP protocol described by Messer.[10]

A 740 base pair (bp) fragment of the TNFB gene which extends from exon 1 to intron 3 and includes the polymorphic NcoI restriction site, was amplified using PCR.

The primers used were: TNF-β L: 5′ CCG TGC TTC GTG CTT TGG ACT A 3′ and TNF-β R: 5′ AGA GCT GGT GGG GAC ATG TCT G 3′.

The amplification product was digested with the restriction enzyme NcoI.[6,10]

The fragments obtained after amplification and digestion were detected by performing an electrophoresis in an agarose gel and staining with the fluorescent dye ethidium bromide.

The comparison of phenotype, genotype and alleles frequencies between patients and controls was studied using $\chi2$ test with Yates' correction.

The relative risk was calculated by Woolf's method with Haldane's modification.

Table 1. MG patients and controls

	MG patients		Controls	
	N	%	N	%
Allele frequencies				
TNFB*1	39	31	58	31.5
TNFB*2	87	69	128	69.6
Phenotype frequencies				
TNFB*1	34	54	51	55.4
TNFB*2	58	92	86	93.5
Genotype frequencies				
TNFB*1/1	5	8	7	7.6
TNFB*1/2	29	46	44	47.8
TNFB*2/2	29	46	42	45.7

Table 2. MG patients with thymic hyperplasia and controls

	Thymic hyperplasia (N=26)		Controls (N=93)			
	N	%	N	%	p	RR
Allele frequencies						
TNFB* 1	28	53.8	58	31.5	p<0.001	2.6
TNFB* 2	24	46.2	128	69.6	p<0.001	0.4
Phenotype frequencies						
TNFB* 1	23	88.5	51	55.4	p<0.005	6.3
TNFB* 2	21	80.8	86	93.5		
Genotype frequencies						
TNFB* 1/1	5	19.2	7	7.6		
TNFB* ½	18	69.2	44	47.8		
TNFB* 2/2	3	11.5	42	45.7	p<0.001	0.2

RESULTS

We did not find significant differences comparing the allele, phenotype and genotype TNFB frequencies in the MG and the control groups (table 1).

When patients were subdivided according to thymic pathology, significant differences were found in the subgroups of MG patients with thymic hyperplasia and MG patients with thymoma.

In the subgroup of MG patients with thymic hyperplasia we found a positive association with TNF*1 allele (p<0.001) and * 1/2 genotype and a negative association with TNFB*2/2 genotype (p<0.001). These results are shown in table 2.

On the other hand we found a positive association between MG patients with thymoma and TNFB*2/2 genotype (p<0.01; RR 5.6) and a negative association with TNFB*1 allele and *1/2 genotype. These results are shown in table 3.

Table 3. MG patients with thymoma and controls

	Thymoma (N=17)		Controls (N=93)			
	N	%	N	%	p	RR
Allele frequencies						
TNFB* 1	4	11.8	58	31.5	p<0.05	3.4
TNFB* 2	30	88.2	128	69.6	p<0.05	0.3
Phenotype frequencies						
TNFB* 1	3	17.6	51	55.4	p<0.01	0.2
TNFB* 2	16	94.1	86	93.5		
Genotype frequencies						
TNFB* 1/1	1	6.7	7	7.6		
TNFB* ½	2	13.3	44	47.8	p<0.01	0.2
TNFB* 2/2	14	93.3	42	45.7	p<0.01	5.6

CONCLUSION

Although the polymorphic NcoI site is an intron of TNFβ, and it is not present in the processed messenger RNA, it was found that homozygotes for either TNF fragment differ in TNF β production of in vitro stimulated peripheral mononuclear cells. In fact TNF β*1 allele is strongly associated with increased TNF β production by PBL in response to PHA. Furthermore, TNF β*1 alleles possess a triplet variation coding for asparagine at amino acid position 26, whereas TNFβ*2 alleles have threonine at this position.[10,11]

TNF β allele might mark a particular immunological responder status that is found in B8/DR3 individuals with an altered immune response to mitogens and suppressor T-cells[12,13] and may contribute in a predisponding manner to the development of autoimmune diseases like MG.

Our results suggest that: TNF β may play a role in the pathogenesis of MG. MG associated with thymoma and thymic hyperplasia are associated with different TNF β alleles: this strengthen the hypotesis that this two form of the disease may have a different pathogenesis.

REFERENCES

1. M.A. Degli Esposti, A. Andreas, F. Christiansen, B. Schalke, E. Albert, R. Dawkins: An approach to the localization of the susceptibility genes for generalized myasthenia gravis by mapping recombinant ancestral haplotypes. Immunogenetics 1992, 35: 355–364
2. G. Webb, D. Chaplin: Genetic variability at human tumor necrosis factor loci. The journal of immunology 1990, 145: 1278–1285
3. R.L. Dawkins, A. Leaver, P.U. Cameron, E. Martin, P.H. Kay, F.T. Christiansen: Some disease-associated ancestral haplotypes carry a Polymorphism of TNF. Human Immunology 1989, 26: 91–974.
4. F. Pociot, L. Briant, C.V. Jongeneel, J. Molvig, H. Worsaae, M. Abbal, M. Thomsen, J. Nerup, A.Cambon-Thomsen: Association of tumor necrosis factor (TNF) and class II major histocompatibility complex alleles with the secretion of TNF-α and TNF-β by human mononuclear cells: a possible link to insulin-dependent diabetes mellitus. Eur. J. Immunol. 1993, 23: 224–231
5. F. Pociot, J. Molvig, L. Wogensen, H. Worsaae, H. Dalboge, L. Baek, J. Nerup: A Tumor necrosis factor beta gene polymorphism in relation to monokine secretion and Insulin-dependent diabetes mellitus. Scand. J. Immunol. 1991, 33: 37–49
6. M.P. Bettinotti K. Hartung, H. Deicher, G. Messer, E. Keller, E. H. Weiss, E. D. Albert: Polymorphism of the tumor necrosis factor beta gene in systemic lupus erythematosus: TNFB-MHC haplotypes. Immunogenetics 1993, 37: 449–454
7. K. Badenhoop, G. Schawarz, H. Schleusener, A.P. Weetman, S. Recks, H. Peters, G.F. Bottazzo, K.H. Usadel: Tumor Necrosis Factor beta gene polymorphisms in Graves' disease. Journal of Clinical Endocrinology and Metabolism. 1992, 74: 287–291
8. M.R. Tola, L.M. Caniatti, I. Casetta, E. Granieri, C. Conoghi, R. Quatrale, V.C. Monetti, E. Paolino, V. Govoni, R. Pascarella, M. Carreras: Immunogenetic heterogeneity and associated autoimmune disorders in myastenia gravis: a population-based survey in the province of Ferrara, northern Italy. Acta Neurol Scand 1994, 90: 318–323.
9. S.H. Chan C.B. Tan, Y.N. Lin, G.B. Wee, M.A. Degli Esposti, R.L. Dawkins: HLA and Singaporean Chinese Myasthenia gravis Int Arch Allergy Immunol 1993, 101: 119–125
10. Messer G., U. Splengler, M.C. Jung, G. Honold, K. Blomer, G.R. Pape, G. Riethmuller, E.H. Weiss: Polymorphic structure of TNF locus: A NcoI polymorphism in the first intron of the human TNF-β gene correlates with a variant amino acid in position 26 and reduced level of TNF-β production. J Exp Med. 1991; 173:209–19.
11. Messer G., Spengler U., Jung M.C., Honold G., Eisenburg J., Sholz S., Albert E.D., Pape G.R., Riethmuller G., Weiss E.H.: allelic variation in the TNF beta gene does not explain the low TNF beta response in patients with primary biliary cirrhosis. Scand J Immunol. 1991, 34: 735–740
12. Hashimoto S., McCombs CC, Michalski J.P.: Mechanism of a lymphocyte abnormality associated with HLA B8-DR3 in clinically healthy individuals. Clin Exp Immunol. 1989, 76:317–23
13. Ambider JM, Chiorazzi N, Gibofsky A. Fotino M., Kunkel H.G: Special characteristics of cellular immune function in normal individuals of the HLA-DR3 type. Clin. Immunol Immunopathol. 1982, 23:269–74.

35

CLINICAL IMMUNOLOGY OF THYMIC TUMORS IN PATIENTS WITH MYASTHENIA GRAVIS

Johan A. Aarli

Department of Neurology
University Clinic
5021 Haukeland Hospital, Bergen, Norway

INTRODUCTION

Approximately 10–15 % of all myasthenia gravis (MG) patients have a thymoma, and 30 - 60 % of all thymoma cases are associated with MG. The clinical manifestations of MG with thymoma are similar to MG with thymic hyperplasia, but the thymoma patients are usually older, and the male:female ratio is about 1:1 compared with 1:2–3 for thymic hyperplasia. Polymyositis and cardiac involvement are uncommon in non-thymoma cases, but are well known in MG with thymoma (Aarli, 1994).

The clinical immunology of thymoma-associated MG comprises both the immune response to acetylcholine receptor protein (AChR) and to striated muscle antigens as well as antigen-non-specific findings. The expression of AChR in neoplastic thymus and the immune response to skeletal muscle serve to differentiate thymoma-associated MG from early onset MG associated with thymus hyperplasia.

THE IMMUNE RESPONSE TO AChR IN MG PATIENTS WITH THYMOMA

AChR antibodies are present in 90 % of all MG patients but in 100 % of patients with thymoma. The mean concentration in thymoma cases is not significantly different from non-thymoma cases with the same age at onset. However, the AChR antibody titres correspond poorly with the severity of the disease.

AChR antibodies are also found in some patients with thymoma who do not have MG. This is not specific to any type of tumor, as it has been reported in non-Hodgkin lymphoma and hamartoma as well as in epithelial tumors (Gilhus et al., 1985). MG may also occur after thymectomy on patients with thymoma (Hassel et al., 1992). Thymoma pa-

Epithelial Tumors of the Thymus, edited by Marx and Müller-Hermelink.
Plenum Press, New York, 1997

tients with AChR antibodies are therefore probably at special risk for subsequent development of MG.

After thymectomy in patients with MG and thymic hyperplasia, the AChR antibody concentration usually falls gradually. This is not so with thymoma. Somnier (1994) reported that the antibody titres did not drop and even rose during the immediate post-thymectomy period, and that this was correlated to an exacerbation of the clinical course. The removal of a thymoma is often associated with a more severe course of the disease. This cannot be related to the size or infiltration of the neoplasms, since it can occur even in patients with small, circumscribed thymic tumors.

The thymic neoplasm usually associated with MG is an epithelial tumor, most often of cortical type. There are several biological differences between normal and neoplastic epithelial cells. Normal cortical thymic epithelium does not present antigen in vitro, while the neoplastic cortical epithelial cells do. The neoplastic cells express a muscle antigen while normal epithelial cells do not (Gilhus et al., 1984). There has been much discussion whether AChR or AChR subunits are present in thymus and in neoplastic thymus tissue. It is the alpha subunit of the molecule which is essential, since it contains the main immunogenic region (MIR). Wheatley and colleges (1993) have demonstrated mRNA for the alpha-subunit of the AChR in the mouse thymus. The alpha subunit has been identified in myoid cells of both normal and MG-associated hyperplastic thymus tissue (Kirchner et al., 1988). Neoplastic thymus does not, however, contain myoid cells. Several investigators have demonstrated the presence of an incomplete alpha subunit in thymomas. Hara and coworkers (1991) demonstrated that the neoplastic epithelial cells from MG thymoma express the alpha-subunit of AChR. Kornstein and co-workers, using reverse transcription followed by the polymerase chain reaction, were also able to demonstrate AChR alpha-subunit mRNA both in thymuses and thymomas from patients with and without MG (Kornstein et al., 1995). Available data suggest that HLA class II-positive epithelial cells from MG-associated thymomas express a 153-kD protein that shares epitopes with the cytoplasmic domain of the AChR. It is not present in thymomas without MG (Geuder et al., 1992). Antibodies cross-reactive between thymoma and AChR or a molecular mimicry between myofibrillary muscle protein and the alpha-subunit of AChR may indicate a paraneoplastic etiology in thymoma-associated MG (Kirchner et al., 1988; Osborn et al., 1992).

Since the neoplastic epithelial cells express an AChR-like protein, the autoimmune process in MG may be initiated by these cells in thymoma cases. Gilhus and co-workers have shown that cultured thymoma epithelial cells can present synthetic AChR peptides to specific HLA-sharing responder T cell lines and clones with comparable efficiency to antigen presenting cells in blood. The responders depended on the specific antigen added. Since neoplastic thymic epithelial cells thus have the capacity to stimulate T cells, it is probable that an autosensitization to AChR also occur in thymoma in vivo (Gilhus et al., 1995). This is analogous to the situation in MG with thymus hyperplasia, since epithelial cells from non-thymoma thymic tissue also present AChR.

THE IMMUNE RESPONSE TO OTHER SKELETAL MUSCLE ANTIGENS

The immune response to AChR is the main pathogenic factor in MG. It is seen in patients with thymoma, in patients with thymus hyperplasia and in patients with MG and thymus involution. The immune response to AChR is therefore not unique to thymoma

MG. The main difference is probably how AChR is presented in the thymoma. It is the immune response to other skeletal muscle antigens that differentiates the thymoma form of MG from the other forms of the disease.

MG patients with thymoma always have, or almost always, in addition to the AChR antibodies, antibodies to other antigens of striated muscle. These antibodies, which are therefore important in the diagnosis of a thymoma, were first demonstrated by Strauss and coworkers in 1960 (Strauss et al., 1960). Such antibodies are detected in around 85 % of thymoma MG patients, but they are almost never detected in patients with young onset and thymus hyperplasia (Aarli et al., 1987). In immunofluorescence (IF) testing, the autoantibodies give a cross-striational staining. They react with heart and skeletal muscle in an identical pattern. Van der Geld and Strauss (1966) demonstrated that they react with the myoid cells of the thymus. They react also with neoplastic epithelial cells (Gilhus et al., 1986; Dardenne et al., 1987; Marx et al., 1992). It has not been possible to define the antigen(s) on the basis of the tissue distribution as revealed by IF techniques. Antigenic material can, however, be isolated by various techniques. Most patients with thymoma-associated MG have antibodies that react with a 0.05 M citric acid (CA) extract of striated muscle (heart as well as skeletal muscle) (Aarli et al., 1981). These antibodies can be demonstrated by several techniques, such as Western blot (WB) or ELISA. When results of IF are compared with WB, it became clear that both tests are concordant when qualitative results are considered. However, there is no relation between titre values, indicating that one technique may detect additional antigen/antibody systems not detected by the other (Kuks et al., 1992). Gilhus has demonstrated that a rabbit antiserum to the CA extract of striated muscle stained the neoplastic, but not normal, thymic epithelium (Gilhus et al., 1984). Accordingly, the thymus epithelial cells may either uncover or develop striated muscle cell epitopes during the process of neoplasia.

These antibodies are of different specificities, but titin is a major antigen (Aarli et al., 1990; Williams et al., 1992). Titin is a giant protein of striated muscle with a molecular weight more than 1 mill. It links the myosin molecule to the Z band. Antibodies to titin are not found in sera from patients with MG and hyperplastic thymus. They are, however, detected in more than 85 % of sera of patients with thymoma-associated MG. These antibodies react with a distinct 30 kD epitope in the I-band part of titin called MGT-30 (Gautel et al., 1993). Animals immunised with titin develop an immune response against the same part of the molecule, which therefore is called the MIR of titin. So far, Marx and coworkers did not detect expression of their titin epitopes in thymomas. (Marx et al., 1992)

About 50 % of patients with MG and thymoma have antibodies which react with a component of the sarcoplasmic reticulum of striated muscle (Mygland et al., 1992). Mygland defined the antigen as the ryanodine receptor (RyR). The ryanodine receptor is a foot protein in the junctional gap between the sarcoplasmic reticulum and the transverse tubules in skeletal muscle. It functions as a calcium release channel during excitation-contraction coupling. Sarcolemmal depolarization activates the dihydropyridine receptor. Subsequently, the ryanodine receptor is activated. Since RyR is a membrane protein, antibody binding may interfere directly with its function. Mygland found that the presence of circulating antibodies to the RyR receptor is associated with a more severe form of thymoma-associated MG (Mygland et al., 1992; 1994). Recent data also show that epithelial cells from MG thymomas express a RyR-epitope (Mygland et al., 1995).

Patients with titin and RyR antibodies usually have a more severe form of the disease (Mygland et al., 1994; Skeie et al. 1995). This reflects that they express an immune response that is related to a thymic tumor. It is not known why patients with thymoma have a more severe form of the disease. It cannot be because the tumor in some cases infiltrate the surrounding tissues. Somnier observed that MG patients with thymoma have myopathic findings on EMG and suggested that the more severe course of the disease is caused by a myopathy of possibly autoimmune origin, coexisting with MG, in these cases (Somnier and Trojaburg, 1993). Weigert, who was the first to publish a case of MG and thymoma (1901), demonstrated lymphocytic infiltration and muscle fibre necrosis both in the heart and deltoid muscle of his patient, obviously much more pronounced than in the lymphorrhages occasionally seen in early onset MG, but minor than corresponding to a full-blown polymyositis.

Patients with MG and thymoma usually have antibodies to several skeletal muscle antigens. Some of these may have a pathogenic significance while others are merely markers of an autoimmune process. It is probable that antigen-presenting cells from these patients alter their pattern of protein processing and presentation to autoreactive T cells, reflecting an epitope spreading. It is still unknown why this process does not occur in early onset MG with thymus hyperplasia.

LATE ONSET MG

MG can have its onset in non-thymoma patients more than 60 years. These patients usually have the same degree of thymus involution as can be found in otherwise healthy old people. Immunologically, they fall into two groups: one which is similar to young onset MG with thymus hyperplasia and one (approximately 30 %) with the same immunological features as found in thymoma-associated MG. Any hypothesis on the immunopathogenesis of thymoma-associated MG must account for how a severe MG can occur in individuals with advanced involution of the thymus.

NEUROMYOTONIA AND RIPPLING MUSCLE DISEASE

In neuromyotonia, there is a generalised muscle stiffness caused by hyperactivity of the peripheral motor nerves. This condition may comprise two apparently related clinical entities, both of them associated with thymoma and MG. Several of the reported patients with acquired neuromyotonia also have associated MG and thymoma. In neuromyotonia, the afflicted muscles are constantly contracting and the electrograhic pattern is characteristic for a neurogenic disorder. Shillito and co-workers have reported that 3 out of 6 such patients had detectable antibodies reacting with voltage-gated potassium channels (Shillito et al., 1995). Serum from the one such patient we have examined contained RyR and MGT30 antibodies.

Rippling muscle disease (RMD) has been reported as a hereditary autosomal dominant disease, but can also occur sporadically. In contrast to neuromyotonia, rippling muscles are electrically silent. Ansevin and Agamanolis (1996) recently described a patient with rippling muscles and MG with thymoma. This patient also had antibodies to AChR and to skeletal muscle. Muscle biopsy revealed interstitial inflammatory infiltrates consisting of plasma cells and T lymphocytes. It is not known whether the presence of MGT30/RyR antibodies is correlated to the MG and thymoma and not primarily to the RMD. It should be noted that plasma exchange leads to improvement, both of neuromyotonia and RMD, and that the rippling disappeared after thymectomy in the patient reported by Ansevin and Agamanolis. This indicates that the rippling phenomenon is mediated by circulating factors.

NON-SPECIFIC IMMUNOLOGICAL FINDINGS

Patients with MG and thymoma have an increase in the number of circulating lymphocytes expressing CD4 and CD8. A substantial number of non-MG patients with thymoma show the same increase. One of the patients reported by Matsui developed MG shortly after surgery (Matsui et al., 1993). It has been suggested that the formation of a thymoma is a part of an immunoregulatory mechanism with a predominance of autoantibody production in genetically predisposed individuals (Somnier, 1994).

In contrast to young onset myasthenia gravis patients with thymus hyperplasia, who have an increased HLA-B8, DR3 frequency, there is no known genetic association in MG with thymoma. In fact, thymoma patients are significantly less often HLA-DR3 positive than is the normal population. The genetic susceptibility to MG in thymoma patients, if any, is therefore different from that seen in patients with early onset and thymus hyperplasia (Spurkland et al, 1991).

REFERENCES

Aarli, JA. Myasthenia Gravis and Thymoma. Chapter 10 in: Handbook of Myasthenia Gravis and Myasthenic Syndromes (ed. R. P. Lisak) Marcel Dekker, New York, Pp.207 - 224, 1994.

Aarli JA, Lefvert AK, Tønder O. Thymoma-specific antibodies in sera from patients with myasthenia gravis demonstrated by indirect hemagglutination. J Neuroimmunol 1981;1:421–427.

Aarli, JA, Gilhus NE, Hofstad H. CA-antibody: an immunological marker of thymus neoplasia in myasthenia gravis? Acta Neurol scand. 1987;76:55–57.

Aarli JA, Stefansson K, Marton LSG, Wollmann RL. Patients with myasthenia gravis and thymoma have in their sera IgG autoantibodies against titin. Clin Exp Immunol 1990;82:284–288.

Anscvin CF, Agamanolis DP. Rippling muscles and myasthenia gravis with rippling muscles. Arch Neurol 1996;53:197–199.

Dardenne, M, Savino, W, Bach, JF. Thymomatous epithelial cells and skeletal muscle share a common epitope defined by a monoclonal antibody. Am J Pathol. 1987;126:194–198.

Gautel M, Lakey A, Barlow PD, Holmes Z, Scales S, Leonard K, Labeit S, Mygland Å, Gilhus NE, Aarli JA. Titin antibodies in myasthenia gravis: identification of a major immunogenic region of titin. Neurology 1993;43:1581–1585.

Geld, HW van der and Strauss, AJL. Autoantibodies and myasthenia gravis: immunological relationship between striated muscle and thymus. Lancet 1966:i:631–637.

Geuder KI, Marx A, Witzemann V, Schalke B, Kirchner T, Müller-Hermelink. Genomic organization and lack of transcription of the nicotinic acetylcholine receptor subunit genes in myasthenia gravis-associated thymoma. Lab Invest 1992;66:452–458.

Gilhus, N. E., Aarli, J. A., Christensson, B., Matre, R.: Rabbit antiserum to a citric acid extract of human skeletal muscle staining thymoma from myasthenia gravis patients. J. Neuroimmunology 1984;34:55–64.

Gilhus NE, Aarli JA, Janzen RWC, Otto HF, Fasske E, Matre R. Skeletal muscle antibodies in patients with a thymic tumour but without myasthenia gravis. J Neuroimmunol 1985;8:69–75.

Gilhus NE, Matre R, Aarli JA, Hofstad H, Thunold S. Thymic lymphoepitheliomas and skeletal muscle expressing common antigen(s). Acta neurol scand 1986;73:428–433.

Gilhus NE, Willcox N, Harcourt G, Nagvvekar N, Beeson D, Vincent A, Newsom-Davis J. Antigen presentation by thymoma epithelial cells from myasthenia gravis patients to potentially pathogenic T cells. J Neuroimmunol 1995;56:65–76.

Hara Y, Ueno S, Uemichi T, Takhashi N, Yorifuji S, Fujii Y, Tarui S. Neoplastic epithelial cells express alpha subunit of muscle nicotinic acetylcholine receptor in thymomas from patients with myasthenia gravis. FEBS letters 1991:279:137–140.

Hassel B, Gilhus NE, Aarli JA, Skogen OR. Fulminant myasthenia gravis and polymyositis after thymectomy for thymoma. Acta neurol scand 1992;85:63–65.

Kirchner T, Tzartos S, Hoppe F, Schalke B, Wekerle H, Müller-Hermelink HK. Pathogenesis of myasthenia gravis. Acetylcholine receptor-related antigenic determinants in tumor-free thymuses and thymic epithelial tumors. Am J Pathol 1988;130:268–280.

Kornstein MJ, Asher O, Fuchs S. Acetylcholine receptor alpha-subunit and myogenin mRNAs in thymus and thymomas. Am J Pathol 1995;146:1320–1324.

Kuks JBM. The thymus and myasthenia gravis. Drukkerij Regenboog, Groningen 1992.

Kuks JB, Limburg PC, Horst G, Oosterhuis HJ. Antibodies to skeletal muscle in myasthenia gravis. Part 3. Relation with clinical course and therapy. J Neurol Sci 1993;120:168–173.

Marx A, Osborn M, Tzartos S, Geuder KI, Schalke B, Nix W, Kirchner T, Müller-Hermelink HK. A striational muscle antigen and myasthenia gravis-associated thymomas share an acetylcholine-receptor epitope. Dev. Immunol. 1992;2:77–84.

Matsui M, Wada H, Ohta M, Kuroda Y. Potential role of thymoma and other mediastinal tumors in the pathogenesis of myasthenia gravis. J Neuroimmunol 1993;44:171–176.

Mygland Å, Tysnes OB, Aarli JA, Flood PR, Gilhus NE. Myasthenia gravis patients with a thymoma have antibodies against a high molecular weight protein in sarcoplasmic reticulum. J Neuroimmunol 1992;37:1–7.

Mygland Å, Tysnes OB, Matre R, Volpe P, Aarli JA, Gilhus NE. Ryanodine receptor autoantibodies in myasthenia gravis patients with a thymoma. Ann Neurol 1992;32:589–591.

Mygland Å, Aarli JA, Matre R, Gilhus NE. Ryanodine receptor antibodies related to severity of thymoma associated myasthenia gravis. J Neurol Neurosurg Psychiat 1994;57:843–846.

Mygland Å., Kuwajima G, Mikoshiba K, Tysnes OB, Aarli JA, Gilhus NE. Thymomas express epitopes shared by the ryanodine receptor. J Neuroimmunol 1995;62:79–83.

Osborn M, Marx A, Kirchner T, Tzartos SJ, Plessman U, Weber K. A shared epitope in the acetylcholine receptor alpha subunit and fast troponin I of skeletal muscle. Is it important for myasthenia gravis? Am J Pathol 1992;140:1215–1223.

Shillito P, Molenaar PC, Vincent A, Leys K, Zheng W, van den Berg RJ, Plomp JJ, Van Kempen GTH, Chauplannaz G, Wintzen AR, van Dijk JG, Newsom-Davis J. Acquired neuromyotonia: Evidence of autoantibodies directed against K+-channels of peripheral nerve. Ann Neurol 1995;38:714–722.

Skeie GO, Mygland Å, Aarli JA, Gilhus NE. Titin antibodies in patients with late onset myasthenia gravis: Clinical correlations. Autoimmunity 1995; 20:99–104.

Somnier FE. Exacerbation of myasthenia gravis after removal of thymoma. Acta Neurol Scand 1994;90:56–66.

Somnier FE, Trojaburg W. Neurophysiological evaluation in myasthenia gravis. A comprehensive study of a complete patient population. Electroencephalogr Clin Neurophysiol 1993;89:73–87.

Spurkland A, Gilhus NE, Rønningen KS, Aarli JA, Vartdal F. Myasthenia gravis patients with thymus hyperplasia and myasthenia gravis patients with thymoma display different HLA associations. Tissue Ant. 1991;37:90–93.

Strauss AJ, Seegal BC, Hsu JC, Burkholder PM, Nastuk WL, Osserman KE. Immunofluorescence demonstration of a muscle binding, complement fixing serum globulin fraction in myasthenia gravis. Proc Soc Exp Biol (NY) 1960;195:184–191.

Weigert C. Patologisch—anatomischhes Beitrag zur Erb´schen Krankheit. Neurolog Zentralblatt 1901;20:594–597.

Wheatley LM, Urso D, Zheng Y, Loh E, Levinson AI. Molecular analysis of intrathymic acetylcholine receptor. Ann NY Acad Sci 1993, 681:74–82.

Williams CL, Hay JE, Huiatt TW, Lennon VA. Paraneoplastic IgG striational autoantibodies produced by clonal thymic B cells and in serum of patients with myasthenia gravis and thymoma react with titin. Lab Invest 1992;66:331–336.

36

MYASTHENIA GRAVIS WITH THYMOMA

H. J. G. H. Oosterhuis and J. B. M. Kuks

Department of Neurology
Academic Hospital to the University Groningen
Postbox 30.001, 9700 RB Groningen, The Netherlands

1. INTRODUCTION

The presence of a thymoma has been recognized as an occurrence beyond statistical probability from the earliest history of myasthenia gravis (MG). After the description by Weigert[1] in 1901 of a patient with a thymoma and lymphorrages in his muscles, considered as metastases of the thymoma, an enlargement of the thymus or a thymoma was mentioned in 28% of the first 250 patients with MG, described until 1912[2]. In large recent series of patients with MG, thymomas occurred in 9 to 16% [3a] and in 20 to 34% of series of thymectomies for MG [4–6].

The incidence of MG in patients with a thymoma was surmised to be 30–40% but in two recent series 59 and 61% were found [7–8]. In epidemiological surveys the incidence of thymomas is lacking except our study in Amsterdam where 19% was found [9].

In general myasthenic signs are more severe in patients with thymoma and especially this category is liable to develop spontaneous crises. Death rates in MG are further influenced by the potential invasive growth of the thymoma and by the association of other malignant diseases such as aplastic anaemia or pancytopenia. These diseases have become more important for the prognosis since the MG itself has become better treatable with immunosuppressive drugs.

We report our experience with 139 patients with MG and thymoma, who comprise 17% of our patients with MG seen between 1960 and 1994.

2. METHODS AND PATIENTS

This series comprises 814 consecutive patients with MG who consulted the first author between 1960 and 1984 and the first or the second author between 1985 and 1994. From 1960 to 1976 these patients were seen in the neurological department of the (former) Wilhelmina Gasthuis in Amsterdam and from 1976 in the neurological department of the Academic Hospital Groningen. About 60% of these patients were in regular treatment, 40% were seen as consultations twice or more in the course of their illness. All patients

Epithelial Tumors of the Thymus, edited by Marx and Müller-Hermelink.
Plenum Press, New York, 1997

who were not in regular treatment were followed by telephone calls and by informations from their neurologists and other physicians.

A follow-up period of at least 3 years was needed for inclusion. Because treatment modalities and diagnostic measures have changed in the last decennia patients were divided into three groups: onset of MG before 1970 (n=284), between 1971 and 1984 (n=261) and from 1985 to 1994 (n=269) in order to enable comparison with patients without thymoma of the same period and of the 3 periods.

The diagnosis of MG was made on the basis of the typical history and fluctuation of clinical signs, confirmed by EMG and/or by a favourable reaction to anticholinesterases (edrophonium, neostigmin, pyridostigmin). Besides all patients with thymomas, 92% of the patients with generalized MG and about 40% of the patients with ocular MG had antibodies to acetylcholine receptors which are highly specific for MG [(10)].

In ocular MG signs had to be confined to the extrinsic eye muscles and/or the palpebral levators, and had to involve both eyes.

The diagnosis of thymoma was made by plain X-rays (n=65), planigraphy including CT-scanning after 1976 (n=46), primary by operation (n=22), primary by autopsy (n=2). In 18 patients the diagnosis of thymoma on X-rays or CT scan was not confirmed by operation or autopsy, but no other diagnosis became more plausible during the follow-up period. A thymoma was excluded in most young patients by thymectomy in older patients by a long follow-up with repeated X-rays combined with the absence of anti-striated muscle antibodies or by autopsy; however the presence of a small silent thymoma is not completely excluded in patients before 1970.

The staging of the thymoma was according to Masaoka [(11)] and was based on the combination of macroscopic (operator) and microscopic (pathologist) data (see table 3).

Patients were classified according to Osserman [(12)] indicating the worst period of their illness.

Treatment of MG was as outlined previously [(3b)]: in short: all patients were treated initially with anticholinesterases, mainly pyridostigmin. In patients with disabling bulbar or generalized signs immunomodulating therapies were given: prednisone and azathioprine, rarely cyclophosphamide or methotrexate since 1970, cyclosporine since 1986. Prednisone was usually started in high dosages once every day (1–1,5 mg/kg) with a gradual change to an alternate day scheme of 0,5 mg/kg/2 days after about half a year and mostly combined with azathioprine (2–3 mg/kg/day). After one year of azathioprine an attempt was made to taper off the prednisone completely. Plasma-exchange was used to prepare the patient for thymectomy, in myasthenic crises and rarely as a long term treatment.

Thymectomy was considered indicated in all patients under the age of 45 year with a generalized MG without thymoma, and in case of a thymoma in all ages. Old age, severe MG or other diseases were relative contra-indications for the operation especially before 1970. In some patients a primary irradiation of the thymoma (4000–5000 rad) was done. If the thymoma was not completely removable, postoperative irradiation was usually given, but exceptions occurred due to the poor general condition of the patient or to the interpretation of the microscopic picture.

3. RESULTS

3.1 Epidemiological Data

Age of onset and type of MG, gender and the presence of thymoma are given in fig. 1.

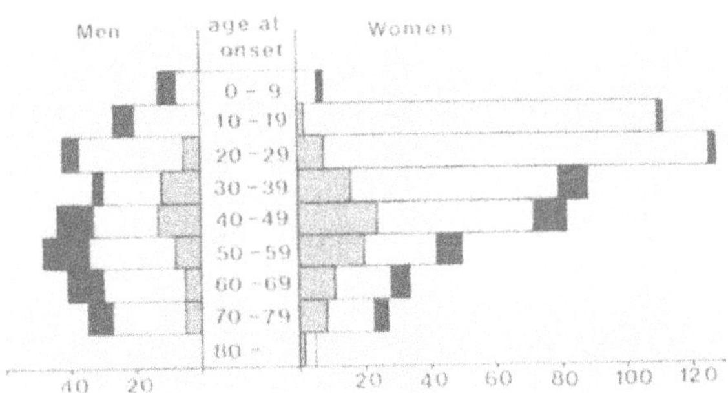

Figure 1. Age of onset and type of MG, gender and the presence of thymoma.

Thymomas were diagnosed in 48 of 284 men and 91 of 530 women, in both groups in17%. Ocular MG had a higher incidence in men than in women, especially in the younger age groups. Thymomas had a somewhat higher incidence in men under the age of 40, and in women over the age, but the difference was not significant (chi square = 1.2, p = 0.25). The highest incidence of thymomas was in 4th and 5th decade in men and the 5th and 6nd decade in women. Only one woman with a thymoma had a purely ocular MG but she wás not followed longer than 3 years. Two patients were mother and daughter; in the latter the detection and operation of the thymoma preceded the signs of MG by 2 years.

The maximum severity of MG was: I Ocular: 0.7%, IIA (mild): 10.8%, IIB (moderate): 44.6%, III: early severe: 10.8%, IV: late severe 32.4%. Comparable frequencies in the non-thymoma patients with onset before 1970 were: ocular: 13.7%, IIA: 14.1%, IIB: 54.4%, III: 1.6%, IV: 16.1%. This implies that the MG in patients with thymoma is "never" alone ocular and more severe than in patients without thymoma.

The latter was also reflected in the higher incidence of bulbar signs in the first 3 months (52/139 in thymomas and 62/250 in non- thymomas, chi square = 5.5, p < 0.02).

3.2 Diagnosis of Thymoma

Thymomas were usually detected by radiological screening because of the MG or by routine radiological examination. In the latter category 17 thymomas were diagnosed and operated in 16 patients before onset of their MG and 2 also thereafter (table 1) with an interval of 1/2 - 28 (!) years (median 3 years).

It was exceptional that the thymoma itself was symptomatic: only in two women a tumor became visible above the clavicula. In most patients the diagnosis thymoma was made within a year of the diagnosis MG, but in 29 patients there was a delay of more than one year. In the period before 1976 when CT scanning was not available, pneumomediastinography was the method of choice to demonstrate a thymoma that was not visible on plain X-rays (AP and 10° oblique sidewards). Since inflation of air could give rise to an exacerbation of the MG, it was often preferred to perform the mediastinal exploration "blindly" in young patients. But also the CT-scan was sometimes insufficient to predict the finding of a small thymoma at operation.

Table 1. Diagnosis thymoma

	–'70	–'84	–'94	**Total**
Preceeding MG	3	5(1)	8(2)	**16(3)**
Within 1 year of MG	21	40	33	**94**
2-5 years after MG	7	7	5	**19**
> 6 years after MG	5	4	1	**10**
X-rays	20	26	19	**65**
Planigraphy or CT scan	6	18	22	**46**
Operation	8	11	3	**22**
Autopsy	1	1		**2**
Tumor in jugulo	1		1	**2**
Unknown			2	**2**
	36	**56**	**47**	**139**

( ) patients with 2 consecutive thymomas

3.3 Clinical Stages of Thymoma

Of the 119 patients in whom the histology of the tumor was known, about half were in stage I and one third in stages III or IV (table 3).

There was no good relation between the time elapsed from the diagnosis thymoma and the stage, even if the group of the pre-MG thymomas was excluded.

Postoperative irradiation was performed in 3 of 5 stage II, 7 of 25 stage III and 4 of 11 stage IVa thymomas, and primary irradiation in 6 patients. In none of these patients a recurrence of the thymoma was seen.

Recurrence after completely removed thymomas was seen in 11 patients (table 2) with primary thymomas in all stages between I and III. The first tumor was diagnosed 5 to 11 years before the onset of MG in 3 patients. Because removal was considered as complete by the surgeon in all cases no postoperative irradiation was given.

The second thymoma was found 4–18 (median 6) years after the first thymomectomy. Unfortunately 7 of the 11 new thymomas were in stage IV at the time of diagnosis. The prognosis in this group of 11 patients was rather poor as 6 died from their second tu-

Table 2. Recurrent thymomas

		Age at	First thymoma		Second thymoma			Follow		
		onset MG	Age	Stage	Age	Stage	Therapy	up until		MG
1	W	35	24	I	35	IV	O+I	42	alive	R
2	M	36	30	III	38	III	O	52	+PR	FR
3	W	37	31	I	36	I	O	42	alive	R
4	W	41	43	I	53	III	IR+Ch	64	+TH	FR
5	W	32	32	I	37	III	O	38	alive	M
6	M	58	64	II	70	IVa	–	74	+TH	R
7	M	40	41	III	46	IVb	IR	46	TH	R
8	W	46	45	I	49	IVa	IR	49	+TH	M
9	W	40	40	III	58	IVa	O+Ch	60	alive	M
10	W	29	30	III	35	IVb	Predn	35	+TH	M
11	W	38	40	III	46	IVa	Predn	46	+TH	FR

Stages according to Masaoka ( ), O = operation, IR = irradiation
Ch = chemotherapy, (F)R = farmacologiacal remission: M = mild
+TH: died by thymoma, +PR: died by complications of prednisone

Table 3. Staging of thymoma (Masaoka[11])

	Diagnosis thymoma				
	Before MG	Within one y	After 2–5 y	After > 6 y	
Operation					
Stage I	9(2)	41(2)	6	4(1)	**60(5)**
Stage IIA	1	9	1(1)		**11(1)**
Stage IIB		4	1		**5**
Stage III	3(1)	19(4)	1	2	**25(5)**
Stage IV	2	4	4	1	**11**
Unknown	1	1			**2**
Autopsy		5[x]	1[xx]	1[xxx]	**7**
No operation		11	2	5	**18**
	16(3)	**94(6)**	**16**	**13(1)**	**139(11)**

( ) recurrent thymoma
[x] 3 patients stage I, one patient stage IIa, 1 patient stage III
[xx] one patient stage IV b
[xxx] one patient stage I

mor and one other from complications of therapy. The MG was well controlled by prednison or in spontaneous remission.

3.4 Associated Autoimmune Diseases and Malignancies

Thymoma associated autoimmune (A-I) diseases (i.e. pure red cell anaemia, pancytopenia, hypo- or hypergamma-globulinemia) were diagnosed in 3 men (6%) and 5 women (5.5%); 6 other associated A-I diseases occurred in 5 men (12.5%) and 15 A-I diseases in 14 women (15%), (table 4).

Table 4. Associated diseases in 139 thymoma patients

	Men (n=48)	Women (n=91)
Pure red cell anemia	1	3[x]
Pancytopenia	1	1
Hypergamma globulinaemia	1	
Hypogamma globulinaemia		2[x]
Hyperthyroidism	1*	4[xx]
Primary hypothyroidism		1
Iliitis terminalis (m.Crohn)		1
Systemic lupus erythematosus	2	2[xx]
Rheumatoid arthritis	1	—
Pernicious anaemia		2
m.Addison		1
Autoimmune hepatitis	1*	
Multiple sclerosis		1
Polymyositis		1
m.Besnier-Boeck (sarcoidosis)		1
Alopecia (sub)totalis	1	
Stomatitis erosiva		1
Malignancies	5	13

[x], [xx], * one patient with both diseases

Table 5. Effects of therapies, final outcome

	Periods of observation			
	–'70	'71–'84	'85–'94	**Totals**
No immuno suppression				
Remission	5(4)	9(9)	5(5)	**19**
Mild	1	7(5)	3(3)	**11**
Moderate	3(1)	2(2)	1(1)	**6**
Died from MG	13(10)	5(4)		**18**
Immuno suppression				
Remission	3(3)	9(9)	25(18)	**37**
Mild	5(2)	7(7)	8(7)	**20**
Moderate	2(1)	5(4)	3(3)	**10**
Died from MG		2(1)		**2**
Died from thymoma	3(2)	7(7)	2(2)	**12**
Died from complications	1(1)	3(2)		**4**
	36(24)	**56(50)**	**47(39)**	**139(113)**

( ) = number of patients who underwent thymomectomy

Malignancies evolved in 10% of the men and 13% of the women.

The mean age at diagnosis of the thymoma was 46 years for the men and 49 years for the women; the mean follow-up period respectively 10.6 and 11.7 years.

In a comparable cohort (patients diagnosed before 1970, mean age at last follow-up 59 years) A-I diseases occurred in 7 of 82 men (8.5%) and 33 of 202 women (16.3%) and malignancies in 4.9% of the men and 7.9% of the women. One obvious difference between the thymoma and the non-thymoma group was the higher incidence of rheumatoid arthritis in the latter (4% in men, 9% in women, general population 1%). The total percentage of A-I diseases and that of malignancies was higher in the thymoma patients than in the comparable group of non-thymoma patients.

3.5 Outcome of Immunomodulating Treatment

The effect of various therapies on the MG at the end of the follow-up period are summarized in the tables.

The effect of anticholinesterases was not considered separately being relatively unimportant as compared with the immunomodulating (I.M.) therapy. No I.M. drugs were given in 60 patients (43%) of whom 6 are listed under: died from thymoma. Of the complete remissions two thirds were dependent upon I.M. therapies, as was the case in patients with mild symptoms. As can been seen from table 5, spontaneous or I.M. induced complete remissions of MG occurred in 40% and a mild MG in another 22%. Twenty patients died from MG, of whom only two under treatment with I.M. (both 100 mg azathioprine); 9 other patients died from the invasion of the thymoma and 3 from thymoma related diseases (pancytopenia in 2, myocarditis with ventricular fibrillation in one (13)), 3 patients died from the complications of I.M. therapy (2 infections by prednisone, one myeloid leukaemia by 6 mercaptopurine) and one older patient died shortly after the irradiation for the thymoma from respiratory insufficiency. There was no difference between men and women but death by MG or thymoma or the complications of treatment was more frequent under the age of 50 years (25/80 vs 10/59 $p < 0.05$).

3.6 Thymomectomy

More than 80% of the patients have been operated upon for removal of the thymoma. The effect of thymomectomy on the course of MG was at best not impressive. Leaving the 16 patients who died of complications of the therapy beyond consideration only 30 patients (24%) went into an acceptable clinical state (19 in remission and 11 mildly affected) while the others continued to need IM drugs (56%), remained in a moderate state (5%) or even died for from MG without IM medication (15%) (table 5). Four of the former 30 patients were not operated vs 20 of the remaining 93 (difference not significant: 50%>p>30%).

Irradiation was given as a single therapy in 6 patients before 1970 without appreciable benefit for the MG.

Removal of a thymoma even caused a deterioration of MG in at least 9 patients who did not receive IM drugs because of a mild clinical state. The MG deteriorated mostly 3–6 months following the operation, and yet dictated the use of IM medication. This deterioration was accompanied by an increase of both antibodies to acetylcholine receptors and to striated muscle as is exemplified in fig 2 [14].

In 80 cases of whom pathological reports were available, a hyperplastic thymus was found in 13 patients, no thymic tissue was detected in 31 while in the remaining 36 patients the thymus was described as involuted (atrophic) (n=19) or normal (n=17). There was no relation between the presence and histology of the residual thymic tissue beside the thymoma and the clinical outcome.

4. COMMENTS

4.1 Methods of Study

This study runs from 1960 until 1994, which implies that important changes took place in the diagnosis of MG (anti-AChR antibodies, single fiber electromyography) in the

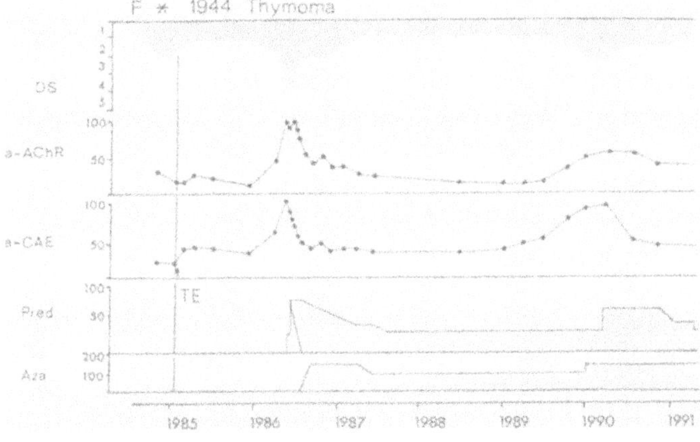

Figure 2. DS: disability scale of myasthenia (1=mild, 4 severe), a-AChR: concentration of antibodies to acetylcholine receptors nmol/L, a-CAE: antibodies to striated muscle, citrate acid muscle extracts with an ELISA method (ref. 14), pred = prednisone mg/2d, aza = azathioprine mg/d, TE = thymectomy.

diagnosis of thymoma (computerized tomography) and in treatment modalities (I.M. therapies, plasma- exchange, artificial respiration). All patients were studied with the same methods and our therapeutic advices did not change appreciably since 1970 when I.M. therapies were given to all patients with moderate and severe signs.

4.2 The Incidence of Thymomas

In the three periods of our study thymomas were diagnosed in respectively 12.7%, 21.5% and 17.5% of the myasthenic patients, with a mean of 17.1% over the whole period. The lower incidence in the first period may be due to the lower sensitivity of the diagnostic procedures, but also to the fact that the first cohort included patients with longstanding disease of whom only had a thymoma. In a recent large series of MG patients followed between 1971 and 1991 in Rome 20% had a thymoma [15]. Some selection bias is not unprobable so that in an epidemiological study the prevalence might be lower.

4.3 Clinical Severity of MG

In the first period (onset until 1970) MG death rate was higher than in the following periods, which should be attributed to the unavailability of prednisone and plasma-exchange. In the second period relatively more patients died from the invasive growth of the thymoma or the thymoma related diseases; the absence of MG-deaths in the last period may be flattered by the shorter follow-up (mean 5.6 year).

As was found in previous studies MG signs in thymoma patients were more severe, with periods of ventilatory insufficiency in 43% versus 15% in non-thymus cases [16]. In this series bulbar signs were relatively more frequent at onset and MG-signs were confined to the ocular muscles in only one patient at 3 years follow-up.

4.4 Other Associated Auto-Immune Diseases

Other associated auto-immune diseases were more frequent in thymoma patients, especially in men, also *extrathymic malignancies* had a higher incidence than the non-thymoma group with the same mean age. The latter was also found in Japan [17].

4.5 The Final Outcome

The final outcome (table 5) includes spontaneous remission in 14% and a mild clinical state in 8% without IM drugs. This compares unfavourably with the outcome in non-thymoma patients [3c]. However the final results of IM therapy, which had to be given in about 75% of thymoma patients, were at least as good as in non-thymoma patients.

4.6 Effect of Thymomectomy

Results in our patient group do not indicate a benificial *effect of thymomectomy* or thymic irradiation on the course of MG, even if a coexistent thymus is removed. In fact this remains difficult to prove or to refute without a randomized clinical trial but this fact has been recognized from the very beginning of thymectomies. Indeed, there were even indications for a clinical and serological deterioration in the year following thymomectomy [14] as was also described by Sommer [18]. Thymomectomy did not prevent the appearance of MG in 16 patients (11.4%).

4.7 Clinical Stages of the Thymoma

At the time of operation (or autopsy) the stage of the thymoma did not correspond with the clinical severity of the MG, which was in agreement with the Roman series [(15)]. The time elapsed between the diagnosis and the operation was not well related to the degree of invasiveness of the thymoma. In general in stage II the tumor could be removed completely with excision of the pleura, but in stage III this was not always possible. No recurrence was seen in the 14 patients who received postoperative radiation therapy because of incomplete macroscopic removal. However in 7 other patients another tumor was detected after complete previous removal suggesting the growth of a second thymoma. No similar cases could be found in literature; only one case was reported of a thymoma emerging after previous removal of a non-tumorous thymus [(19)]. The question remains whether the second tumours should be considered as metastases not detected at the time of the first operation or as really new tumours in aberrant thymic tissue. In the latter case the intriguing - but merely hypothetical - point rises that these patients might be genetically susceptible of developping a thymoma. However finding most recurrent thymomas in stage IV favours the probability that we are dealing with the metastases of the primary tumour. The recurrence of thymomas in 6 other patients only were found after incomplete removal without postoperative irradiation.

REFERENCES

1. Weigert C. Pathologisch-anatomischer Beitrag zur Erbschen Krankheit (Myasthenia Gravis), Neurologischen Zentralblatt 1901, 20:597–601
2. Starr MA. Myasthenia Gravis J Nerv Ment Dis. 1912, 39:721–731
3. Oosterhuis HJGH. Myasthenia gravis Churchill Livingstone Edinburgh 1984 a.28; b. 206–207; c. 62–67
4. Keynes G . Investigations into thymic disease and tumour formation. BR J Surg XLII 1955, 449–462
5. Mulder DG, Hermann Chr, Keesey J and Edwards H. Thymectomy for Myasthenia Gravis Am J Surg 1983, 146, 61–65
6. Maggi G, Casadio C, Cavallo A, Cianci R, Molinatti M and Ruffini E. Thymectomy in Myasthenia Gravis: results of 662 cases operated upon in 15 years. Eur J Cardiothorac Surg 1989, 3: 504–509
7. Monden Y, Uyama T, Taniki T, Hashimoto J, Fujii Y, Nakahara K, Kawashima Y and Masaoka A . The characteristics of thymoma with Myasthenia Gravis: a 28 year experience. J Surg Onc 1988, 38, 151–154
8. Levasseur P, Menestrier M, Gaud C, Dartevelle P, Julia P, Rojas-Miranda A, Navajas M, Le Brigand H and Merker M. Thymomas et maladies associées. A propos d'une serie de 255 thymomas opérées, Rev Mal Respir. 1988, 5, 173–178.
9. Oosterhuis HJGH. Diagnosis and differential diagnosis. In: Myasthenia Gravis. Eds De Baets M and Oosterhuis HJGH. CRC Press Boca Raton 1993, 208–209.
10. Limburg PC, The TH, Hummel-Tappel E, Oosterhuis HJGH. Anti-acetylcholine receptor antibodies in Myasthenia Gravis. Journal of the Neurological Sciences 1983, 58: 357–370.
11. Masaoka A, Monden Y. Nakahara K, Tamioka T. Follow-up study of thymomas with special reference to their clinical stages. Cancer 1981, 48, 2485–2492.
12. Osserman KE and Genkins G. Studies in Myasthenia Gravis: a review of a twenty year experience in over 1200 patients. Mt Sinai J Med 1971, 38, 497–537.
13. Jongste MJL de, Oosterhuis HJGH, Lie KL. Intractable ventricular tachycardia in a patient with giant cell myocarditis, thymoma and Myasthenia Gravis. International Journal of Cardiology 1986, 13, 374–378.
14. Kuks JBM, Limburg PC, Horst G. Oosterhuis HJGH. 1993 Antibodies to skeletal muscle in Myasthenia Gravis. Part 3 Relation with clinical course and therapy Journal of the Neurological Sciences 1993, 120: 168–173.
15. Palmisani MT, Evoli A, Batocchi AP, Provenzano C, Tonali P. Myasthenia Gravis associated with thymoma: clinical characteristics and long-term outcome. Eur Neurol 1993, 34: 78–82.
16. Oosterhuis HJGH. Myasthenia Gravis. A review: Clinical Neurology and Neurosurgery 1981, 83: 105–135.

17. Monden Y, Kyama T, Kimura S and Tanaki T. 1991 Extrathymic malignancy in patients with Myasthenia Gravis Eur J Cancer 1991, 27: 745–747.
18. Sommer FE. Exacerbations of Myasthenia Gravis after removal of thymomas. Acta Neurol Scand 1994, 90: 56–66.
19. Husain F, Ryan NJ, Hogan GR, Gonzalez E 1990. Occurrence of invasive thymoma after thymectomy for Myasthenia Gravis: report of a case. Neurology 1990, 40: 170–171.

37

REPRODUCIBILITY OF A HISTOGENETIC CLASSIFICATION OF THYMIC EPITHELIAL TUMOURS

Pauline M. Close,[1*] Thomas Kirchner,[2] Cornelius J. Uys,[1] and Hans Konrad Müller-Hermelink[1]

[1]Department of Anatomical Pathology
University of Cape Town and Groote Schuur Hospital
Cape Town, South Africa
[2]Institute of Pathology
University of Würzburg
Würzburg, Germany

INTRODUCTION

A histogenetic classification of thymic epithelial neoplasms proposed by Müller-Hermelink and co-workers has been shown by a number of recent studies to be of clinical and prognostic value. Reproducibility is an important criterion for the acceptance of any new classification for general diagnostic use. The reproducibility of this classification was tested on 51 cases of thymic epithelial neoplasia, by comparing results obtained by pathologists working from published criteria only with results obtained by the pathologists who developed the classification. In 78% of cases there was complete concordance of results. Analysis of the 22% discordant cases showed that this discordance was due to a degree of subjectivity in determining cut-off points between categories adjacent to each other in the morphologic spectrum of thymic epithelial neoplasia (medullary *vs* mixed, cortical *vs* well-differentiated thymic carcinoma). In terms of the important clinical distinction between benign (medullary and mixed) thymomas and those with more aggressive biological behaviour (cortical types and well-differentiated thymic carcinoma), the degree of reproducibility was 96%. The high degree of reproducibility of this histogenetic classification of thymic epithelial neoplasms should facilitate its acceptance and use in routine diagnostic pathology.

---

* Address for correspondence: Dr. P. M. Close, Department of Anatomical Pathology, University of Cape Town Medical School, Anzio Road, Observatory 7925, Cape Town, South Africa. Tel: 021 406 6413; fax: 021 686 1613.

Epithelial Tumors of the Thymus, edited by Marx and Müller-Hermelink.
Plenum Press, New York, 1997

There is as yet no widely accepted histological classification of thymic epithelial neoplasms which satisfactorily fulfills the criteria of a sound scientific basis, clinical relevance and reproducibility. The traditional histopathological classification divides thymomas into epithelial, lymphocytic, mixed epithelial and lymphocytic, and spindle cell types.[1–3] This classification lacks a sound scientific basis and is poorly reproducible. Previous studies using this classification have concluded that histologic type is of little value in predicting prognosis and that the various syndromes associated with thymoma may occur with any histologic type.[2–5] The distinction between thymoma and thymic carcinoma has traditionally been made on the basis of the presence or absence of cytological features of malignancy.[6–8]

Müller-Hermelink and co-workers have proposed a histogenetic classification of thymomas based on similarities between neoplastic thymic epithelial cells and the corresponding cell types in normal thymus.[9–11] They have also recognised a distinctive type of low grade well-differentiated thymic carcinoma (WDTC)[12] which is related to cortical thymoma. There is increasing evidence for the clinical and prognostic value of this classification[13–18] but there have as yet been no published studies of its reproducibility. This is an important aspect of the acceptance of any new classification for general diagnostic use. The purpose of this study therefore was to assess the reproducibility of this histogenetic classification of thymic epithelial tumours.

MATERIALS AND METHODS

Cases of thymoma were obtained over a 35 year period (1957–1992) from surgical biopsy and postmortem material from the records of the Department of Anatomical Pathology, University of Cape Town Medical School. Only cases in which the blocks were available were included in this study. The total number of cases studied was 51. These cases included biopsies and surgical resections of thymic epithelial tumours. Clinical information was obtained from hospital records and from the records of the Cardiothoracic Surgery Unit and the Department of Radiation Oncology. Intra-operative assessment of the degree of local invasiveness of the tumours was recorded. Clinical staging according to the Masaoka system was possible in 48 of the 51 cases. Correlation of clinical behaviour with histologic subtype was not included in this study of the reproducibility of histogenetic classification. A duplicate set of sections was cut from all blocks. Sections were cut at 3–4μ and stained with haematoxylin and eosin. The Müller-Hermelink histogenetic classification of thymomas was used. Cases were classified independently, without prior discussion of the cases, by PMC and CJU in Cape Town (using published criteria only[10–12]) and TK in Würzburg, Germany. The following five categories of thymic epithelial tumour were used: medullary, mixed, predominantly cortical, cortical and well-differentiated thymic carcinoma. Typical examples of each category are shown in Figures 1 and 2.

In order to become familiar with the criteria for histogenetic classification of thymomas, PMC and CJU went through all the cases once before the second and final analysis when the results of classification were recorded. On a date and time decided in advance, the results of classification by PMC and CJU in Cape Town and TK in Germany were exchanged by fax and the concordance was analysed.

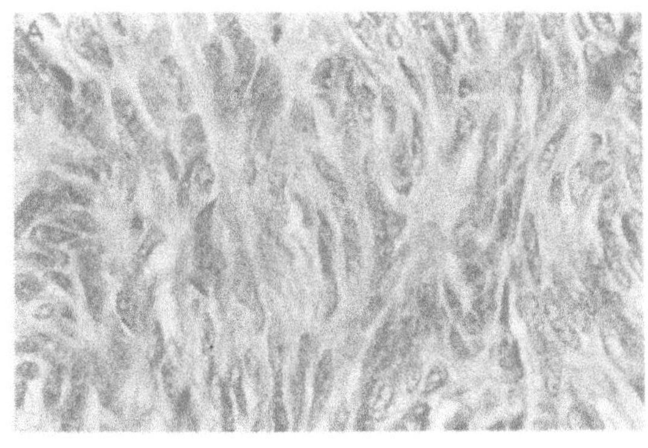

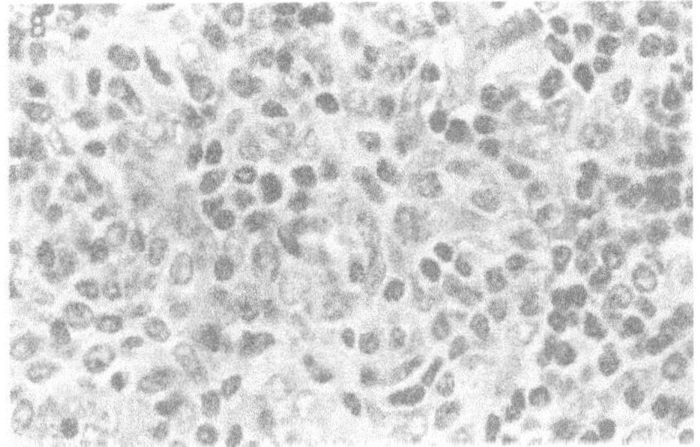

Figure 1. Benign thymomas. A: Medullary type of thymoma showing spindle cell morphology of thymic epithelial cells and paucity of lymphocytes. B: Mixed thymoma with epithelial cells of intermediate type and numerous lymphocytes.

RESULTS

The patient group consisted of 25 males and 25 females. In one referred case no clinical information was obtainable. The age range was 10 - 82 years. Thirteen patients had symptoms of myasthenia gravis.

The results of histogenetic classification of these cases are compared in Table 1.

In 40/51 (78%) cases there was complete concordance of results of classification. In 11/51 (22%) cases, there were varying degrees of discordance (Table 1).

Table 1. Comparison of classification of thyomas in Cape Town and Würzburg

Type of thymoma	Cape Town PMC/CJU	Würzburg TK
Medullary	4	7
Mixed	17	12
Predominantly cortical	2	3
Cortical	17	15
WDTC and epidermoid CA	10	13
Unclassifiable	1	1
Total cases	51	51

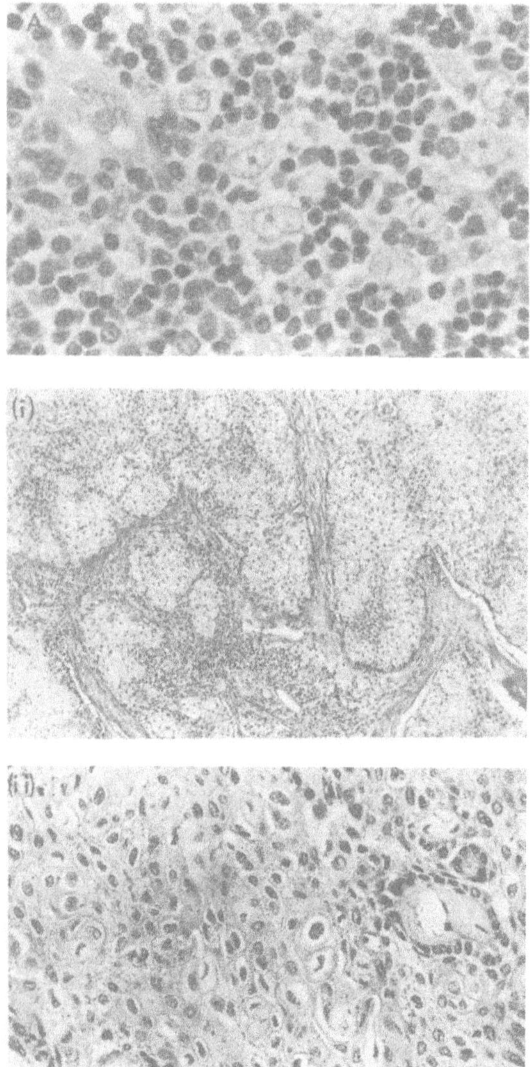

Figure 2. Malignant thymic epithelial tumours. A: Cortical type of thymoma with numerous lymphocytes and cortical-type thymic epithelial cells, with large vesicular nuclei, distinct nucleoli and pale cytoplasm. B: Well-differentiated thymic carcinoma. (i) Low magnification showing organoid, lobular growth pattern and paucity of lymphocytes. (ii) Higher magnification to show characteristic epithelial cells with folded, crumpled nuclei resembling koilocytes, with perinuclear halos. Note perivascular epithelial palisading.

In terms of the distinction between benign (medullary and mixed) thymomas and aggressive (cortical types and WDTC) thymomas, the degree of reproducibility was 96% (49/51 cases). (Table 2).

Analysis of the discordant cases showed that there were 4 main areas which affected reproducibility of this classification:

1. Medullary *vs* mixed thymoma. (3 cases). All three cases were classified by TK as medullary and by PMC/CJU as mixed. However one case was classified as "mixed, predominantly spindled" and medullary thymoma was considered. This case reflects lack of clarification of cut off points for mixed cases.

Table 2. 96% concordance

Benign	Aggressive
medullary	predominantly cortical
mixed	cortical
	WDTC

2. Cortical *vs* mixed thymoma. (2 cases). Both cases were classified by TK as cortical and by PMC/CJU as mixed, however there was debate about both cases with cortical thymoma being favoured initially by PMC on account of nuclear morphology. Preservation of cytological detail was poor in one case.
3. Cortical *vs* predominantly cortical thymoma. (3 cases). Two cases were classified by TK as predominantly cortical and by PMC/CJU as cortical while the case classified by PMC/CJU as predominantly cortical was called "lymphocyte depleted cortical thymoma" by TK.
4. Well-differentiated thymic carcinoma with cortical areas *vs* cortical thymoma with epidermoid differentiation. (3 cases). All 3 cases were classified by TK as WDTC and by PMC/CJU as cortical thymoma. In one case the biopsy was so small that the accuracy of classification was doubtful. In the other 2 cases PMC/CJU noted epidermoid foci and considered the possibility of WDTC. These cases illustrate the difficulty in establishing the cut off point between cortical thymoma and WDTC.

DISCUSSION

The criteria for histogenetic classification of thymic epithelial tumours as published by Müller-Hermelink and co-workers were found to be relatively easy to learn and apply. Clinicopathological studies[12–18] have shown that biological behaviour of thymic epithelial tumours correlates with two lines of differentiation. One line comprises medullary and mixed thymomas. The other line includes cortical thymomas, predominantly cortical thymomas and well-differentiated thymic carcinomas, which are more often invasive and associated with myasthenia gravis than medullary and mixed thymomas. Thus mixed thymomas, even with cortical areas, should be differentiated from true cortical types of thymoma. In most cases little difficulty was experienced in assigning thymic epithelial tumours to one of five histological categories and the clinically important distinction between benign and aggressive types of thymoma was readily made with a high degree of reproducibility. However, certain problem areas were encountered and these are discussed in more detail below with suggestions for improvement of the classification for general use.

Mixed *vs* Cortical and Medullary Thymomas

The main difficulty here is in establishing and reliably reproducing cut-off points in areas where there is a spectrum of morphology. If >75% of the tumour consists of either medullary or cortical areas it should be assigned to these categories. Criteria for adequate sampling (eg one block/cm greatest tumour diameter) should be laid down. Area to area variability within thymic tumours means that small biopsies may not be representative and cannot be relied upon for accurate classification and prognostication.

Cortical *vs* Predominantly Cortical Thymoma

We found the term "predominantly cortical thymoma" confusing and support the alternative term "organoid" thymoma proposed by Harris et al[18] as this conveys the characteristic morphology of these tumours which show prominent cortico-medullary differentiation closely resembling normal thymus.

Cortical Thymoma *vs* WDTC

Cortical thymoma and WDTC form a morphologic spectrum and these tumours not infrequently contain both cortical thymoma-like areas and areas resembling WDTC. Kirchner et al[12] have recommended that tumours should only be classified as WDTC if they contain a clear-cut predominance (> 50%) of areas of WDTC. In practice this distinction is somewhat subjective, can be difficult and is clearly dependent on adequate tumour sampling. The extent of morphologic overlap between cortical thymoma and WDTC also poses a challenge in developing acceptable terminology for this group of closely related thymic epithelial tumours.

Lymphocyte-Poor Tumours

Medullary thymomas, lymphocyte depleted cortical thymomas and WDTC all contain very few lymphocytes and this may cause difficulty in classification. In medullary thymomas the presence of abundant pericellular reticulin, the salt and pepper pattern of nuclear chromatin and the absence of perivascular palisading are very helpful in making the distinction from WDTC, which contains little reticulin, has haloed, folded nuclei and shows perivascular palisading. The cytologic features of of WDTC are very characteristic, and unlike squamous carcinoma at other sites.[12] The cells resemble dysplastic or koilocytic cervical epithelium with nuclear folding and perinuclear halos.

In summary, we found this classification to be highly reproducible in making the important clinical distinction between benign thymomas (medullary and mixed) and those with more aggressive biological behaviour (cortical types and well-differentiated thymic carcinoma). The high degree of reproducibility of this histogenetic classification of thymic epithelial neoplasms should facilitate its acceptance for general diagnostic use.

ACKNOWLEDGMENTS

We gratefully acknowledge the support of the Cancer Association of South Africa and the Medical Research Council of South Africa, the expert technical assistance of Rochelle Barnard and the photographic expertise of Beverley Seymour.

REFERENCES

1. Levine GD, Rosai J. Thymic hyperplasia and neoplasia: a review of current concepts. *Hum. Pathol.* 1978; **9**; 495–515.
2. Salyer W R, Eggleston J C. Thymoma. A clinical and pathological study of 65 cases. *Cancer* 1976; **37**; 229–249.
3. Lewis JE, Wick MR, Scheithauer BW et al. Thymoma: A clinicopathologic review. *Cancer* 1987; **60**; 2727–2743.

4. Gray GF, Gutowski WT. Thymoma: a clinicopathologic study of 54 cases. *Am J Surg Pathol* 1979; **3**; 235–249.
5. Kornstein M. Controversies regarding the pathology of thymomas. *Path Annu* 1992; part 2 1–15.
6. Snover DC, Levine GD, Rosai J. Thymic carcinoma. Five distinctive histological variants. *Am J Surg Pathol* 1982; **6**; 451–470.
7. Wick MR, Weiland LH, Scheithauer BW et al. Primary thymic carcinomas. *Am J Surg Pathol* 1982; **6**; 613–630.
8. Kuo T, Chang J-P, Lin F-J, Wu W-C et al. Thymic carcinomas: Histopathologial varieties and immunohistochemical study. *Am J Surg Pathol* 1990; **14**; 24–34.
9. Marino M, Müller-Hermelink H K. Thymoma and thymic carcinoma. Relation of thymoma epithelial cells to the cortical and medullary differentiation of thymus. *Virchows Arch [Pathol Anat]* 1985; 407;119–149.
10. Müller-Hermelink HK, Marino M, Palestro G. Pathology of thymic epithelial tumours. In: Müller-Hermelink HK, ed. *Current Topics in Pathology: The Human Thymus*. Berlin, Springer-Verlag, 1986:208–268.
11. Kirchner T, Müller-Hermelink HK. New approaches to the diagnosis of thymic epithelial tumors. *Progress in Surgical Pathology* 1989; **10**; 167–189.
12. Kirchner T, Schalke B, Buchwald J et al. Well-differentiated thymic carcinoma. An organotypical low-grade carcinoma with relationship to cortical thymoma. *Am J Surg Pathol* 1992; **16**; 1153–1169.
13. Pescarmona E, Rendina EA, Venuta F et al. The prognostic implication of thymoma histologic subtype. A study of 80 consecutive cases. *Am J Clin Pathol* 1990; **93**; 190–195.
14. Pescarmona E, Rendina EA, Venuta F et al. Analyis of prognostic factors and clinicopathological staging of thymoma. *Ann Thorac Surg* 1990; **50**; 534–538.
15. Kirchner T, Schalke B, Marx A et al. Evaluation of prognostic features in thymic epithelial tumours. *Thymus* 1989; **14**; 195–203.
16. Close PM, Uys CJ. Thymic pathology: 32 years' experience in Cape Town. Presented at the 3rd Meeting of the European Association for Haematopathology. Würzburg, Germany 7–11 October 1990. (Abstract)
17. Kuo TT, Lo SK. Thymoma: a study of the pathologic classification of 71 cases with evaluation of the Müller-Hermelink system. *Hum Pathol.* 1993; **24**; 766–771.
18. Quintanilla-Martinez L, Wilkins EW, Ferry JA, Harris NL. Thymoma - Morphologic subclassification correlates with invasiveness and immunohistologic features. A study of 122 cases. *Hum Pathol* 1993; **24**; 958–969.

38

MORPHOLOGY OF THYMIC REMNANTS REMOVED AFTER VIDEO-ASSISTED THORACOSCOPIC EXTENDED THYMECTOMY IN PATIENTS WITH THYMOMATOUS MYASTHENIA GRAVIS

R. Scelsi,[1] M. Paulli,[1] U. Gianelli,[1] M. T. Ferro',[2] M. Longoni,[2] L. Novellino,[2] and G. Pezzuoli[2]

[1]Department of Human Pathology
University of Pavia and Research Unit
Pathology Section, I.R.C.C.S. Policlinico S. Matteo
Pavia, Italy
[2]Division of Neurology and Surgery
Policlinico S. Marco Zingonia
Bergamo, Italy

SUMMARY

On a total of 67 patients with Myasthenia Gravis (MG) that had a Video-Assisted Thoracoscopic Extended Thymectomy (VATET) for removal of the thymus gland and cervical and anterior mediastinal fat tissue, 12 revealed a thymoma. Nine patients with capsulated non-invasive thymoma were studied for detection of thymic remnants in cervical and pre-pericardial fat tissue. Six out of nine subjects showed thymic remnants that in half of them demonstrated lymphoid follicular hyperplasia Immunohistochemical characterization of atrophic thymic remnants showed small T-lymphocytes (CD1a; CD3) and rare epithelial cells (EMA; Cytokeratin and LN3).Thymic remnants with lymphoid follicular hyperplasia showed germinal centres positively stained for LN1 (CDw75). Since the last alteration has been considered an important cause of failure of surgical treatment of MG, an accurate investigation and removal of all possible thymic remnants together with the proper thymus may be performed.

INTRODUCTION

Myasthenia gravis (MG) is an autoimmune disease in which the thymus gland is the site for triggering and self-maintenance of auto-immune reactions to acetylcholine recep-

Epithelial Tumors of the Thymus, edited by Marx and Müller-Hermelink.
Plenum Press, New York, 1997

tors. Pathologic changes in the thymus have been found in 75% to 85% of MG patients and about 70% of cases showed a "thymic lymphoid follicular hyperplasia" (1–2). Furthemore, 15% has developed thymomas (2,16). In thymomatous and non-thymomatous MG, the persistence of neuro-muscular symptoms after thymectomy may be related to pathology of residual thymic tissue outside the capsule of the proper thymus (4–9–12–13).

Therefore the entire thymus has to be removed along with the thymoma and a wide surgical removal of involved structures together with all thymic remnants in the extra-thymic cervical and mediastinal fat tissue is required (5–6). In the past, different surgical approaches for an extended thymectomy with or whitout sternotomy have been proposed (5–6–15). Recently, a Video-Assisted Thoracoscopic Extended Thymectomy without sternotomy (VATET) has been introduced (10). In the present study we report the results of a topographic and morphofunctional investigation of thymic remnants in cervical and mediastinal fat tissue from 9 MG patients with non-invasive thymoma that had a VATET.

PATIENTS AND METHODS

From January 1994 through February 1996, 12 patients with thymomatous MG on a total of 67 MG patients underwent VATET for extended thymectomy. All patients were discharged from hospital within 6 days after surgery. Normal and thymomatous thymic lobes were isolated and removed through a cervical incision. Cervical pretracheal and anterior mediastinal (bilateral pre-pericardial) fat tissue was removed separately, weighed and investigated by light microscopy for thymic remnants.

The removed tissue was reduced in blocks (1.5X1.5 cm), fixed in 10% buffered formaldehyde and paraffin embedded. Sections were stained with haematoxylin-eosin, Giemsa, periodic acid-Schiff and Gomori's silver impregnation for reticulin. On the ground of gross and microscopic findings, the tumors were classified as non-invasive and invasive thymomas; histopathological subtypes were classified according to Lewis (7) and Muller-Hermelink (8). Lymphoid follicular hyperplasia of thymic tissue was defined by the presence of expanded lymphoid follicles (1).

Immunohistochemistry was performed on paraffin sections using the streptavidin-peroxidase methods (14), using the following antisera and monoclonal antibodies: 010 (CD1a) (courtesy of Dr. Boumsell, Hopital Saint Louis, Paris, France); EMA (epithelial membrane antigen), cytokeratin, S-100 protein, CD34; CD3 and L-26 (CD20) (Dako, Glostrup, Denmark); MT2 (CD45RA),LN3 (HLA-DR), LN2 (CD74), LN-1 (CDw75), MT 1 (CD43), UCHL-1 (CD45RO) (Biotest, Frankfurt am Main, Germany). Reaction products of immunostaining were developed by immersion of sections in 3–3′ diamino benzidine hydrochloride/H202 or 3-amino-9 ethylcarbazole/H202 solutions.

RESULTS

In the present series 3 patients had invasive thymoma and they were discharged from the study. Nine patients with thymomatous MG had capsulated thymoma. Histological type of thymoma and association with thymic remnants in cervical and pre-pericardial regions are shown in Table 1. Morphological studies revealed thymic remnants in cervical and/or pre-pericardial fatty tissue in 6 out of 9 patients. Thymic remnants appeared as rounded or enlongated islands composed predominantly of T-lymphocytes that expressed the CD1a, CD3 and, variably, the CD43 antigens; we noticed few scattered CD20 (L-26)

Table 1. Histology and distribution of thymic remnants in thymomatous MG

Case	Thymoma	Thymic remnants	
		Cervical fat	Prepericardial fat
1	cortical	(involution) ++	(involution)+
2	mixed	–	–
3	cortical	(involution) ++	–
4	medullary	–	–
5	medullary	–	–
6	cortical	(lymphoid hyperplasia) ++	–
7	cortical	–	(involution) +
8	cortical	(lymphoid hyperplasia) ++	(lymphoid hyperplasia) ++
9	mixed	(lymphoid hyperplasia) +	(lymphoid hyperplasia) ++

positive B-lymphocytes whereas the anti-cytokeratin, anti-EMA and LN3 (HLA-DR) antibodies reacted with intermingled epithelial cells. Three out of the cases showed thymic remnants with numerous germinal centres that strongly stained with the monoclonal antibody LN1 (CDw75). A minority of the B-follicles showed secondary changes with areas of hyalinazation and, occasionally, follicular atrophy. In all cases the anti-CD 34 showed the presence of numerous blood vessels of small-to medium size diameter. Thymic remnants were detected in both cervical and pre-pericardial fat tissue in 3 patients with cortical and mixed thymoma. Thymic remnants in cervical fat only were detected in 2 cases of cortical thymoma. In one case they showed involution and in the other showed lymphoid follicular hyperplasia. Involuted thymic remnants seen in the pre-pericardial fat only were detected in a case with cortical thymoma. In 2 patients with medullary thymoma no thymic remnants have been observed. In all cases no thymomatous transformation of thymic remnants was seen.

DISCUSSION

Thymectomy is still important in the surgical treatment of MG, but the success of the treatment is strongly linked to complete removal of all thymic tissue. Previous surgical and anatomic studies had shown that thymus is widely distributed in the neck and mediastinal adipose tissue (5,6) and that aberrant thymic tissue may occur as widely scattered foci in the mediastinal fat tissue extending from cervical pretracheal region to the diaphragm (4,9). The presence of remnants in cervical areas can be explained by the close embrionic and developmental relationship between thymus and foregut (3). In anterior mediastinal fat, they probably represent a residual coat of subcapsular cortical cells of the proper thymus during the physiological thymic involution.

Previous reports indicated that 37% of patients with thymomatous and non-thymomatous MG had extracapsular thymic remnants in cervical and prepericardial regions. These remnants may undergo involution or pathological changes such as true hypertrophy and lymphoid germinal centre hyperplasia, just like the proper thymus gland (13). In the present series, thymic remnants both in cervical and prepericardial fat tissue were seen in half of the MG patients with non-invasive thymoma. They were generally considered atrophic, consisting of small T-(CD1a and CD3) lymphocytes and rare epithelial cells, other than in 3 cases which showed lymphoid follicular hyperplasia with numerous germinal centres positively stained for the MoAb LN1, (CDw75).

The persistence of these structures has been considered an important cause of failure of surgical treatment of MG (12). Germinal centres are not normally present in the thymus gland; yet 70 % of patients with MG and thymic abnormalities show this form of thymic lymphoid hyperplasia (11). The presence of expanded follicles in our series furtherly emphasizes the importance of removing all extrathymic fat tissue in order to avoid every possible cause of recurring disease (5–9–13). Thymomas arising in undescended thymuses or in submandibular, paratracheal and intrathyroid ectopic thymuses are reported (11), but thymomatous transformation of thymic remnants was not observed at yet.

REFERENCES

1. Castleman B The pathology of the thymus gland in mysthenia gravis. Ann NY Acad Sci 135, 496–5o5; 1966
2. Beghi E, Antozzi C, Batocchi AP Prognosis of myasthenia gravis: a multicenter follow-up on 844 patients. J Neurol Sci 106, 213–220;1991
3. Gilmour JR The embriology of the parathyroid glands, the thymus and certain associated rudiments. J Pathol Bacteriol 45, 507–510; 1937
4. Fukai I, Funato Y, Mizuno T, Hashimoto T, Masaoka A Distribution of thymic tissue in the mediastinal adipose tisssue. J Thorac Cardivasc Surg 101, 1099–1122; 1991
5. Jaretzky A, Wolff M Maximal thymectomy for myasthenia gravis. J Thorac Cardivasc Surg 96, 711–716; 1988
6. Jaretzky A, Penn AS, Younger DS, Wolff M, Rowland LP Maximal thymectomy for myasthenia gravis. J Thorac Cardivasc Surg 95, 747–757; 1988
7. Lewis JE, Wick MR, Scheithauer BW Thymoma. A clinicopathologic review. Cancer 60, 2727–2743; 1987
8. Muller-Hermelink HK, Marino M, Palestro G Pathology of thymic epithelial tumors Curr Top Pathol 75, 207–268; 1986
9. Masaoka A, Nagaoka Y, Yotake Y Distribution of thymic tissue at the anterior mediastinum. J Thorac Cardivasc Surg 4, 747–716; 1975
10. Novellino L, Longoni M, Spinelli L, Pezzuoli G Extended thymectomy without sternotomy performed by cervicotomy and thoracoscopic technique in the treatment of myasthenia gravis. Int Surg 79, 378–381; 1994
11. Rosai J, Levine GD Tumors of the thymus. In Atlas of tumor pathology. Second series. Fasc 13. Washington DC 1976 Armed Forced Institute of Pathology
12. Rosenberg M, Jauregui WO, De Vega ME, Roncoroni AS Recurrence of thymic hyperplasia after thymectomy in myasthenia gravis. Its importance as a cause of failure of surgical treatment. Am J Med 74, 78–82; 1983
13. Scelsi R, Ferro MT, Scelsi L, Novellino L, Mantegazza R, Cornelio F, Porta M, Longoni M, Pezzuoli G. Detection and morphology of thymic remnants after VATET in patients with myasthenia gravis Int Surg 80, 126–131; 1995
14. Shi Z.R., Itkowitz S.H.& Kin Y.S.. A comparison of three immunoperoxidase techniques for antigen detection in colorectal carcinoma tissues. Journal of Histochemistry, 32, 219–229, 1988.
15. Sugarbaker DJ Thoracoscopy in the management of anterior mediastinal masses: Ann Thorac Surg 56, 653–656;1993
16. Wilkins EW, Edmunds LH, Castleman B Cases of thymoma at the Massachussets general Hospital J Thorac Cardivasc Surg 52, 322–330;1966

CORE NEEDLE BIOPSY OF ANTERIOR MEDIASTINUM MASSES

M. Boaron,[1] S. Artuso,[1] N. Lacava,[1] N. Santelmo,[1] M. Sartini,[1] V. Poletti,[2] A. Cancellieri,[3] and G. Baruzzi[3]

[1]Divisione di Chirurgia Toracica
[2]Divisione di Pneumologia
[3]Servizio di Anatomia e Istologia Patologica
Ospedale Maggiore, Bologna, Italia

In the vast majority of anterior mediastinal masses a biopsy is necessary in order to plan the treatment. A number of techniques are available and the choice and sequence of them are related to the size, morphology, localization, clinical diagnosis, age of the patient and skill of the operator and of the pathologist.

In our experience core needle biopsy of mediastinal neoformations by a large bore needle proved to be advantageous since it is effective, safe, quick, painless, and performed on an outpatient basis.

In 1974 we began to carry out transthoracic needle biopsies in most instances with 21G thin needles. In case of large masses close to the chest wall we have occasionally employed cutting needles (Silverman, Vim, Menghini) chosen at random (1).

Since the eighties all patients with thoracic masses have undergone CTscan, and the imaging diagnosis of mediastinal masses have become reliable, so we have standardized the use of cutting needles under fluoroscopic guidance for the large clinically primary growths of the anterior mediastinum, and of fine needles under CT guidance or by the Wang technique (2) in the case of deep or small lesions and secondary lymphnode growths.

Based on the favourable previous experience,we have chosen to employ cutting needles in selected patients, as histology is more reliable than cytology expecially for mediastinal primary tumors (3, 4 ,5,). The fluoroscopic guidance makes the procedure simpler, faster, less expènsive and feasible in an operatory room, that is fully equipped to cope with any complication.

PATIENTS AND METHODS

154 consecutive patients have undergone 167 core biopsies by Menghini needles for clinically primary anterior mediastinum tumors, whose size exceeded 4 cm, which were

Epithelial Tumors of the Thymus, edited by Marx and Müller-Hermelink.
Plenum Press, New York, 1997

closer than 3 cm to the chest wall, and could easily be observed using two plane fluoroscopy. Most of them were large or bulky masses, often stuck to the chest wall.

The age of patients ranged from 1 to 94 years, the male/female ratio was 53/47.

All patients had been investigated by CT scan before the biopsy.

Severe respiratory insufficiency and previous pneumonectomy when ventilated lung had to be passed through were considered the only contraindication.

The Superior Vena Cava Syndrome in the presence of a large mediastinal mass was considered a formal indication; 23 of our patients were in such condition and we had to puncture a number of them in a half- sitting position as they were unable to bear the supine position.

Premedication has been done with Atropine only.The procedures were performed in an operatory room, under local anesthetic except in the case of children who undewent a general anesthesia.

We have routinely employed a 1.8 mm disposable Menghini needle *, fitted with a home made blunt steel obturator, which is exchanged for the original one when the needle has reached the lesion. Smaller bore (mm1.2,1.4,1.6,) Menghini needles have been occasionally utilized in the paediatric age, in conditions of poor coagulation, when ventilated lung had to be deeply passed through.

A rotating C arm X ray apparatus was utilized for a two plane approach.

Up to three punctures were performed until a macroscopically good specimen was obtained.

When it proved impossible to obtain a good core sampling we have utilized the fragments for smear examination whose results are not our present concern.

After the procedure the patients were kept under observation for about four hours and discharged if asymptomatic, after a chest X ray had excluded any complication. Most patients anyway spent their first postoperative night in the hospitals from which they had been referred to our department.

All the specimens were formalin-fixed and routine processed for paraffin embedding. 3 μm sections were cut and stained with haematoxylin/eosin (H&E) for histologic examination. Immunohistochemical studies, using the avidin-biotin-peroxidase complex method by Hsu et al. (6) as well as histochemical procedures were performed when the cases were deemed problematical and to subclassify Hodgkin's and non Hodgkin's lymphomas.

All the biopsies have been revised by the same pathologists :AC & GB

We considered that a definite diagnosis was achieved if the material submitted to the laboratory allowed the pathologist to meet all the minimal diagnostic criteria that are recognized as reliable when dealing with histological sections.

The diagnoses of malignancy and lymphoma without further definition were considered non-diagnostic.

RESULTS

A definite pathological diagnosis of the lesion has been obtained in 122/167 biopsies (73%), 9 of which have been repeated once, four twice.

* Hepafix®, B. Braun, Melsungen, Germany.

Table 1. Results of 167 core needle biopsies on 154 patients

Patients	154	% of patients	% of biopsies
Biopsies	167	1.1	
Definite diagnoses	122	79	73
Inadequate specimen	45	21	27

In 45 cases the specimen were inadequate (27%). The main reasons were: massive necrosis, sampling outside the target mass, or lacking of pathological tissue in stone-like lesions, most of which were Hodgkin's lymphomas that needed a surgical biopsy (Tabs 1,2).

Disagreement between the definite diagnosis of the reviewers and the original one was recorded in 2 cases of lymphoma, all biopsied before 1988, belonging to the large cell with sclerosis category, described by Perrone et al. in 1986 (7), and in a case whose initial diagnosis of thymoma was converted into "lymphoblastic lymphoma".

In all the 49 patients who underwent a subsequent surgical biopsy or resection, the diagnoses were confirmed (Tab 3).

Of the 45 patients where needle biopsies had been unsuccessful , 10 were submitted to mediastinoscopy, 7 to anterior mediastinotomy, 5 to Video-Assisted Thoracoscopy,7 to explorative mini-thoracotomy, 1 to a resective procedure, 15 were lost to follow up (Tab 4).

No death was recorded in this series. Two relevant complications were observed:

1. an acute haemopericardium with cardiac tamponade, probably due to puncture of the aortic root in a young woman: the procedure was interrupted, a pericardial catheter was placed under ultrasonography guidance. After the tamponade had been relieved by subtracting blood three times amounting to 140cc, the patient did well.
2. an acute Superior Vena Cava Syndrome with caval trombosis was attributed to a minimal intralesional haemorrhage which anyway increased caval compression

Table 2. Histologic definite diagnoses of needle biopsies in 154 patients

Hodgkin's lymphoma	23
Non Hodgkin's lymphoma	32
Thymic carcinoma lymphoepithelioma-like	2
Thymoma	21
Angioleiomyomatosis	1
Angiosarcoma	2
Embryonal rabdomyosarcoma	2
Yolk sac tumor	1
Seminoma	1
Mediastinal goiter	1
Follicular carcinoma in mediastinal goiter	1
Inflammatory pseudotumor with atypical mycobacteria	1
Metastatic carcinoma	31
Sarcoidosis	2
Wegener disease	1
Total definite diagnoses	122

Table 3. Needle biopsy diagnoses verified by surgical procedures

Hodgkin's lymphoma	7/23
Non Hodgkin's lymphoma	5/32
Lymphoepithelioma like thymic carcinoma	2/2
Thymoma	18/21
Angioleiomyomatosis	1/1
Angiosarcoma	2
Embryonal rabdomyosarcoma	2/2
Seminoma	1/1
Mediastinal goiter	1/1
Follicular carcinoma in mediastinal goiter	1/1
Metastatic carcinoma	7/31
Sarcoidosis	2/2
Number of verified needle biosies	49/122

over the critical caliber. The patient was put on Heparine and recovered within 48 hours.

Pneumothorax was the most common complication being observed in 16 cases (8.5%) five of which required drainage (3%).

8 patients (4.7%) presented mild haemoptysis.

A minimal haemothorax was observed in 6 cases (6.5%), none of which required treatment.

Transient hypotension from vago-vagal reflex, observed in 12 cases (7.1%), and acute pain, probably referable to a minimal PNX, are probably responsible for some poor samplings and for the decision of some patients not to undergo a further puncture after an unsatisfactory biopsy.

No patient suffered from any significant complication after being discharged.

None of the 23 patients who presented a SVCS at the moment of the biopsy had any complication connected with this condition (Tab 5).

The incidence of failed sampling was clearly related in our series to the operators' experience, whilst no relation was observed in the rate of complications.

DISCUSSION

Needle biopsy is the least traumatic invasive sampling technique. Fine needles employed through the percutaneous or transbronchial way give excellent results for the diag-

Table 4. Biopsy technique in 45 failed needle biopsies

Mediastinoscopy	10
Ant. mediastinotomy	7
V.A. thoracoscopy	5
Explor. mini thoracotomy	7
Surgical resection	1
Unknown procedure	15

Table 5. Complications in 167 core needle biopsies on 154 patients

	No. of patients	% of patients	% of biopsies
Haemothoraces	6	3.8	3.5
Pnx (untreated)	11	7.1	6.5
Pnx (drained)	5	3.2	2.9
Haemophtysis	8	5.2	4.7
Vago-vagal hypotension	12	7.7	7.1
Acute SVCS	1	0.06	0.06
Haemopericardium	1	0.06	0.06
Death	0	0	0

nosis of epithelial neoplasms, especially for the secondary ones whose primary is known. Aspiration cytology is usually unsuitable for the cell typing of primary mediastinal tumors with particular regard to lymphomas and to a lesser extent thymomas, whilst the large specimens provided by cutting needles allow excellent histological and immunocytochemical definition (3,4,5,8).

The risk of puncture, when a large lesion is close to the chest wall, is usually minimal regardless of the caliber of needles. The slight risk of injury to the mammary vessels is minimized by keeping two cm away from the sternal edge or by ultrasonography or CT guidance.

To further minimize the risk of mammary or intercostal vessel damage we have provided the Menghini needles with a blunt obturator. The risk of intralesional haemorrhage can be related to the needle size, but in our series we have recorded only one case of symptomatic intralesional haemorrage whilst, in six more patients, a minimal increase of the lesion size, demonstrated by a postoperative chest X ray, had no clinical consequences.

The large bore needles increase the risk of haemothorax, haemoptysis and pneumothorax in comparison with fine needles, but we are convinced, based on this series, that in selected patients, on account of the short intrapulmonary passage, the risk is still trivial compared with the advantages of this technique.

We have chosen the Menghini needles because of the optimal external / internal diameter ratio, and the previous experience of tissue tearing whilst withdrawing "sleigh needles", which could be dangerous in the mediastinum.

We initially decided to employ fluoroscopic guidance due to the favourable prior series and the scarce availability of the CT, but even when CT became more available we utilized it almost only for fine needle aspiration of small and deep mediastinal lesions.

Fluoroscopic guidance is easier, faster, less expensive and allows the operator to work in a fully equipped operatory room and to take the biopsy under direct control. We are convinced that in cases of large lesions close to the chest wall the main advantage of CT guidance is the possibility of avoiding necrotic areas. CT is also an advantage for less experienced operators who can check the needle position before starting the biopsy. In the light of this experience we utilize CT or ultrasonography guidance as a second choice and for the training of residents.

Like other authors we have observed a close relationship between the general and specific experience of the operator and the quality of samples(9). On the contrary the incidence of PNX and haemothoraces seems to be unrelated to the skill of the operators as the most important factor seems to be the depth of ventilated lung parenchyma to be passed through. Other complications and specifically the only two remarkable ones happened to senior surgeons who are generally more self confident and aggressive.

Conversely to the restrictive criteria proposed by the American Thoracic Society with regard to the indications and contraindications to transthoracic biopsies(10),we should note that in our series the indication was extended even to very sick patients and that the limited number of complications, particularly severe ones, is directly linked to the selection of patients with large lesions close to the chest wall.

Risks, morbidity and limitations of this procedure must be compared with those of mediastinoscopy, mediastinotomy and Video-Assisted Thoracoscopic Surgery, which are most commonly employed in such patients.

Mediastinoscopy has a 90% diagnostic rate, requires an experienced surgeon, is contraindicated in the Superior Vena Cava Syndrome, and can be dangerous in the presence of massive mediastinal invasion.

Mediastinotomy has a 100% diagnostic rate and a low surgical risk, but in these patients the need for opening the pleura and thoracic drainage is common.

VATS has a 100% diagnostic rate, but is much more expensive than the other techniques and usually requires one lung ventilation.

All these procedures are usually performed under general anaesthesia, which can be a problem on account of the presence of caval or tracheobronchial compression, both quite common in large or bulky mediastinal tumors.

In conclusion, based on the reports of the literature (8) and on our series, we believe that the transthoracic puncture should be considered the first choice for the sampling of tumors of the anterior mediastinum, and the employment of cutting needles should be considered for large clinically primary masses.

The best technique of guidance is still a matter of debate and is obviously related to the experience of the operator: fluoroscopy and ultrasonography are probably the most simple, fast and inexpensive methods and give the opportunity to follow the progression of the needle into the mass. When feasible, ultrasonography enables the visualization of the mediastinal structures. In the presence of small lesions or diffuse necrosis and when simpler techniques have failed, CT guidance should be employed.

REFERENCES

1. M. Boaron, G. Mattioli, G. Ravasi, L. Zingo "Needle Biopsy of Endothoracic Neoformations:A Five-Year Experience" J.Surg.Oncol. 1978:10: 55–59.
2. Wang K.P. "Staging of Bronchogenic Carcinoma by Bronchoscopy".Chest 1994:106: 588 - 593.
3. Chong-Jen Yu, Pan-Chyr Yang, Dun-Bing Chang, Huey-Don Wu, Li-Na Lee, Yung-Chie Lee, Hsong Kuo, Kwen-Tay Luh. "Evaluation of Ultrasonically Guided Biopsies of Mediastinal Masses" Chest 1991:100:399 -405
4. Pan-Chyr Yang, Yung Chie Lee, Chong-Jen Yu, Dun-Bin Chang, Huey-Dong Wu, Li-Na Lee, Sow-song Kuo, Kwen-Yai Luh. "Ultrasonography Guided Biopsy of Thoracic Tumors". Cancer 1992:&):2553–2560
5. Andersson T., Lindgren P.G., Elvin A."Ultrasound guided tumour biopsy in the anterior mediastinum. An alternative to Thoracotomy and mediastinoscopy."Acta Radiol. 1992:33:423–427.
6. Hsu S.M., Raine L., Fanger H."Use of avidin-biotin peroxidase complex (ABC) in immunoperoxidase technique: a comparison between ABC and unlabelled antibody (PAP) procedures.J. Isthochem.Cytochem. 1981:29:577–580.
7. Perrone T., Frizzera G.,Rosai J."Mediastinal diffuse large cell lymphoma with sclerosis. A clinicopathologic study of 60 cases."Am. J. Surg. Pathol. 1986:10:176–191.
   Herman S.J.,Holub R.V., Weisbrod G.L., Chamberlein G.W."Anterior mediastinal masses: utility of transthoracic needle biopsy."Radiology 1991:180:167 - 170
8. Zafar N., Moinuddin S."Mediastinal Needle Biopsy"Cancer 1995:76:1065 - 1068.
9. Powers C., Silverman J., Geisinger K., Frable W." Fine-needle Aspiration Biopsy of the Mediastinum". Am.J.Clin. Pathol. 1996:105: 168 -173
10. Sokolowski J.W., Burgher L.W., Jones F.L., Patterson J.R., Selecky P.A. " Guidelines for percutaneous transthoracic needle biopsy" Am. Rev.Respir. Dis. 1989;140:255–256

40

CYCLIN-DEPENDENT KINASE 6 (PLSTIRE) EXPRESSION IN NORMAL THYMUS, THYMOMAS, AND T-CELL LYMPHOBLASTIC LYMPHOMA

Marco Chilosi,[1] Claudio Doglioni,[2] Maurizio Lestani,[1] Fabio Menestrina,[1] Serena S. T. Pedron,[1] Alice Benedetti,[1] Luca Morelli,[1] Vittorio Rucco,[1] and Giovanni Pizzolo[3]

[1]Istituto di Anatomia Patologica
Università di Verona
[2]Anatomia Patologica
Ospedale Civile di Feltre, Italy
[3]Cattedra di Ematologia
Università di Verona

Different benign and malignant processes should be included in the differential diagnosis of a patient presenting with a mediastinal mass, depending on the age and clinical features. These include thymoma, T-cell lymphoblastic lymphoma/leukemia, thymic follicular hyperplasia, true thymic hyperplasia, and others. Thymomas are mediastinal neoplasms arising from thymic epithelial cells that exhibit heterogeneous morphology and, in most cases, are admixed with various proportions of non-neoplastic cortical thymocytes [1–5]. The histological diagnosis of thymoma is usually based on the recognition of neoplastic epithelial cells, but some diagnostic problem can be encountered in cases with abundant lymphoid component, especially when only small tissue fragments (e.g. by mediastinoscopy) or cytological material are available. Immunohistochemistry can provide some help in difficult cases by demonstrating more precisely the presence of epithelial cells using cytokeratin-specific antibodies[6]. An extremely precise characterization of cortical thymocytes can be obtained by immunophenotypic demonstration of several membrane, cytoplasmic or nuclear antigens such as CD1, coexpressed CD4 and CD8 antigens, cytoplasmic CD3 and nuclear Terminal deoxynucleotydil transferase (TdT)[7]. Unfortunately, this thymocyte antigenic repertoire is identical or very similar in all thymic lesions including normal thymus, hyperplastic thymus, thymoma and most lymphoblastic lymphomas. Gene rearrangement analysis of the T-cell receptor can provide definitive

Epithelial Tumors of the Thymus, edited by Marx and Müller-Hermelink.
Plenum Press, New York, 1997

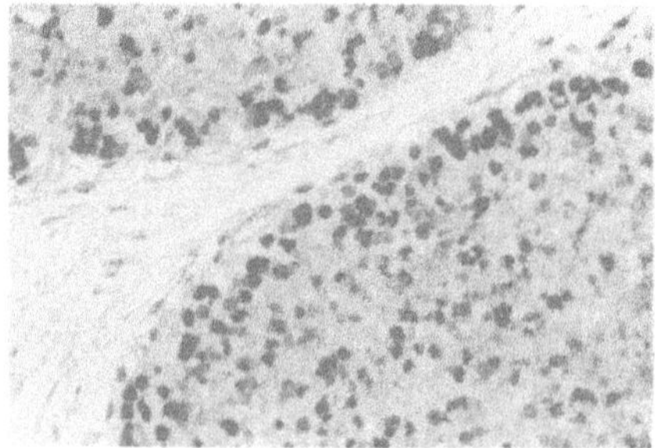

Figure 1. Infant thymus. A minority (10–15%) of cdk6 immunostaining cortical thymocytes is demonstrated, mainly located in the subcapsular zone. LSAB-immunoperoxidase on formalin-fixed, paraffin embedded sections.

proof of T-cell clonality and can be of paramount diagnostic utility in difficult cases[8], providing that high numbers of fresh cells are available, which is not always the case, especially in Fine-Needle Aspiration (FNAB) preparations.

In a recent study on the expression of various molecules regulating the cell-cycle in the human thymus, we observed a striking difference of expression of the cyclin-dependent kinase 6 (cdk6, PLSTIRE) between normal and neoplastic cortical thymocytes (Chilosi, submitted). Cdk6 is the earliest inducible member of the cdk family in human T lymphocytes, first appearing in mid-G1, prior to the activation of any other cdk, and independently of the key T cell progression factor IL-2 [9,10]. Cdk6 is one of the targets of $p16^{ink4A}$ and $p15^{ink4B}$, two highly homologous cdk-inhibitors that exert their inhibitory function by directly binding cdk in the absence of any cyclin, thus specifically interfering with the formation of catalitically active kinase complexes [11]. Interestingly, these cdk-inhibitors ($p16^{ink4A}$ and $p15^{ink4B}$) are encoded by two genes (MTS1 and MTS2) that are frequently deleted in T-cell leukemias (up-to 77% of T-ALL cases according to different series) [13–18]. Cdk6 shows a striking differential expression among normal tissues, being detected at high levels only in T lymphocytes[19].

According to our findings, cortical thymocytes in normal and hyperplastic thymic samples exhibited low proportions of cdk6 expressing cells (10–15%), whereas neoplastic samples (T-cell lymphoblastic lymphoma and leukemia, 13 cases) were characterized by very high proportions of cdk6 reacting cells (up to 100%) (Table I). In normal thymus cdk6 immunoreactive cells appear as large blasts mainly located in the outer cortex (fig.

Table I. Expression of CDK6 revealed by immunohistochemical analysis in normal and pathologic samples of lymph node, bone marrow and thymus

Sample	N° of samples	CDK6 reacting cells	%
React. lymph node	4	paracortical areas	1–5
Normal bone marrow	10	blasts	<1
Fetal thymus	1	cortical thymocytes	10–15
Infant thymus	4	cortical thymocytes	10–15
Hyperplastic thymus	4	cortical thymus	10–15
Thymoma (cortical)	4	thymocytes	<10
Thymoma (mixed)	3	thymocytes	10–30
T-LBL (mediast.)	4	T-blasts	90–100
T-LBL (lymph node)	1	T-blasts	90–100
T-ALL (bone marrow)	8	T-blasts	90–100

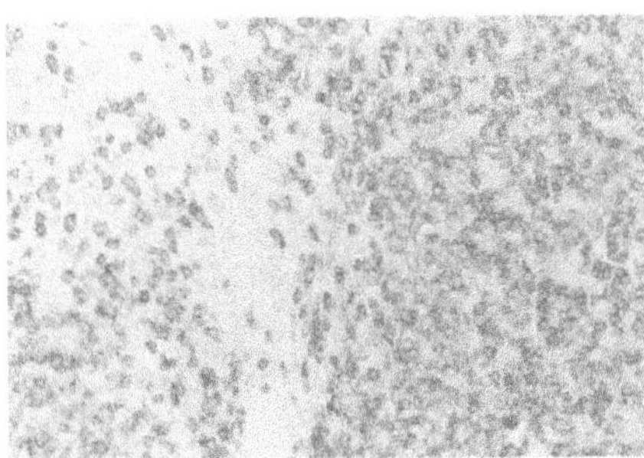

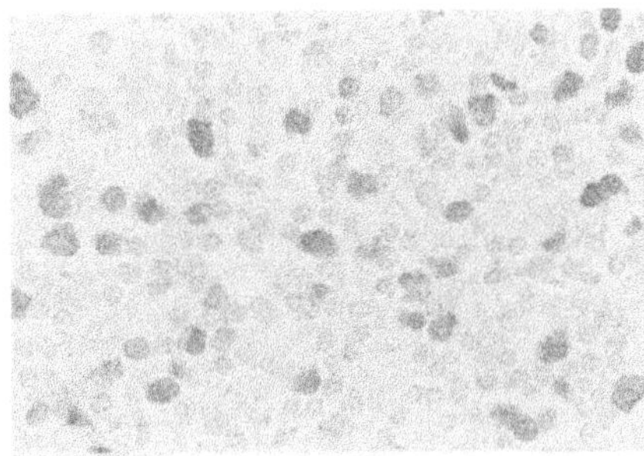

Figure 2. Thymoma with a rich lymphoid component. (*Left*) CD1a immunostaining demonstrates the "cortical" immunophenotype of lymphoid-looking cells. (*Right*) only a small proportion of lymphoid cells exhibit nuclear and cytoplasmic immunostaining for cdk6. LSAB-immunoperoxidase on formalin-fixed, paraffin embedded sections.

1), probably corresponding to immature subcapsular thymocytes[20]. Interestingly, in all thymoma samples of the cortical type (according to the Marino and Muller-Hermelink classification) [4, 21] in our series (4 cases) the proportions of cdk6 expressing thymocytes were similar to those observed in normal thymic cortex (10–15%) (fig. 2), thus confirming that lymphoid cells in thymoma are in fact normal thymocytes growing in an abnormal microenvironment [1–3]. Thymomas of the mixed type were characterized by higher figures of cdk6+ thymocytes (up to 30%), especially in areas where the lymphoid component was relatively scanty, but this frequency is still much lower than in T-lymphoblastic lymphoma (figs. 3 and 4).

These findings are relevant for several reasons. First, the restricted expression of cdk6, mainly observed in the subcapsular subset of cortical thymocytes in the normal thymus, suggests that this cyclin-dependent kinase is a key molecule in the control of the cell cycle during the early phases of T-cell ontogeny, thus expanding the previous information available on the role of this cdk in peripheral T cells [10]. Second, it is possible to speculate that in neoplastic thymocytes cdk6 overexpression significantly contribute to deregulation of G1 checkpoint in concert with cdk-inhibitors' deletion or other genetic anomaly. Finally, the observed difference of cdk6 expression between non-neoplastic cortical thymocytes (low proportions of cdk6+ cells as observed in normal thymic cortex and thymomas) and neoplastic T lymphoblasts (up to 100% cdk6+ neoplastic thymocytes) could improve the diagnostic accuracy of FNAB analysis of mediastinal masses, since cytologic false positive diagnosis of a lymphocyte predominant thymoma as a malignant lymphoma can

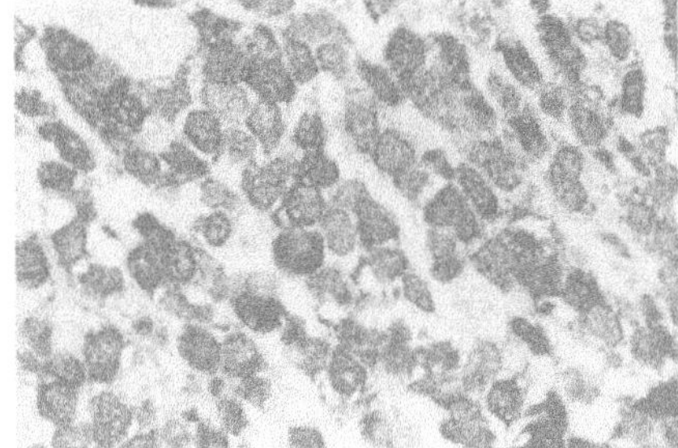

Figure 3. T-lymphoblastic lymphoma, mediastinal mass. The large majority of neoplastic cells show nuclear and cytoplasmic cdk6 immunostaining. LSAB-immunoperoxidase.

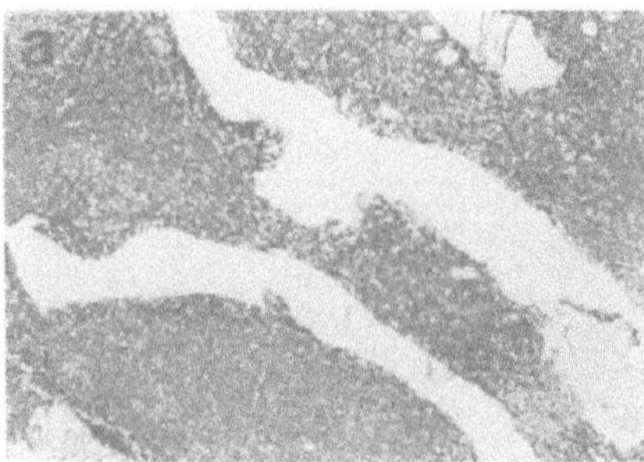

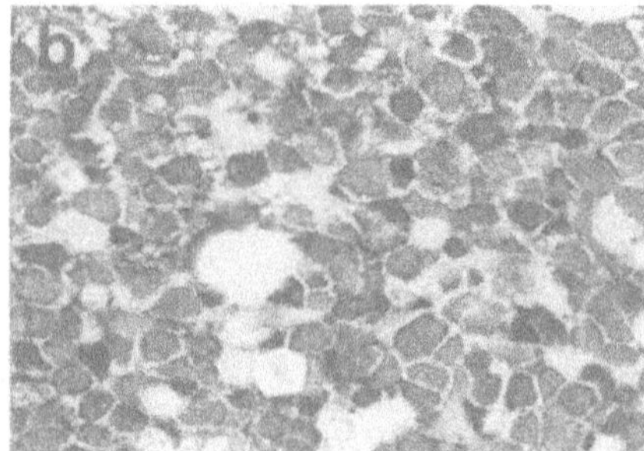

Figure 4. T-cell lymphoblastic leukemia, paraffin section from a bone marrow trephine biopsy. Strong nuclear and cytoplasmic cdk6 immunoperoxidase in the majority of neoplastic cells. LSAB-immunoperoxidase. Different magnifications in a) and b).

occur[23]. The immunohistochemical analysis of cdk6 can be easily performed on routinely processed material and cytological smears, and can represent a simple and reliable method to distinguish neoplastic from non-neoplastic cortical thymocyte populations, thus expanding the panel of antibodies recognizing fixative resistant epitopes which are relevant in the differential diagnosis of thymic neoplasms (Table II).

SAMPLE IMMUNOSTAINING

The immunohistochemical analysis for cdk6 was performed on formalin-fixed (<24 h fixation) paraffin-embedded tissue samples. Briefly, sections were deparaffinized in xylene, rehydrated, washed in PBS, immersed in 0.01M, citrate buffer, pH 6, and irradiated in a microwave oven for 5 min at 750 W (three times), and 10 min at 600 W (once). The sections were then kept for 15 min at room temperature before further PBS washing and immunostaining. Cdk6 immunostaining was performed using an affinity-purified rabbit polyclonal antibody (CDK6 - C-21, Santa Cruz Biotechnology, Santa Cruz, CA) raised against a peptide corresponding to amino acid residues 306–326 mapping at the carboxy terminus of cdk6. Antibody localization was effected by a peroxidase-avidin-biotin method (LSAB-immunoperoxidase, Dako Glostrup, Denmark) with 3–3′-diaminobenzidine as chromogen.

Table II. Antibodies recognizing fixative resistant (using antigen retrieval) epitopes useful as markers in the differential diagnosis of thymic neoplasms

Antibody	Specificity	Reference
CD1	CT	22
CD8	CT, CTL	–
TdT	CT	7
CD20	B-cells	5
Keratin	Epithelial cells	6
Cdk6	CT subset	this study

CT: cortical thymocytes; CTL: cytotoxic lymphocytes.

REFERENCES

1. Chilosi M, Iannucci AM, Pizzolo G, Menestrina F, Fiore-Donati L, Janossy G: Immunohistochemical analysis of thymoma. Evidence for medullary origin of epithelial cells. Am J Surg Pathol 8:3O9–318,1984
2. Chilosi M, Iannucci A, Fiore-Donati L, Tridente G, Pampanin M, Pizzolo G, Ritter M, Bofill M, Janossy G: Myastheniagravis:immunohistologicalheterogeneityinmicroenvironmentalorganization ofhyperplastic and neoplastic thymusessuggesting differentmechanisms oftolerance breakdown. J Neuroimmunol 11:191–204,1986
3. Chilosi M, Iannucci A, Menestrina F, Lestani M, Scarpa A, Fiore-Donati L, Tridente G, Di Pasquale B, Pizzolo G, Palestro G, Janossy G: Immunohistochemical evidence of active thymocyte proliferation in thymoma. Its possible role in the pathogenesis of autoimmune disease. Am J Pathol 128:464–470,1987
4. Kirchner T, Muller-Hermelink HK. New approaches to the diagnosis of thymic epithelial tumors. Prog Surg Pathol 10:167–189,1989
5. Chilosi M, Castelli P, Martignoni G, Pizzolo G, Montresor E, Facchetti F, Truini M, Mombello A, Lestani M, Scarpa A, Menestrina F: Neoplastic epithelial cells in a subset of human thymomas express the B cell-associated CD20 antigen. Am J Surg Pathol 16:988–997,1992
6. Battifora H, Sun TT, Bahu RM, Rao S. The use of antikeratin antiserum as a diagnostic tool: thymoma versus lymphoma. Hum Pathol 11:635–641,1980
7. Chilosi M, Pizzolo G. Review of Terminal deoxynucleotidyl transferase: Biological aspects, methods of detection, and selected diagnostic applications. Appl Immunohistochem 3:209–221,1995
8. Scarpa A, Chilosi M, Capelli P, Bonetti F. Menestrina F, Zamboni G, Pizzolo G, Palestro G, Fiore-Donati L, Tridente G: Expression and gene rearrangement of the T-cell receptor in human thymomas. Virchows Arch B (Cell Pathol) 58:235–239,1990
9. Meyerson M, Harlow E. Identification of G1 kinase activity for cdk6, a novel cyclin D partner. Mol Cell Biol 14:2077–2086,1994
10. Lucas JJ, Szepesi A, Modiano JF, Domenico J, Gelfand EW. Regulation of synthesis and activity of the PLSTIRE protein (cyclin-dependent kinase 6 (CDK6)), a major cyclin D-associated CDK4 homologue in normal human T lymphocytes. J Immunol 154:6275–6284,1995
11. Hall M, Bates S, Peters G. Evidence for different modes of action of cyclin-dependent kinase inhibitors: p15 and p16 bind to kinases, p21 and p27 bind to cyclins. Oncogene 11:1581–1588,1995
12. Ohnishi H, Kawamura M, Ida K, Sheng XM, Hanada R, Nobori T, Yamamori S, Hayashi Y. Homozygous deletions of p16/MTS1 gene are frequent but mutations are infrequent in chidhood T-cell acute lymphoblastic leukemia. Blood 86:1269–1275,1995
13. Hatta Y, Hirama T, Miller CW, Yamada Y, Tomonaga M, Koeffler HP. Homozygous deletions of the p15 (MTS2) and p16 (CDKN2/MTS1) genes in adult T-cell leukemia. Blood 85:2699–2704,1995
14. Hebert J, Cayuela JM, Berkeley J, Sigaux F: Candidate tumor-suppressor genes MTS1 ($p16^{INK4}$) and MTS2 ($p15^{INK4B}$) display frequent homozygous deletions in primary cells from T- but not from B-cell lineage acute lymphoblastic leukemias. Blood 84:4038–4044,1995
15. Okuda T, Shurtleff SA, Valentine MB, Raimondi SC, Head DR, Behm F, Curcio-Brint AM, Liu Q, Pui C-H, Sherr CJ, Beach D, Look AT, Downing JR: Frequent deletion of $p16^{INK4a}$/MTS1 and $p14^{INK4b}$/MTS2 in pediatric acute lymphoblastic leukemia. Blood 85:2321–2330,1995
16. Quesnel B, Preudhomme C, Philippe N, Vanrumbeke M, Dervite I, Lai JL, Bauters F, Wattel E, Fenaux P: p16 gene homozygous deletions in acute lymphoblastic leukemia. Blood 85:657–663,1995
17. Cayuela JM, Hebert J, Sigaux F: Homozygous MTS1 ($p16^{INK4}$) deletion in primary tumor cells of 163 leukemic patients. Blood 85:854,1995
18. Takeuchi S, Bartram CR, Seriu T, Miller CW, Tobler A, Janssen JWG, Reiter A, Ludwig W-D, Zimmermann M, Schwaller J, Lee E, Miyoshi I, Koeffler HP. Analysis of a family of cyclin-dependent kinase inhibitors: p15/MTS2/INK4B, p16/MTS1/INK4A, and p18 genes in acute lymphoblastic leukemia of childhood. Blood 86:755–760,1995
19. Tam SW, Theodoras AM, Shay JW, Draetta GF, Pagano M: Differential expression and regulation of cyclin D1 protein in normal and tumor human cells: association with Cdk4 is required for cyclin D1 function in G1 progression. Oncogene 9:2663–2674,1994
20. Janossy G, Bofill M, Trejdosiewicz LK, Willcox HNA, Chilosi M. Cellular differentiation of lymphoid subpopulations and their microenvironments in the human thymus. In: Muller-Hermelink, ed. The human thymus. Histopathology and pathology. Berlin: Springer-Verlag,1986: 89–125
21. Marino M, Muller-Hermelink HK. Thymoma and thymic carcinoma. Relation of thymoma cells to the cortical and medullary differentiation of thymus. Virchows Arch A (Pathol Anat) 407;119–149,1985
22. Krenàcs L, Tiszalvicz L, Krenàcs T, Boumsell L. Immunohistochemical detection of CD1a antigen in formalin-fixed and paraffin-embedded tissue sections with monoclonal antibody 010. J Pathol 171:99–104,1993
23. Powers CN, Silverman JF, Geisinger KR, Frable WJ. Fine-needle aspiration biopsy of the mediastinum. A multi-institutional analysis. Am J Clin Pathol 105:168–173,1996

41

OUR APPROACH IN THE PREPARATION FOR THYMECTOMY IN MYASTHENIA GRAVIS

Jose M. Ponseti,* Eloy Espín, Jose M. Fort, Carlos Vicens, and Manuel Armengol

Myasthenia Gravis Unit
Department of Surgery
Hospital General Vall d'Hebron
Universidad Autonoma de Barcelona, Spain

Thymectomy, first performed by Sauerbruch in 1912, became a major treatment in myasthenia gravis although no prospective study of its value has ever been made (1–5). Since the first thymectomies, postoperative myasthenic crisis, has been one of the most important and feared postoperative complications, with a mortality rate ranging from 15%-33,3% in the 1950s to a current 3% (6–9).

No effective medical treatment for post-thymectomy myasthenic crisis existed until 1935, when Walker (10) demonstrated the benefits of physostigmine. Physostigmine and its derivatives have since become basic in the preoperative and postoperative treatment of myasthenic crisis . Later, the suspicion of its autoimmune ethiology led some authors to use steroids (11). As soon as overwhelming evidence of is autoimmune origen was reported in the early 70´s, other immunosuppressive agents (12–14) were introduced (i.e. Azathioprine in Europe and Cyclosporine in USA), with clear benefit.

Plasmapheresis (15–19) is also used in patients with myasthenis crisis, and as a method for preparation for patients undergoing thymectomy.

Recently, high-dose IV gammaglobulin has been used in patients with myasthenia gravis as primary treatment (20–23) as well as for preparation for thymectomy (24,25).

To date, no prospective or retrospective studies have been reported evaluating the effectiveness of preoperative preparation of patients with myasthenia gravis undergoing thymectomy. Our own review on the literature concerning the results of thymectomy in 4137 patients with myasthenia gravis between 1958 and 1992 did not clarify either the criteria for selecting patients for pre-thymectomy preparation or the most suitable agent (4,5,26–32).

* Correspondence: Jose Mª Ponseti, M.D., F.A.C.S., Department of Surgery, Hospital General Universitario Vall d'Hebron, Universitat Autonoma de Barcelona, Pg Vall d'Hebron 119-129, 08035 Barcelona, Spain. Tel. 34-3-4-183400.

Epithelial Tumors of the Thymus, edited by Marx and Müller-Hermelink.
Plenum Press, New York, 1997

In view of the need for clear criteria for the selection of patients for preoperative preparation for thymectomy, as well as for an evaluation of the relative effectiveness of the drugs currently available, we made a historical review of our cases over a 28-year period to compare the postoperative results of different forms of pre-thymectomy preparation.

MATERIAL AND METHODS

The Myasthenia Gravis Functional Unit of the Vall d'Hebron General and University Hospital of Barcelona has treated from 1967 to 1995 a total of 361 patients with myasthenia gravis. The male/female ratio was 2/3. Age ranged from 4 to 67 yr. (39 ± 16)., similar to other series, which reflect a high incidence in young patients and a female to male predominance.

Of our original group of 361 patients with myasthenia gravis, 329 (91,1%) underwent surgery; 88 (26,7%) of the surgical patients had thymoma and 241 (73,3%) did not have thymoma. The distribution by Osserman grade of the thymectomized patients was: 9 grade I with only ocular symptoms, 67 grade II-A (mild generalised myasthenia with ocular symptoms), 144 grade II-B (generalised and bulbar symptoms), 97 grade III (respiratory disturbances), and 12 grade IV (late respiratory symptoms). All surgical patients had age under 55 (mean age 36,92 ± 16,34 years), 219 (66,5%) were females and 110 (33.5%) males. All the 32 patients not surgically treated had grade I disease, age over 55, and no thymoma.

Surgical approach was always through a median sternotomy .and in cases of thymoma a more radical technique was used.

Preparation for thymectomy varied over the 28-year period. Between 1967–1984 cholinesterase inhibitors were given at minimum dosage before surgery, pyridostigmine bromide every 4 to 6 hours was commonly used and discontinued 12 hours before surgery (160 cases). The cholinesterase inhibitor was restarted when the postoperative refractory period concluded at 1/3 the initial dosage. In the 1975–1990 period we used high-dose prednisone every other day (100 mg/48 h) starting 10–20 days before surgery and throughout the postoperative period until the dosage could be tapered off (87 cases). In 1984 and during a short period, patients were prepared with plasmapheresis (10–20 L of plasma exchange) every other day for 10–14 days and underwent surgery 5–10 days after concluding plasmapheresis (1 case). Since 1986 intravenous immunoglobulins at high doses (i.,e., 400 mg/kg/day for 5 consecutive days) was given before surgery, allowing patients to be scheduled for surgery 24 h. later (81 cases).

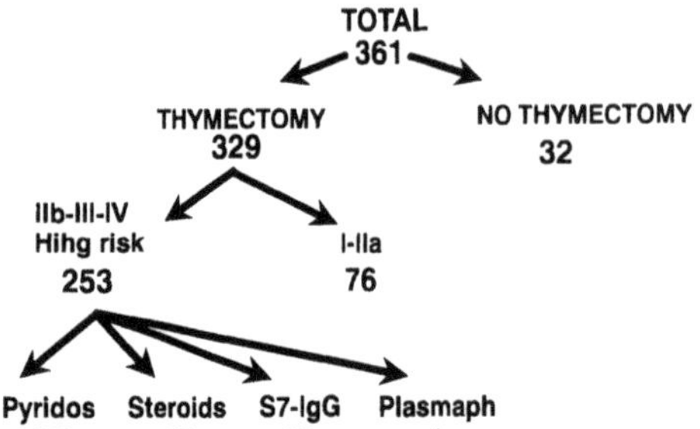

Figure 1. Distribution of patients by the type of preoperatory preparation.

Table 1. Clinical characteristics of the high risk patients distributed by the type of pre-thymectomy preparation

	PYRIDOSTIG.	STEROIDS	S7- IgG
YEARS	1967-1984	1975-1990	1986-1995
CASES	121	65	66
AGE M (SD)	33 (14)	43 (19)	39 (15)
SEX M/F	33/88	26/39	22/44
T. EVOL. M (SD)	23 (41)	22 (40)	17 (42)
THYMOMA Y/N (%)	27/94 (22)	31/34 (48)	14/52 (22)
BULBAR (%)	51 (42)	40 (61)	52 (78)
RESPIRATORY (%)	70 (58)	25 (39)	14 (22)

In our group those patients who experienced respiratory failure were intubated when intubation criteria were met. Tracheostomy was performed if intubation was required for more than 10 days. Of the 329 patients who underwent thymectomy, 252 high risk patients (Osserman grades II-B, III and IV, with bulbar and/or respiratory symptoms) were selected for the final study. Seventy-six patients with grade I and II-A disease were excluded because respiratory complications were uncommon and one patient prepared with plasmapheresis was excluded because of the small number.

This selection criteria gave us a final study group of 252 high risk patients which was further divided into three differents groups according to the type of preoperative treatment recieved: the pyridostigmine, the steroid and the immunoglobulin groups (Fig 1) which roughly correlate with three chronologically different phases.

The pyridostigmine group (1967–1984) included 121 patients pre-medicated with cholinesterase inhibitors. The steroid group (1975–1990) contained 65 patients pre-medicated with prednisone every other day. The immunoglobulin group (1986–1995) included 66 patients pre-medicated with high-dose IV immunoglobulin. (Table 1)

RESULTS

Comparative statistical analysis were all performed with the SPSS package.

Of the 252 high-risk patients who underwent thymectomy, 119 (47,2 %) patients experienced postoperative myasthenic crisis; (Fig. 2) ; 57 (22,6 %) of these patients required

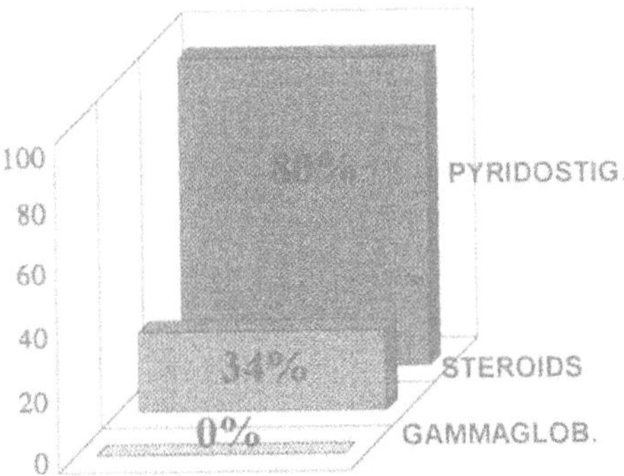

Figure 2. Percentage of patients that experienced postoperative myasthenic crisis distributed by the type of preoperative preparation.

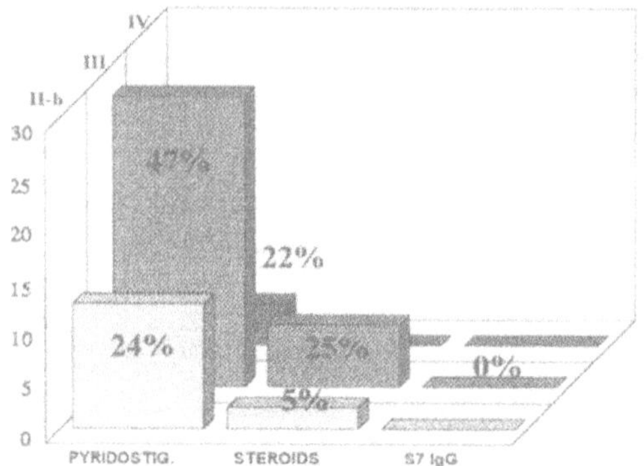

Figure 3. Postoperative mechanical ventilation according to the Osserman classification and the type of preparation.

intubation and mechanical ventilation (Fig. 3) and 30 (12 %) of these patients eventually required tracheostomy(Fig. 4). Postoperative complications included 27 cases of atelectasis, 18 patients with pneumonia, 2 mediastinitis and 4 wound infections. There were no operative deaths.

In the pyridostigmine group (n=121), 97 (80,1%) patients experienced postoperative myasthenic crisis with bulbar symptoms or impaired respiratory function. Forty-eight (39,6%) required intubation and mechanical ventilation and 25 (20,6%) tracheostomy. Twenty-two patients had atelectasis, 14 pneumonia and 3 wound infections. The mean intensive care unit stay was 4.78 days and the mean hospital stay was 14,78 days, mainly explained because the need for intubation and the occurrence of complications.

In the steroid group (n=65) the overall results were better. Twenty-two (33,8%) patients had myasthenic crisis, 9 (13,8%) patients required intubation, and 5 (7,6%) tracheostomy. Postoperative complications occurred in only 10 cases (4 pneumonia, 5 atelectasis and 1 wound infection). The mean intensive care unit stay was 5,37 days and the mean hospital stay was 12,43 days. (Fig. 5)

In the immunoglobulin group (n=66), no patient had postoperative myasthenic crisis or symptoms of respiratory failure, no patient required intubation or tracheostomy, and no complications were detected. Mean intensive care unit stay was 0,67 days and the mean hospital stay was 4,2 days (Fig. 6).

The rate of occurrence of postoperative complications varied significantly ($p<0.001$) between the pyridostigmine, steroid, and immunoglobulin groups, respectively: myasthenic crisis, 80.1%, 33.8% and 0%; intubation 39.6%, 13.8% and 0%; and tracheostomy, 20,6%, 7.6% and 0%. The duration of the ICU and hospital stays differed significantly between the pyridostigmine (4,7±0,4 and 14,7±0,7 days, respectively) and steroid (5,3± 1,9

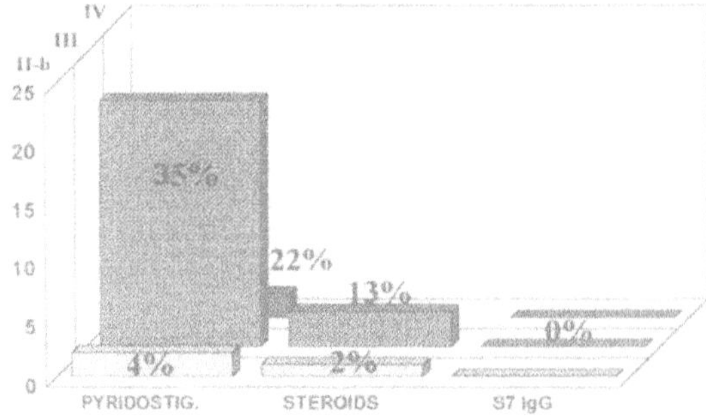

Figure 4. Postoperative tracheostomy according to the Osserman classification and the type of preparation.

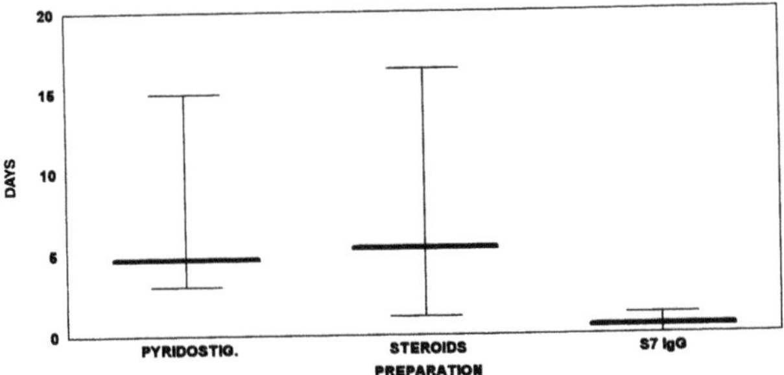

Figure 5. Mean intensive care unit stay.

and 12,4±1,4 days) groups compared with the immunoglobulin group (0,67±0,1 and 4,2±0,3 days) all showed p<0,001 values. (Table 2)

DISCUSSION

Since thymectomy was introduced in the treatment of myasthenia gravis, thymectomy, is accepted as the therapy that shows the largest number of remissions, decreasing symptoms, lowering incidence of myasthenic crisis and mortality in the clinical course of myasthenia gravis (11).

The surgical problems have centered on the approach, extension of the excision, and preoperative preparation of the patient in order to prevent and lessen postoperative myasthenic crisis.

The group of Mount Sinai, NY (4), advocates the less traumatic transcervical approach to thymectomy as a means of reducing postoperative morbidity, a technique rejected by most surgeons because the thymus resection is often incomplete. The transsternal approach is thought to be safer because it enables extended thymectomy; and it also is suitable for the enlarged and maximum thymectomy techniques now being studied (33,34).

Post-thymectomy myasthenic crisis, which causes important complications, is characterized by an immediate postoperative phase (6–48 hours) during which muscular strength decreases progressively, accompanied by refractoriness to anticholinesterase

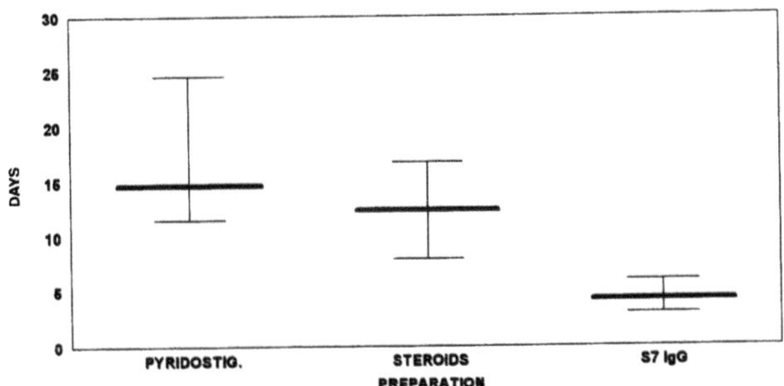

Figure 6. Mean in-hospital stay.

Table 2. Summary of results of postoperative myasthenic crisis, complications, intubations, tracheostomy and mean of in-ICU and in-hospital stay according to the type of preparation

	PYRIDOSTIG	STEROIDS	S7 IgG
YEARS	1967 - 1984	1975 - 1990	1986 - 1995
CASES	121	65	66
CRISIS (%)	97 (80)	22 (34)	0 (0)
ATELECTASIA	22	5	0
PNEUMONIA	14	4	0
INFECTION	5	1	0
GI.TUBE FEEDING	48 (39)	19 (29)	0 (0)
INTUBAT. (%)	48 (39)	9 (14)	0 (0)
TRACHEOT.(%)	25 (21)	5 (8)	0 (0)
IN-ICU STAY	4,78	5,37	0,6
IN-HOSPITAL STAY	14,78	12,43	4,22
MORTALITY	0	0	0

medication. Under this situation, the patient sometimes must undergo intubation and if the need for mechanical ventilation continues, tracheostomy should be performed.

The intubation of a patient who lacks muscular strength to remove pulmonar secretions is not free of complications and often leads to atelectasis with the needing of repeated tracheal aspirations and the predisposition to respiratory infections which increases refractoriness to anticholinesterase agents, thus creating a vicious cycle of postoperative complications. In these cases, tracheostomy may help to break this cycle, but a new intervention in an area adjacent to the mediastinal field implies a risk of communication of the two surgical compartments with a possible mediastinal contamination by tracheal secretions, producing mediastinitis, one of the most feared complications.

As late as 1992, "intubation and reintubation" were reported as being required frequently in the postoperative period of thymectomy (Kirschner) "*there is no moral victory in early extubation if a crash reintubation is necessary shortly thereafter*" (39). The physicians responsible for the postoperative care of thymectomized patients have long sought a good preoperative pharmacological preparation as a mean of preventing postoperative oscillations in muscular strength and myasthenic crises, and thus intubation and tracheostomy, which in the past have been responsible for most of the morbidity and mortality that accompany thymectomy.

When surgeons first began to operate on the thymus, the only medications available were anticholinesterase agents. Treatment of these patients required close observation during the postoperative period and was accompanied by frequent respiratory failure and need for reintubation, making complications a common part of the postoperative time of these patients.

Our results from the 1967–1984 period in patients treated with pyridostigmine showed that 80% of high-risk patients undergoing thymectomy had postoperative myasthenic crisis, 39% required intubation for respiratory failure, and 21,% needed tracheostomy. In 1990 Molnár and Szobor (9) recommended preoperative treatment with anticholinesterase agents and cited intubation and tracheostomy rates of 80% and 13%, respectively. Other authors who use anticholinesterase agents systematically intubate their patients for the first few postoperative days to prevent respiratory complications (29).

Evidence of an autoimmune origin of myasthenia gravis (40,41) supported by the finding of anti-acetylcholine receptor antibodies (15) was the basis for treating the disease with ACTH and prednisone (5,11,28,33,42). Corticosteroid treatment now is considered a standard in myasthenia gravis, and constitute the most commonly used treatment for myasthenia gravis, but they also show the largest array of potential side effects. Improvement usually begins in 2 to 4 weeks with a maximal benefit realized after 6 to 12 months or more.

Prednisone soon was introduced as a prethymectomy treatment and the results were frankly promising. We used prednisone (100 mg every other day) from 1975 to 1990 and achieved a very significant decrease in the occurrence of post-thymectomy myasthenic crises (34%), intubation (15%), and tracheostomy (9%). Nonetheless, the post-thymectomy period, although much improved, remained precarious.

The immunosuppressive agent azathioprine, and cyclosporine are not indicated for pre-thymectomy preparation because the high risk of surgical infection. Its use in myasthenia gravis are mostly in patients for whom corticosteroids are contraindicated, in those with an insufficient response with corticoids, or as a help in reducing dose of steroids.

In 1977 plasmapheresis was introduced as a treatment for myasthenic crisis and as a technique for potentiating immunosuppressive medication in high-risk patients (16–19). Plasmapheresis also is useful in preparing patients for thymectomy. It acts reducing the number of circulating antibodies and improves both muscular strength and tolerance to surgery. Removal by centrifugation or filtration of 12 to 15 liters of the patient's plasma and its substitution with albumin (6–8 procedures on alternate days) produces spectacular improvement in many patients. Nonetheless, the side effects of plasmapheresis, short duration of its therapeutic effect, gradual decline in its effectiveness, and a rebound effect curtail turns it usefulness.The beneficial effects of this technique are temporary, lasting only few weeks, and are not free of complications, which can be dramatic as pulmonary embolism The development of new semiselective filters (Immusrba TR-350®) to eliminate antibodies so that the patient's plasma can be reused has not alleviated these problems (43–48). As in our case , the only one prepared with plasmapheresis was also the unique patient that needed blood transfusions during the operation and in the postoperative recovery time because of coagulating alteration which is a complication of plasmapheresis.

The results reported in 1984 by Gadjos et al, (20) using intravenous administration of high-dose gammaglobulin (400 mg/kg/day x 5) introduced a new option into the treatment of myasthenic crisis and the pre-thymectomy preparation of patients (21,23,24,26,48–50).

In our group of 137 patients given gammaglobulin, 83 received it as pre-treatment for thymectomy, 66 of them in the high-risk disease group because of bulbar symptoms or impaired respiratory function. Of the high-risk patients, none had a postoperative myasthenic crisis, none required intubation or tracheostomy, nor experienced either side effects or related morbidity.

Even that the mode of action of high-dose immunoglobulins in myasthenia gravis is still unknown, (i.e. it has no consistent effect on the measurable amount of acetylcholine receptor antibody) several hypotheses have been proposed : competition of immunoglobulins with antibodies for receptors on the neuromuscular plate, that the infusion of large amounts of gammaglobulin may reduce antibody production by means of a negative feedback mechanism, and that the idiotypes or immunoactive proteins present in the gammaglobulin may mediate directly between the antibody and immunoglobulin idiotypes and anti-idiotypes (49,52–60).

Our review of the bibliography disclosed the absence of any generally accepted criteria for pre-thymectomy preparation of the myasthenic patient, but the general tendency seemed to be to prepare patients with high-risk disease. Likewise, no pre-thymectomy treatment is accepted at all specialized centers, although anticholinesterase agents, prednisone, plasmapheresis, and immunoglobulin are the treatments most often used. After reviewing our cases, we conclude that patients with myasthenia gravis grade II-B, III and IV should all receive treatment before thymectomy. Intravenous high-dose immunoglobulin is the optimal preoperative preparation because it sharply reduces morbidity and produces shorter ICU and hospital stays. The expense of this medication is easily compensated by the patient's increased safety and reduced care requirements.

REFERENCES

1. Perlo VP, Poskenzer DD, Schwab RS, Viets H, Osserman KO, Genkins G. Myasthenia gravis: Evaluation of treatment in 1,355 patients. Neurology 1966; 16: 431–442.
2. Buckingham JM,Howard FM Jr, Bernatz PE. The value of thymectomy in myasthenia gravis: a computer-assisted matched study. Ann Surg 1976; 184:453–458.
3. Olanow CW, Wechsler AS, Sirotkiin-Roses M. Thymectomy as primary therapy in myasthenia gravis. Ann NY Acad Sci. 1987; 505: 595–606.
4. Papatestas AE, Genkins G, Kornfeld P, Eisenkraft JB, Fagerstrom RP, Pozner J, Aufses AH: Efects of thymectomy in Myasthenia Gravis. Ann Surg. 1987; 206: 79–88.
5. Otto TJ, Strugalska H. Surgical treatment for myasthenia gravis. Thorax 1987; 42: 199–204.
6. Galofre M, Ponseti JM. Timectomia en la miastenia gravis. Barcelona Quirurgica 1971; 15: 449–453.
7. Osserman KE. Myasthenia Gravis. Grune & Stratton. NY. 1958; 165–183.
8. Viets HR. Myasthenia Gravis. The second international symposium proceedings. Charles C Thomas Publisher, Bannerstone House, Springfiie, Illinois, USA. 1961; 637–652.
9. Molnár J, Szobor A. Myasthenia gravis: effect of thymectomy in 425 patients. A 15-year experience. Eur J Cardio-thorac Surg 1990; 4: 8–14.
10. Walker MB: Treatment of myasthenia gravis with physostigmine. Lancet 1934;1: 1200–1201
11. Oosterhuis HJ. Observations of the natural history of myasthenia gravis an the efect of thymectomy.Ann NY Acad Sci 1981 ; 377 : 678–690.
12. Martens HG, Balzereit F, Leipert M. The treatment of severe myasthenia gravis with immunosuppressive agents. Eur Neurol 1969; 2: 321–339.
13. Ponseti JM, Galofre M. Prespectivas actuales en el tratamiento de la miastenia gravis. Med Clin (Barc) 1972; 58: 308–313.
14. Mertens HG, Hertel G, Renther P, et al: Effect of immunosuppressive drugs(azathioprine). Ann NY Acad Sci 1981; 377: 691–699.
15. Patrick J, Lindstrom J: Antiimmune response to acetylcholine receptor. Science 1973; 180:871–872.
16. Dau PC, Lindstrom CK, Cassel CK, Denys EH, Shev EE, Spitler LE: Plasma pheresis and immunosuppessive drog therapy in myasthenia gravis. N Engl J Med 1977; 1134–1140.
17. Dau PC: Plasmapheresis and the Immunobiologi of Myasthenia Gravis. Houghton Mifflin, Boston 1979
18. Ponseti JM. Miastenia gravis y timoma. Rev Neurol. 1975 ;3 : 279–287.
19. Ponseti JM, Plasmaferesis en el tratamiento de la miastenia gravis. Med Clin (Barc) 1983; 80: 121–122.
20. Gajdos P, Outin H, Elkharrat D, Brunel D, Rohan-Chabot P, Raphael JC, Goulon M, Goulon-Goeau C, Morel E: High-dose intravenous gammaglobulin for myasthenia gravis. Lancet 1984; 406–407.
21. Fateh-Moghadam A, Wick M, Besinger U, Geursen RG: High-dose Intravenous gammaglobulin for myasthenia gravis: Lancet 1984; 848–849.
22. Ippoliti G, Cosi V, Piccolo G, Lombardi G,Mantegaz R. High-dose intravenous gammaglobulin for myasthenia gravis. Lancet 1984; 2: 809
23. Devathasan G, Kneh YK,Chng PN. High-dose intravenous gammaglobulin for myasthenia gravis Lancet 1984; 2: 809–810.
24. Arsura EL, Bick A, Brunner G, Namba T, Grob D: High-dose intravenous immunoglobulin in the managment of myasthenia gravis: Arch Intern Med 1986; 146: 1365–1368.
25. Bonaventura I, Ponseti J, Español T, Matias-Guiu J, Codina-Puiggros A. High-dose intravenous gammaglobulin therapy for myasthenia gravis. J Neurol 1987; 234: 363.
26. Szobor A. Crises in Myasthenia Gravis. Hafner Publishing Company, NY. 1970; 39–42.
27. Grob D, Brunner NG, Namba T: The natural course of myasthenia gravis and effect of therapeutic measures. Ann NY Acad Sci 1981; 377: 652–669.

28. Rodriguez M, Gomez MR, Howard FM, Taylor WF: Myasthenia gravis in children: long-term fallow-up. Ann Neurol 1983; 13: 504–510.
29. Pradas J, Illa I, Tratamiento de la miastenia gravis: Sant Pau 1984; 5: 24–39.
30. Cooper JD, Al-Jilaihawa AN, Pearson FG, Humphrey JG, Humphrey HE. An improved Technique to facilitate transcervical thymectomy for myasthenia gravis. Ann Thorac Surg. 1988; 45: 242–247.
31. Mulder DG, Graves M, Herrmann C. Thymectomy for Myasthenia Gravis: Recent Observations and Comparisons With Past Experience. Ann Thorac Surg 1989; 48: 551–555.
32. Ponseti JM. Contribucion al estudio de la miastenia gravis. Valor de la espirometria como indice de recuperacion. Resumen de Tesis Doctoral. Universidad Autónoma de Barcelona, 1977
33. Jaretzki III J, Penn AS, Younger DS, Wolff M Olarte MR, Lovelace RE, Rowland LP, "Maximal" thymectomy for myasthenia gravis. J Thorac Cardiovasc Surg 1988 ; 95 : 747–757.
34. Kornfeld P, Merav A, Fox S, Maier K. Haw reliable are imaging procedures in detectin residual thymus after previus thymectomy. Ann NY Acd Sci 1993 ; 681 :575–576.
35. Fischer JE, Grinvalski HT, Nussbaum MS, Sayers HJ, Cole RE, Samaha FJ. Aggressive surgical approach for drug-free remission from myasthenia gravis. Ann Surg 1987;205:496–503
36. Hankins JR, Maye RF, Satterfielt JR, Turney SZ, Attar S, Sequeira AJ, Thompson SW, McLaughlin JS. Thymectomy for myasthenia gravis: 14-year experience. Ann Surg 1985;201:18–25.
37. Olanow CW, Wechsler AS, Roses AD. A prospective study of thymectomy and serum acetylcholine receptor antibodies in myasthenia gravis. Ann Surg 1982; 196:113–121.
38. Papatestas AE, Genkins G, Kornfeld P, Eisenkraft JB, Fagerstrom RP, Pozner J,Aufses AH. Effects of thymectomy in myasthenia gravis. Ann Surg 1987; 201: 79–88.
39. Kirschner PA. Myasthenia gravis and other parathymyc syndromes. Chest Sur Clin N A. 1992 ;2. 1. 183–201.
40. Simpson JA: Myasthenia gravis: A new hypothesis. Scott Med J. 1960; 5: 419–436.
41. Nastuk WL, Plescia OJ, Osserman KE: Changes in serum complement activity in patients with myasthenia gravis. Proc Soc Exp Biol Med 1960; 105: 177–184.
42. Maggi G, Casadio C, Cavallo A, Cianci R, Molinatti M, Ruffini E. Thymectomy in myesthenia gravis: Resutls of 662 cases operated upon in 15 years. Eur J Cardio-thorac Surg. 1989; 3: 504–511.
43. Sato T, Nishimiya J, Arai K, Anno M, Yamawaki N, Kuroda T, Inagaki K. Selective removal of anti-acetylcholine receptor antibodies in sera patients with myasthenia gravis in vitro with a new immunosorbent. In: Oda T, ed. Therapeutic Plasmapheresis (III). Stuttgart-New York: Schattauer, 1983; 565–568
44. Heininger K, Gaczkowski A, Hartung HP Toyka KV, Borberg H. Plasma separation and imunoadsorption in myasthenia gravis. Therapeutic Plasmapheresis (V) Ed. Shattauer. 1985; 3–10.
45. Passalacqua S, Splendiani G, Sturniolo A, Costanzi S, Barbera G, Bartoccioni E, Evoli A, Scoppetta C, Adorno D, Di Guilio S, Casciani CU. Immunosorbent treatment in myasthenia gravis. Apheresis. Alan R. Liss Inc. 1990; 285–288.
46. Kawanami S, Mori S, Uchida T, Nagasawa H, Shirotani T, Naito S, Shibuya N. Therapeutic Plasmapheresis (IX) ICAOT Press. Cleveland. 1991; 318: 167–171.
47. Avanzi G, Marconi G. Semiselective Immunoadsorption of Anti-AChR abs on TRyptophan Column in Myasthenia Gravis. Clinical Experience in 32 Patients. Transfus. Sci. 1993; 14: 17–21.
48. Stricker RB, Kwiatkowska BJ, Habis JA, MacLeod DE, Kiprov DD. Response to plasmapheresis following failure of intravenous gammaglobulin in patients with Myasthenia Gravis and Guillain-Barre Syndrome. J Clin Apheresis 1993; 8: 733.
49. Ferrero B, Durelli I, Cavallo R, Dutto A, Aimo G, Pecchio F, Bergamasco B. Therapies for exacerbation of Myasthenia Gravis. The mechanism of action of intravenous high-dose immunoglobulin G. Ann NY Acd Sci 1993; 681: 563–566.
50. Arsura EL, Bick A, Bruner NG, Grob B. Effects of repeated doses of intravenous immunoglobulin in myasthenia gravis. Am J Med Sci 1988; 295: 438–443.
51. Fort JM, Ponseti JM. Altas dosis de globulina gamma intravenosa en el tratamiento de la miastenia gravis. Med Clin (Barc) 1988; 91: 325–328.
52. Zweiman B. Theoretical mechanisms by which immunoglobulin therapy might benefit myasthenia gravis. Clin Immunol Immunopathol. 1989; 53: 83–91
52. Ponseti JM. Miastenia Gravis. Manual Terapéutico. Springer-Verlag Ibérica. Barcelona.1995 ; 139–145.
54. Drachman DB. Myasthenia Gravis. N Engl J Med 1994; 330: 1797–1810.
55. Edan G, Landgraf F. Experience with intravenous immunoglobulin in myasthenia gravis : a review. J Neurol Neurosurg Psychiatry1994;57(Supplement):55–56.
56. Stricker RB, Kwiatkowska BJ, Habis JA, Kiprov DD. Myasthenic Crisis: Response to Plasmapheresis following failure of intravenous γ-Globulin. Arch Neurol 1993;50:837–840.

57. Sanders DB, Scoppetta C. The treatment of patients with myasthenia gravis.In Myasthenia Gravis and Myasthenic Syndromes. Edited by Sanders DB. Neurologic Clinics 1994;12 :343–368
58. Blasczyk R, Westhoff U, Grosse-Wilde H: Soluble CD4, CD8, and HLA molecules in commercial immunoglobulin preparations. Lancet 1993; 341: 789–790.
59. Lam L, Whitsett CF, McNicoll JM, Hodge TW, Hooper J: Immunologically active proteins in intravenous immunoglobulin. Lancet 1993; 342: 678.
60. Ahlberg R, Yi Q, Pirskanen R, Martell G, Swerup C, Rieber P, Riethmüller G, Holm G, Lefvert AK. Clinical improvement of Myasthenia Gravis by treatment with a chimeric ant-CD4 monoclonal antibody.Ann NY Acd Sci 1993; 681: 552–555.

42

ONSET OF MYASTHENIA GRAVIS AFTER THYMECTOMY FOR THYMOMA

F. Tezzon,[1] M. G. Passarin,[1] T. Zanoni,[1] G. Furlan,[2] and G. Ferrari[1]

[1]Department of Neurology
[2]Department of Thoracic Surgery
Ospedale Civile Maggiore, Verona

Myasthenia Gravis (M.G.) is an autoimmune disease with antibodies directed against the skeletal muscle acetylcholine receptor (AChR) (4). Although the production of AChR antibodies is due to B lymphocytes, there is evidence that T cells are involved in the autoantibody response. (4,18).

A role for T cells in the etiology of M.G. is suggested by the well known high incidence in myasthenic patients of pathological changes in the thymus, either a thymoma or the presence of germinal centres called hyperplasia (3). These have the appearance and phenotypic characteristics of germinal centers in reactive lymph nodes. Lymphocytes in the thymus and peripheral blood appear to be sensitized to muscle in M G patients (16). Muscle-like myoid cells are present in the thymus gland and also Ach-reactive T cells in the thymus tissue from M G patients with and without thymoma have been described (10,16). In 1939 Blalock (2) reported the remission of generalized M. G. in a 21 year old woman after removal of the cystic remains of a thymic tumor. Since then, thymectomy has been used to treat M G and was utilized to treat thymoma with and without M. G. (9).

Although no prospective controlled study on the possible effectiveness of thymectomy has been conducted, there is now a general consensus that patients between puberty and 60 years of age with generalized M.G..H would benefit from thymectomy (1).

From the literature it is known that aproximately 10–20 % of patients with M.G. have a thymoma and one third - 50 % of patients with thymoma have M.G, the percentage is variable from neuromuscular centres or thoracic surgery clinics (15). Myasthenic patients with thymoma show different clinical characteristics as compaired with other myasthenic patients: thymoma is associated with more severe disease,poor response to thymectomy, increased risk of operative mortality (5,14). Rarely, the onset of M G may be after thymectomy (11). The current study reports the incidence of M G in 83 patients with thymoma; of particular interest are 4 patients who developed M G after total thymectomy for removal of a thymoma.

Epithelial Tumors of the Thymus, edited by Marx and Müller-Hermelink.
Plenum Press, New York, 1997

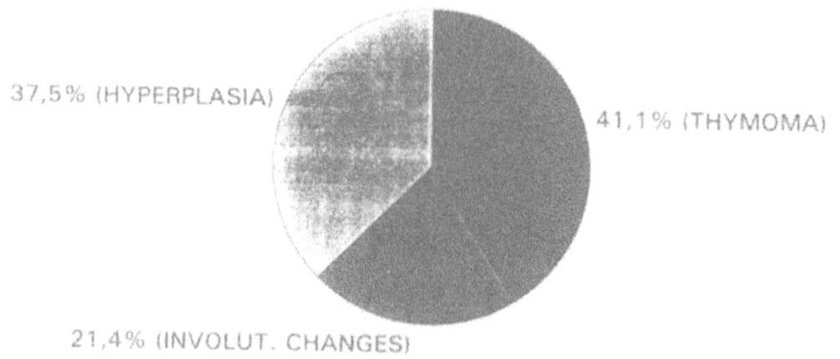

MATERIALS AND METHODS

In our series of 160 myasthenic patients, 56 underwent thymectomy, with a sternal splitting surgical approach and with the most complete resection including the tumor, the thymus gland, and the surrounding fatty tissue as well. Thymectomy was performed also in 64 non myasthenic patients with thymoma. In 4 patients from this group M G appeared after thymomectomy. The diagnosis of M.G. was performed according to clinical, pharmacological and neurophysiological criteria. Severity of the disease was graded according to Osserman (13). Radiological examination of the mediastinum by chest X-rays and axial tomography and,from 1978, by computerized tomography.

RESULTS AND DISCUSSION

The distribution of the thymic pathological findings from the 56 myasthenic patients submitted to thymectomy is shown in Fig.1. 23 resulted the myasthenic patients with thymoma, including 4 patients with onset of MG after thymectomy.

The incidence of M G in the patients with thymoma resulted 27.7 % and the incidence of myasthenic patients with thymoma in the myasthenic group was 14.4 %.

It has been known from many years that a thymoma can remain "dormant" for a long time before the onset of M.G. and clinical M.G. can first appear or be exacerbated after thymectomy (17).

Therefore, we use to evaluate muscle weakness and fatigability with the response to edrophonium and electromyographic examination in every patient before mediastinal operation. In the majority of our myasthenic patients with thymoma, M. G. was already present when the tumor was first detected but in a few patients mild M.G. was in that occasion recognized. In 4 patients thymomectomy was performed prior to the onset of weakness.

Their clinical features are summarized in Table 1. First of all, the onset of M. G. was not during or immediately after excision of thymoma, but delayed. The course was particularly severe in 3 patients. In patient 1 the discovery of thymoma was occasionally made during aorto-coronaric by-pass, without any radiological evidence on X-rays.

The appearance of M. G. after thymomectomy has been reviewed some years ago by Namba et al. (11) who described 7 new cases in addition to the 26 already published by others. More recently other case reports have been described (6,12,17). The latency between thymomectomy and onset of M.G. ranged from some weeks to many years.

The relationship between thymoma, thymomectomy and M.G is not fully known; our data confirm previous reports where in the presence of a thymoma M.G. is more se-

Table 1. Clinical features of patients with onset of M G after thymomectomy

	Patient			
	1	2	3	4
Age	50	33	38	37
Sex	M	F	M	M
Thymoma	invasive	capsulated	capsulated	invasive
Latency of M G onset	2 months	2 months	3 years	6 months
Course of M G	severe	severe	mild/moderate	severe
Therapy	steroids AZA, P. E. I. G. i. v.	steroids AZA, P. E.	steroids	steroids AZA

vere and little influenced by surgical excision of the tumor (5). A beneficial effect of surgery is often to be awaited on long time (15); in the meantime an adequate immunosuppression may be necessary to counteract possible clinical exacerbations. Exacerbations after thymomectomy have been repeatedly described as well as the onset of M. G. A direct and immediate causal relationship between thymoma and M.G. seems to be excluded if we consider the long interval between the two events. Loss of suppressor activity (8), autoimmune paraneoplastic syndrome (7) or persistence in a peripheral pool of autoreactive T lymphocytes (11) have been proposed as possible mechanisms in a causal relationship between thymoma and M.G. In every case, thymomectomy is necessary to remove the potentially malignant and invasive tumor (9).

REFERENCES

1. Beghi E, Antozzi C, Batocchi A P, Cornelio F, Cosi V, Evoli A, Lombardi M, Mantegazza R, Monticelli M L, Piccolo G, Tonali P, Trevisan D, Zarrelli M. 1991. Prognosis of Myasthenia gravis: a multicenter follow-up study of 844 patients. J Neurol Sci.106:213–220.
2. Blalock A, Mason M F, Morgan H J,Raven S S.1939. Myasthenia gravis and tumors of the thymic region: report of a case in which the tumor was removed. Ann Surg.110:544–561.
3. Castleman B.1966. The pathology of the thymus gland in Myasthenia Gravis.Ann N Y Acad Sci.135:496–505.
4. Drachman D B.1994. Myasthenia Gravis. N Engl J Med.330:1797–1810.
5. Durelli L, Maggi G, Casadio C, Ferri R, Rendine S, Bergamini L. 1991.Actuarial analysis of the occurrence of remissions following thymectomy for Myasthenia Gravis in 400 patients. J Neurol Neurosurg Psych. 54:406–411.
6. Hassel B, Gilhus N E, Aarli J A, Skogen O R. 1992. Fulminant Myasthenia Gravis and polymyositis after thymectomy for thymoma. 85:63–65.
7. Holfeld R.1980. Myasthenia Gravis and thymoma: paraneoplastic failure of neuromuscular transmission. Lab Invest. 62:241–243.
8. Kuroda Y, Ken-ichiro O, Neshige R, Shibasaki H. 1993. Exacerbation of Myasthenia Gravis after removal of a thymoma having a membrane phenotype of suppressor T cells. Ann Neurol. 15:400–402.
9. Maggi G, Casadio C, Cavallo A, Cianci R, Molinatti M, Ruffini E. 1991. Thymoma: results of 241 operated cases. Ann Thorac Surg 51:152–156.
10. Muller-Hermelink H K, Marx A, Gender K, Kirchner T. 1993. The pathological basis of thymoma-associated Myasthenia Gravis. Ann N Y Acad Sci. 681:56–65.
11. Namba T, Brunner N G, Grob D. 1978. Myasthenia Gravis in patients with thymoma with particular reference to onset after thymectomy. Medicine. 57:411–432.
12. Neau P, Robert R, Pourrat O, Patte F, Gil R, Lefevre J P. 1988. Myasthenie survenant après ablation d'un thymome. La Presse Med. 17:391–392.

13. Osserman K E, GenkinsG.1971. Studies in Myasthenia Gravis: review of a twenty-year experience in over 1200 patients. Mt Sinai J Med. 38:497–537.
14. Palmisani M T, Evoli A, Batocchi A P, Provenzano C, Tonali P. 1993. Myasthenia Gravis associated with thymoma: clinical characteristic and long term outcome. Eur Neurol. 34:78–82.
15. Papatestas A E, Genkins G, Kornfeld P, Eisenkraft J B, Fagerstrom R P, Pozner J, Aufses A. H. 1987. Effects of thymectomy in Myasthenia Gravis. Ann Surg. 206:79–88.
16. Sommer N, Willcox N, Harcourt G C, Newsom-Davis J.1990 Myasthenic thymus and thymoma are selectively enriched in acetylcholine receptor-reactive T cells. Ann Neurol.28:312–319.
17. Somnier F E. 1994. Exacerbation of Myasthenia Gravis after removal of thymomas. Acta Neurol Scand. 90:56–66.
18. Wekerle H. 1993. The Thymus in Myasthenia Gravis. Ann N Y Acad Sci. 681:47–55.

43

ASPECTS OF CLINICAL PREPARATION OF THYMECTOMY IN MYASTHENIC CASES WITH OR WITHOUT THYMOMA AND THE CLINICO-BIOLOGICAL FOLLOW-UP OF THE THYMECTOMIZED PATIENTS

Paolo Confalonieri,[1] Renato Mantegazza,[1] Carlo Antozzi,[1]
Lorenzo Novellino,[2] Giuseppe Pezzuoli,[2] Maria Teresa Ferro',[3]
Manlio Sgarzi,[1] and Ferdinando Cornelio[1]

[1]Divisione Malattie Neuromuscolari
Istituto Nazionale Neurologico "Carlo Besta"
Milano, Italy
[2]Divisione di Chirurgia Generale
Policlinico S. Marco
Zingonia, Italy
[3]Divisione di Neurologia
Policlinico S. Marco
Zingonia, Italy

1. INTRODUCTION

Several uncontrolled studies performed since the 1950s proved that thymectomy is effective in Myasthenia Gravis (MG). MG is an autoimmune disease characterized by muscle weakness and fatigability in which autoantibodies (AntiAChR-Ab) are targeted to the acetylcholine receptor (AChR) at the neuromuscular junction.[1] Aim of surgery is to remove the site of autoantigen sensibilization and self-sustainment of the autoimmune response. Previous studies showed that the efficacy of thymectomy is positively correlated with the time from diagnosis, young age and absence of thymoma.[2,3,4] Furthermore, over the last two decades there has been considerable debate on the best surgical technique in terms of tolerability and clinical outcome.[5,6] Transcervical thymectomy, a relatively easy procedure with minimal postoperative morbidity,[7] may fail to remove the entire gland and miss ectopic thymic tissue often present in the neck and mediastinum.[8] In this regard, transsternal thymectomy is required to remove all thymic tissue and is now accepted as the technique associated with the higher remission rate in MG.[9] Extended transsternal thymectomy (ETT) combines the removal of thymus and fat tissue from the pericardic and cervical regions in which functional thymic

Epithelial Tumors of the Thymus, edited by Marx and Müller-Hermelink.
Plenum Press, New York, 1997

remnants may persist, usually in the space from the thyroid gland to the diaphragm, between the two phrenic nerves.[10] Since the extended approach requires a median sternotomy, ETT is a major surgical procedure which may limit the indication of thymectomy in patients with bulbar or ocular MG, and in patients in which surgical morbidity may have detrimental effects on patients' condition. Moreover, a median sternotomy is sometimes not easily accepted by female patients for aesthetical reasons.

We report the protocol for the clinical preparation of MG patients to thymectomy, and the immuno-biological and clinical follow-up. We also review the preliminary data obtained using the mini-invasive video assisted thoracoscopy extended thymectomy (VATET) without sternotomy as an effort to improve the surgical technique.

2. PATIENTS AND METHODS

75 myasthenic patients, 54 females (72%) and 21 males (28%), were submitted to thymectomy between February 1994 and February 1996; Age at onset and age at thymectomy are reported in table 1.

Diagnosis of MG was established according to clinical, pharmacological and electrophysiological criteria.

Patients were studied according to a clinico-biological protocol designed for a complete evaluation of immunological aspects as well as the assessment of VATET efficacy (table 2). Since pre-surgical clinical conditions are considered of critical importance for the post-thymectomy clinical course,[11] our patients were treated as listed in table 3 to avoid any bulbar or respiratory compromise before surgery (figure 1); at the time of surgery 37.3% of patients were treated with anticholinesterase drug and 55.8% of patients with steroids, either alone (41.3%) or in association with azathioprine, cyclophosphamide or cyclosporine (14.5%) (table 3).

Mediastinic evaluation was performed by contrast enhanced computerized tomography (CT) or nuclear magnetic resonance (NMR).

The surgical procedure begins with a transverse cervical incision and a revision of the peri-thyroid space. Afterwards, the sternum is drawn upward by a lifter to obtain the best visualization of the mediastinum. A double lumen tube was used to allow the separate ventilation of each lung. The video-assisted thoracoscopic technique requires the insertion of three trocars in either the left or right pleural cavity to introduce the videocamera and the surgical instruments. After a complete isolation, the thymus and fat tissue are removed through the cervical incision (figure 2).

Table 1. Features of MG patients included in the study

Whole MG population	75 (66 VATET; 9 ETT)
Females	54 (72%)
Males	21 (28%)
Age at thymectomy	
Whole MG population	34 ± 14 yrs[a]. (range 13-37)
thymomatous patients	48 ± 15 yrs.
non-thymomatous patients	29 ± 11 yrs.
Age at onset	
Whole MG population	31 ± 14 yrs. (range 9-72)
thymomatous patients	46 ± 15 yrs.
non-thymomatous patients	26 ± 10 yrs.

[a] Mean ± standard deviation.

Table 2. Clinico-biological protocol for thymectomy evaluation

1. Pre-thymectomy	Clinical evaluation
	Anti-AChR, anti-titin, anti-ryanodine receptor Abs
	Lymphocyte phenotype[a]
	TCR repertoire
	Lymphokine dosage (IL-2, IFN-γ,TNF-α)
	Radiology (CT scan)
2. Thymectomy (on thymus)	Histology & immunotyping
	Lympho/thymocyte phenotype as at point 1
	TCR repertoire
3. Post-thymectomy (schedule)	As at point 1 (CT scan at the end of follow-up)
	2, 6, 12, 24, 36 months

[a] Performed by FACS analysis only in non-immunosuppressed patients.

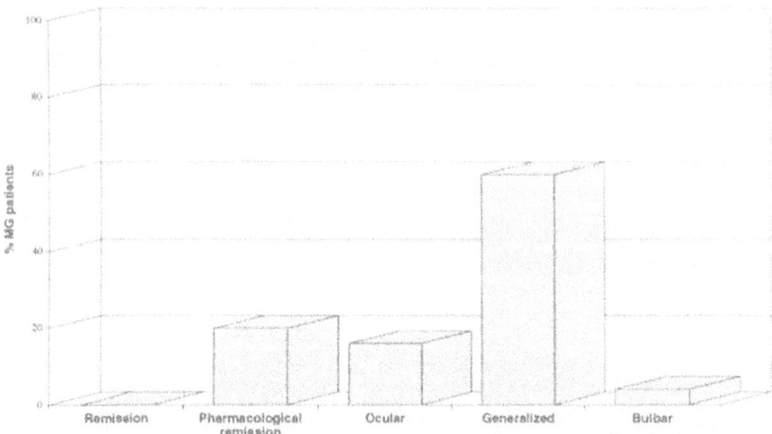

Figure 1. Clinical state of MG patients before surgery.

Table 3. T therapy at thymectomy

No therapy	2	(2.6%)
Anti-AChE[a]	28	(37.3%)
Anti-AChE + Prednisone	19	(25.3%)
Anti-AChE + Prednisone + Azathioprine	4	(3.3%)
Anti-AChE + Azahioprine	3	(4.0%)
Prednisone	12	(16.0%)
Prednisone + Azathioprine	5	(6.6%)
Prednisone + Cyclophosphamide	1	(1.3%)
Prednisone + Cyclosporine	1	(1.3%)

[a] AChE = anticholinesterase inhibitors.

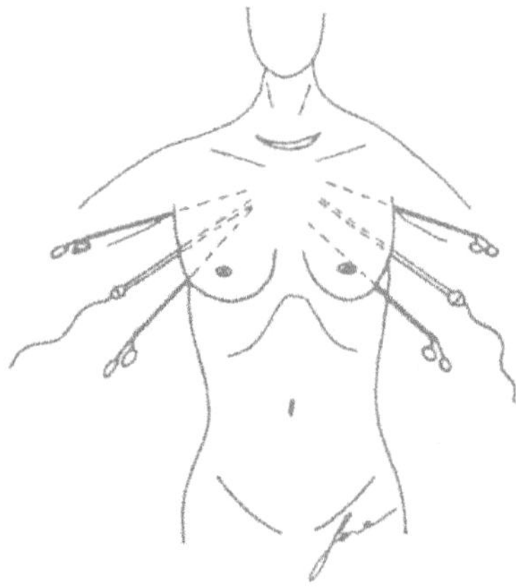

Figure 2. Schematic drawing of the applied VATET procedure.

The removed tissue is then separated into the thymus gland, the pericardic fat and perithyroid fat and weighted separately. Specimens are either fixed in 10% formalin or frozen in liquid nitrogen. Histopathological examination is performed by Hematoxylin-Eosin, Giemsa and modified Gomori Silver impregnation for reticulin staining. Hyperplasia is definied by the presence of lymphoid follicles, usually not seen in normal adult thymus; thymic involution by the degree of fatty replacement; thymoma was classified according to Muller-Hermelink criteria.[12]

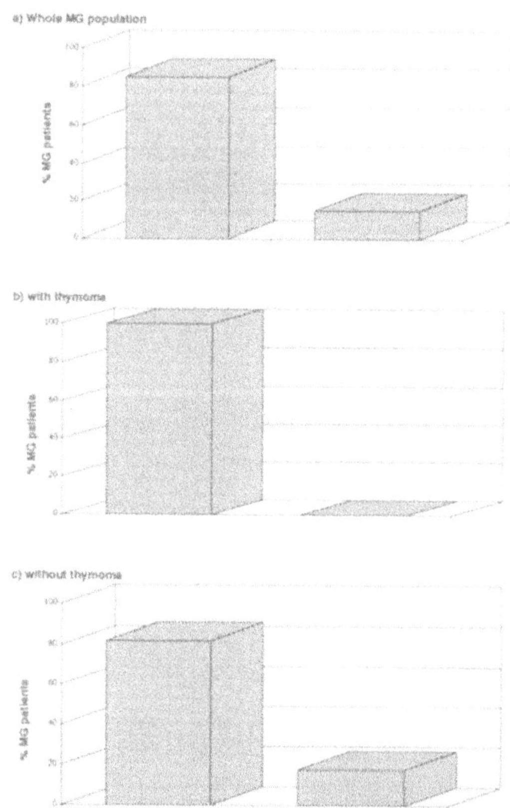

Figure 3. Positivity or negativity for antiAChR serum autoantibodies in various populations of MG patients.

Clinical evaluation was planned at 2, 6, 12, 24 and 36 months after thymectomy (table 2), by objective measurement of muscle strength and fatigability according to a previously reported MG score;[13] the following clinical categories were identified: remission (no myasthenic symptoms without drug treatment for at least one year); pharmacological remission (no myasthenic symptoms with drug treatment); ocular, generalized, bulbar or respiratory classes defined according to the score obtained.

3. RESULTS

Seventy-five consecutive MG patients were underwent thymectomy, either by VATET (66 patients) or ETT (9 patients), at the same institution.

Determination of AntiAChR-Ab was performed as described.[14] AntiAChR-Ab were detectable in 85% of MG patients; none of the patients with thymoma was seronegative (figure 3). Autoantibodies against the striated muscle protein titin were present in 73% of patients with thymoma and in 13% of patients without thymoma (figure 4).

The histopathological examination showed thymic hyperplasia in 58.3%, involuted thymus in 19.4% and thymoma in the remaining 22.3% (figure 5).

Four (26.6%) thymomas showed infiltration of the capsula or neighboring tissues. A thymoma was suspected in 42% of patients while in 58% radiologic signs of thymic hyperplasia or involution were found (figure 5).

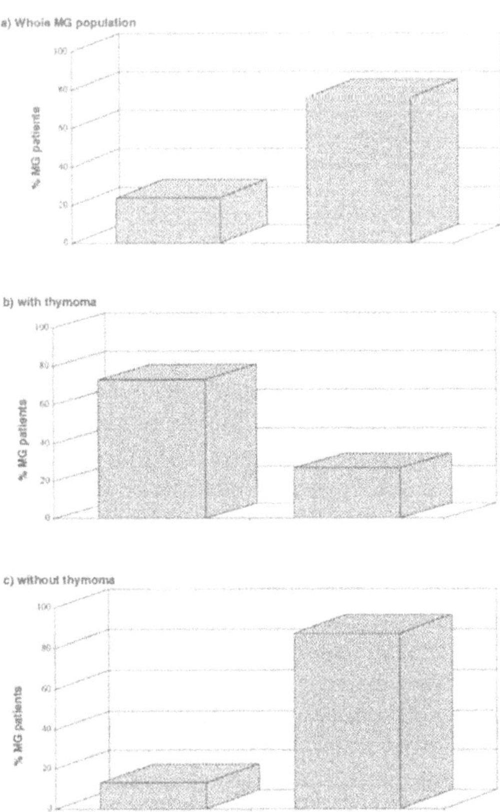

Figure 4. Absence or presence of anti-titin serum autoantibodies in various populations of MG patients.

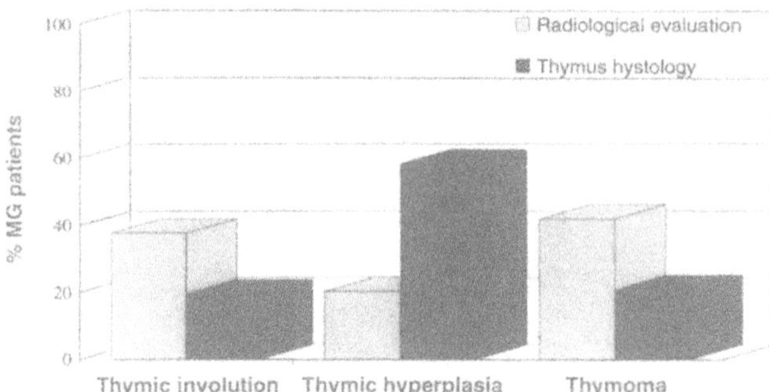

Figure 5. Radiological versus histological diagnosis of thymic alterations in MG patients.

The wet weight of the removed tissue was 58.2±41.1 grams (mean± S.D.); the amount of tissue was comparable with that removed by conventional ETT: 59.6±42.4 grams. A more detailed analysis of the tissue removed by VATET showed a mean thymic weight of 34.9±27 grams, mean pericardial fat of 22.9±18 grams and perithyroid fat: 0.746±21 grams.

The post-operative hospital stay was shorter in VATET patients compared to the small number of myasthenics treated by ETT: 7.07±2.12 days (mean± S.D.) versus 11.6±6.18, respectively; a t-Test (1 tail) revealed a t-value of 7.95, $p = 0.0001$.

The mean clinical follow-up of thymectomized MG patients was 8±4.5 months. Twenty-eight patients had a follow-up of at least 12 months and were evaluated for a preliminary outcome study. As reported in figure 6, 17 patients (60.7%) showed a significant clinical improvement and 39.3% remained clinically stable at the end of follow-up.

Clinical evaluation at one year showed that more than 70% of patients were symptom-free (remission 17.9%, pharmacological remission 53.6%); no patient had bulbar muscles impairment; 28.6% were classified as ocular (3.6%) or generalized (25%) MG patients (figure 7).

4. DISCUSSION

The complete and sustained remission is believed the most reliable endpoint on which evaluate the efficacy of thymectomy.[15, 9] Over the last decades several variables were considered relevant to the prognosis of thymectomized patients, including age at onset, sex, time from disease onset to surgery, maximal severity of the disease before surgery, need for immunosuppressive treatment and thymic hystology. Indeed, the presence of thymoma and the incomplete removal of thymic tissue may affect the clinical outcome after thymectomy.[9,16,4] The median sternotomy with extended "maximal" thymectomy is necessary to obtain both the complete removal of thymic tissue and ectopic isles at the neck and pericardium. The procedure is invasive and often badly accepted by young myasthenic females because of disfiguring scars. We present a series of 66 myasthenic patients who underwent thymectomy between 1994 and 1996 using the mini-invasive video assisted thoracoscopic extended thymectomy (VATET) without the need for sternotomy.

All patients underwent VATET successfully. We had no mortality, no morbidity, no injuries of the phrenic or recurrent laryngeal nerves, and no post-operative myasthenic crisis. The observed percentages of thymic involutions, hyperplasias and thymomas were comparable to those reported in other series.[9, 17] We observed 40% of discordance between the pre-thymec-

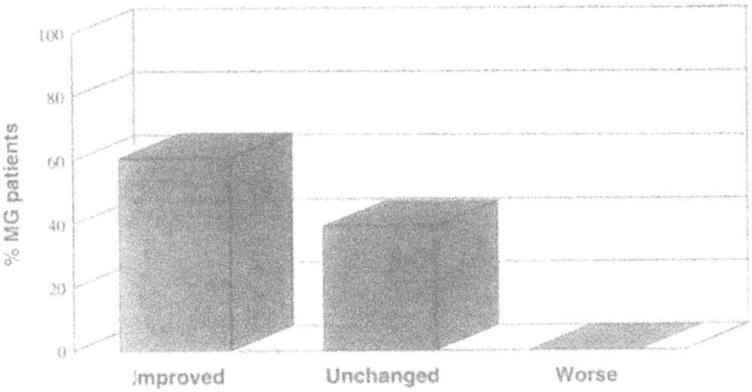

Figure 6. Clinical outcome in 28 patients with a follow-up of at least a year after thymectomy.

tomy radiological evaluation and thymic histology (figure 5). In 48.3% of cases a thymoma was suspected by CT scan but not confirmed histologically while 3.4% of thymuses considered normal or hyperplastic by CT were later histologically diagnosed as thymomas. This observation suggests the need for a more accurate evaluation of pre-thymectomy radiological studies by trained radiologists. In this regard, serological testing for anti-titin antibodies might be of consideral help in the pre-surgical screening of patients.

It is worth noting that the amounts of thymic tissue removed by ETT and VATET were comparable. This aspect must be emphasized since the efficacy of thymectomy correlates also with the amount of thymic tissue removed,[9] including the complete removal of pericardic and perithyroid fat. Furthermore, histological analysis revealed the presence of scattered lymphoid hyperplastic tissue in the fat tissue of the anterior mediastinum in 42% of cases. This finding is of critical relevance because the incomplete removal of even microscopical active thymic tissue might hamper the success of thymectomy. Either hyperplastic/involuted thymuses or thymomas could be removed by this technique as showed by a 164 gram thymoma operated by VATET. An intercostal incision was performed in this case to allow the removal of the solid mass otherwise impossible through the cervical incision. On the basis of these data we think that VATET is as radical as the classical ETT approach. Moreover, VATET is recommendable for the reduced invasivity and absence of disfiguring scars (figure 8).

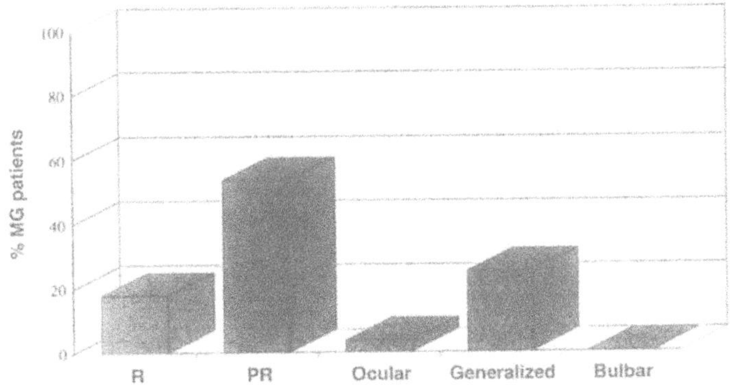

Figure 7. Remission of residual myasthenia gravis at one year after thymectomy.

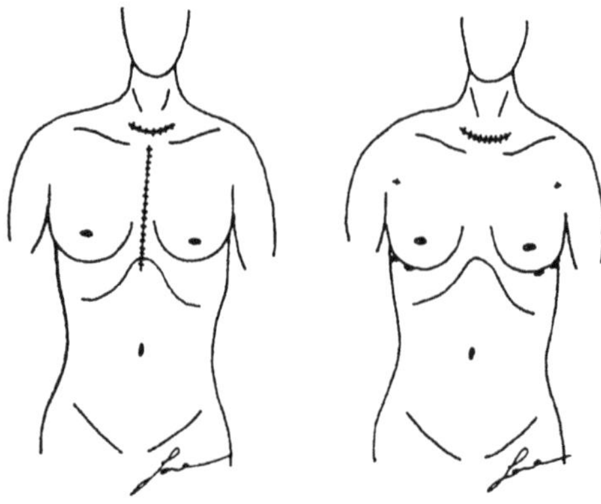

Figure 8. Reduced invasivity and absence of significant scar formation in VATET (*right*) as compared with ETT (extended transsternal thymectomy, *left*).

compared with pre-thymectomy clinical status, 60.7% of our patients had a significant improvement and no patients showed signs of clinical deterioration. These findings, even though preliminary, suggest a good response to VATET; this is particularly important since the disease usually shows a fluctuating course during the first years from the onset.

The proposed mini-invasive technique shortened the time of hospital stay when compared to ETT with sternotomy, thus improving the acceptance of a surgical therapy, and was able to further minimize the risks associated with hospitalization.

Serological assays of anti-AChR and titin Ab may be of help in the diagnostic screening of thymomas before surgery. In fact, anti-AChR Ab were present in 100% of our MG patients with histologically proven thymoma; interestingly, anti-titin Ab were found in 72% of patients with histologically proven thymoma compared to 13% in patients without thymoma.

In conclusion, VATET is a mini-invasive approach suitable for the extended thymectomy in large series of myasthenic patients. We propose VATET as a radical, safe, and reliable technique with a minor impact on the psychological aspects of young female MG patients. The low morbiliity associated with VATET suggests a re-evaluation of the indications to thymectomy. A mini-invasive approach could be more easily proposed to ocular MG cases and to older MG patients, in which a strategic therapy able to influence the natural history of the disease is still indicated.

REFERENCES

1. Drachman DB: Myasthenia Gravis. N Engl J Med 1994, 330:1797–1810
2. Perlo VP, Arnason B, Poskanzer D, Castleman B, Schwab RS, Osserman KE, Papatestas A, Alpert L and Kark A: The role of thymectomy in the treatment of myasthenia gravis. Ann NY Acad Sci 1971, 183:308
3. Mulder DG, Graves M, Herrmann C: Thymectomy for myasthenia gravis: recent observations and comparisons with past experience. Ann Thorac Surg 1989, 48:551
4. Beghi E, Antozzi C, Batocchi AP, Cornelio F, Cosi V, Evoli A, Lombardi M, Mantegazza R, Monticelli ML, Piccolo G, Tonali P, Trevisan D and Zarelli M: Pregnosis of myasthenia gravis: a multicenter follow-up study of 844 patients. J Neurol Sci 1991, 106:213–220
5. Masaoka A & Monden Y: Comparison of the results of transsternal simple, transcervical simple, and extended thymectomy. Ann N Y Acad Sci 1981, 755–765
6. Papatestas AE, Genkins G & Kornfeld P: Comparison of the results of the transcervical and transsternal thymectomy in myasthenia gravis. Ann N Y Acad Sci 1981, 766–778
7. Papatestas AE, Genkins G, Kornfeld P: Effects of thymectomy in myasthenia gravis. Ann Surg 1987, 206:79–88

8. Jaretzki A III, Bethea M, Wolff M, Olarte MR, Penn AS, Rowland LP: A rationale approach to total thymectomy in the treatment of myasthenia gravis. Ann Thorac Surg 1977, 24: 120–130
9. Jaretzki A III, Penn AS, Younger DS, Wolff M, Olarte MR, Lovelace RE and Rowland LP: "Maximal" thymectomy for myasthenia gravis. J Thorac Cardiovasc Surg 1988, 95: 747–757
11. Mulder DG, Hermann C, Buckberg GD: Effect of thymectomy in patients with myasthenia gravis. Am J Surg 1974, 128:202–205
12. Marino M, Muller-Hermelink HK: Thymoma and thymic carcinoma. Relation of thymoma epithelial cells to the cortical and medullary differentiation of thymus. Virchows Arch A Pathol Anat Histopathol 1985, 407:119–149
13. Mantegazza R, Antozzi C, Peluchetti D, Sghirlanzoni A and Cornelio F: Azathioprine as a single drug or in combination with steroids in the treatment of myasthenia gravis. J Neurol 1988, 235:315–453
14. Gotti C, Mantegazza R and Clementi F: new antigen for antibody detection in myasthenia gravis. Neurology 1984, 34:374–377
15. McQuillen MP: Symposium on therapeutic controversies: myasthenia gravis-thymectomy. Trans Am Neurol Assoc 1978, 103:283–286
16. Engel AG: Disturbances of neuromuscular transmission: acquired autoimmune myasthenia gravis. Myology. Edited by Engel AG & Franzini-Armstrong C. Mc Graw Hill, 1995, vol.2, chapter 68, pp. 1769–1797
17. Hankins JR, Mayer RF, Satterfield JR, Turney SZ, Attar S, Sequeira AJ, Thompson BW, McLaughlin JS Thymectomy for myasthenia gravis: 14-year experience. Ann Surg 1985, 201:618–625

44

LONG-TERM PROGNOSIS OF PATIENTS WITH THYMOMA-ASSOCIATED MYASTHENIA GRAVIS

B. C. G. Schalke, I. Schmitt, A. Marx, K. Toyka, and H. K. Müller-Hermelink

Department of Neurology
Department of Pathology
University of Würzburg
Josef Schneider Str., D-97080 Würzburg
University of Regensburg
Dep. of Regensburg
Universitätsstr. 84, D-93042 Regensburg

Pathogenesis of myasthenia gravis (MG) is heterogeneous, however it is not possible to distinguish between myasthenia gravis associated with lymphofollicular hyperplasia (LFH) in the thymus or thymoma only by clinical signs and symptoms. In paraneoplastic MG pathogenesis can be clearly distinguished from MG associated with LFH. Not only the morphological finding in the thymus and thymoma is different, but there also seems to be no genetic predisposition and no significant therapeutic effect of thymomectomy on the clinical course of MG in the thymoma patients, whereas an association with the HLA typ A1/B8/DR3 and a therapeutic effect of thymectomy is shown in MG patients with LFH (7). Long term prognosis of patients with thymoma associated MG could be influenced by several factors e.g. thymoma morphology, thymic remnant, tumor size and infiltration or invasion into adjacent organs, operation technique, post- or preoperative radiation, chemotherapy, and recurrence of tumor. 30 years ago long term prognosis was mainly limited by the poor outcome of thymoma associated myasthenia gravis, because many of these patients suffered or even died from myasthenic crisis, today this should no longer be the case because of the better immunosuppressive and supportive therapies.

PATIENTS AND METHODS

We analysed retrospectively the data of thymoma patients with paraneoplastic, acquired MG, operated between 1971 and 1990. Tumors and the thymic remnant were classified or reclassified if possible according to the criteria of Müller-Hermelink and

Epithelial Tumors of the Thymus, edited by Marx and Müller-Hermelink.
Plenum Press, New York, 1997

Kirchner (1,2). Most of the patients were regulary or by invitation seen in the MG ambulance. If the patient deceased, or could not come a questionnaire was send to the patient and/or the family doctor. Thymoma recurrences were registered till 1994.

Severity of myasthenic symptoms at the onset was classified according to the Osserman classification (5). For better comparison follow up was classified according to Perlo et al. (6). Consumption of acetylcholinesteraseinhibitors, immunosuppressive drugs, side effects, secondary disorders and malignancies, thymoma recurrences, postoperative and supportive therapies, and causes of death were documented.

RESULTS

72 patients with thymoma were entered into the study. Thirtyfive of the patients were female (f) and 37 were male (m). The age at the time of operation was between 14 and 77 years (median 50years) with normal age distribution and no peaks at different ages.

At time of making the diagnosis 71 patients could be classified according to the Osserman classification. 2 patients (2.82%, 1f,1m) did not have any myasthenic symptoms at the time of thymomectomy (Osserman: 0). They developed myasthenic symptoms 4 respectively 10 years after thymomectomy. At the time of operation 75% of the patients had a severe MG with involvement of the bulbar muscles (Osserman IIb, III, IV). In two patients follow up stopped in 1976 and 1988, no further data could be included.

In 50% of the cases thymomectomy was carried out within 3 months after the first occurrence of myasthenic symptoms, in 83% the preoperative time was up to 18 months, the other12 patients had a preoperative duration of MG between 22 months and 17 years.

Immunosuppression (> 3 months) was started in 35 patients before the operation, 17 recieved azathioprine alone, 11 cortisone or ACTH, and 7 patients a combination of azathioprine and cortisone.

A significant finding was that only 11% of the patients with cortical and 14 % with predominant cortical thymomas were without immunosuppressive pretreatment (p=0.0038), whereas 100% of the patients with medullary, 53% with a well diff. thymic carcinoma, and 37% with a mixed thymoma had such preoperative treatment.

Only patients with cortical and mixed thymomas developed a postthymomectomy or pure ocular MG (p=0.021). Severe myasthenic symptoms (Osserman III+IV) were found in 74% of patients with a well differentiated thymic carcinoma or cortical thymoma, and in the 2 patients with medullary thymoma.

Anemia was diagnosed in 9 patients. In one case the patient developed aplastic anemia after initial thymomectomy and again he developed aplastic crisis after reoperation 10 years later for local recurrence of thymoma. Autoimmune Hashimoto´s thyreoiditis was

Table 1. Osserman classification at the time of thymomectomy

Type	No.	(%)	Male/female
0	2	(2.8)	1/1
II	2	(2.8)	2/0
IIa	13	(18.3)	11/2
IIb	20	(28.2)	9/11
III	25	(35.2)	10/15
IV	9	(12.7)	4/5

seen in 3 and goitre in 8 patients, 3 patients had gastritis, 2 arthritis, and 1 developed alopecia areata and loss of all his finger and toe nails within 2 weeks. These non malignant secondary disorders, except aplastic crisis did not influence long term prognosis significantly.

A second malignancy was diagnosed in 11 of 71 patients (1x rectum carcinoma, 2 x urothelial carcinoma, 1 x IgA plasmocytoma, 1 x bronchial carcinoma, 1 x gastric cancer, 2 x breast cancer, 1 x thyroid carcinoma, 1 x bowel cancer, 1 x adeno carcinoma of corpus uteri). In one case breast cancer was diagnosed and treated 9 years before myasthenic symptoms started. Another patient already had myasthenic symptoms for 10 years and was treated for 5 years with azathioprine before bowel carcinoma was diagnosed and treated. The second malignancy was diagnosed 4 x within the 5 years and 5 x between 6 and 18 years (median 9.96 years) after thymomectomy. 9 of these patients recieved azathioprine therapy for 3 to 18 years (median 7.9 years). The frequency of secondary malignancies was not significantly increased, compared to the normal population.

Reclassification of the thymoma was possible in 67 patients. More than 50% of the operated patients had a cortical and predominant cortical thymoma, 25% had a well differentiated thymic carcinoma and only 18% a mixed and 3% a medullary thymoma. The age distribution for all histological subtypes was normal.

In 64 cases it was possible to evaluate invasion and infiltration into adjacent organs, 23 tumors were macroscopically encapsuled and showed no microscopical capsuleinvasion. In 19 thymomas microscopically capsuleinvasion, and in 22 tumors an infiltration into adjacent organs like fat, pleura, lung, pericardium, midriff, lymphnodes, or vena cava was seen macroscopically as well as microscopically. In 3 patients with organinfiltration metastatic spread into the pleura was already present at the time of operation.

The frequency of surgical stage 2 +3 of thymoma according to Masaoka (4) (2 = invasion of capsule and mediastinal connective tissue and 3 = invasion of contiguos organs pericard, pleura, lung, main vessels) was significantly higher in male patients (16 men (52%), 6 women (18%), p = 0,0062).

Well differentiated thymic carcinomas showed infiltration in 11 of 16 cases (69%), cortical thymomas only in 8 of 28 cases (29%), this difference was significant (p= 0.0014). Complete encapsulation was found in 12 of 28 (42%) patients with cortical thymomas and 2 of 6 (33%) with the predominant cortical thymoma. In the combined group of mixed and medullary thymomas no capusle disruption was seen.

Extended operation of the tumor, thymic remnant, and mediastinal fat and connective tissue was macroscopically complete in 69/72 cases, in 3 patients operation was incomplete because of inoperable pleural implants of thymoma tissue at the time of operation.

14 patients with assumed curative operation recieved postoperative radiation therapy (40–60gy) of the upper mediastinum. Therapeutic indication for this was infiltration in 7 cases and capsule invasion in 5 cases. Although grade of invasion or infiltration was not

Table 2. Thymoma histology

Histology	no	%	F/M	Untreated(%)
Carcinoma	17	25	8/9	18
Cortical thym.	28	42	15/13	53
Pred.cort. thym.	8	12	1/7	13
Mixed thym.	12	18	7/5	7
Medullary thym.	2	3	2/0	0

Table 3. Causes of death

Myasthenia associated:	1 x myasthenic crisis, 2 x tracheobronchitis/sepsis
Thymoma associated:	2 x abdominal metastasis, 1 x diffuse metastatic spread into the lung, 1 x meningeosis carcinomatosa, 1x aplastic crisis
Non MG or thymoma associated:	2 x urothelial-carcinoma, 1 x plasmocytoma, 1 x bronchial carcinoma, 3 x cardiac failure

clear, 2 cases recieved radiation therapy, 1 patient came into complete long term remission, 10 years later the other patient developed a recurrence of thymoma, he died after palliative reoperation from aplastic crisis.

Because of pleural implants at the time of operation curative operation was not possible in 3 patients, 2 of these patients recieved postopertive radiation (60 and 70 gy) and subsequently developed postradiation pneumonitis. One year later metastatic spread into the lung and 28 months later into the mediastinum was diagnosed in one patient, the other patient developed after 3 years induration of the right lung, he died 8 months later, the reason was not clear, autopsie wasn't allowed. The third patient recieved polychemotherapy (Bleo-CHOP) for 1 year, he was in remission, after that he developed metastatic spread into the pleura and lung, it was not possible to stop this by different types of combined chemotherapies, he died 6 years after thymomectomy.

Recurrence of tumor was diagnosed in 11 of 72 (15.3%) or 9 of 69 in group of the patients with complete operation after of 1 to 14 years (on average 7.2 years) after initial thymomectomy. 3 of 24(12.5%) patients with an encapsuled thymoma developed metastasis. Five patients with recurrence of tumor died from metastasis after an average survival time of 11.3 years. In one case the patient died 14 years after thymomectomy from myasthenic crisis, autopsie proved local metastasis.

It is interesting that 9 of 10 patients with recurrence of tumor had a duration of myasthenic symptoms shorter than 3 months before thymomectomy, and that none of those 11 patients pretreated before thymomectomy with cortisone, and only 2 of 17 patients pretreated with azathioprine developed recurrence of tumor after the operation. Radiation therapy before operation to reduce the size of thymoma was carried out in one patient, because the primary tumor was inoperable, however 10 years later he developed diffuse miliary metastatic spread into the lung, he died 11 years after thymomectomy.

In the group of patients with tumor recurrence primary histology of the tumor at the time of operation was 3 x carcinoma, 6 x cortical thymoma, 1 x predominant cortical thymoma, 1 x mixed thymoma.

7 of 11 patients with tumor recurrence had severe myasthenic symptoms before thymomectomy (Osserman III), 2 had only a mild generalized MG (Osserman IIa), and 1 patient a generalized MG with bulbar signs (Osserman IIb), 1 patient was free of MG

Table 4. Survial rate in association to the grade of tumor invasion

Grade of invasion	≤ 3 years	≤5 years	≤10 years
Encapsuled	95.5% (20)	71.6% (15)	33.4% (7)
Capsule invasion	100% (16)	87.5% (14)	50% (8)
Organ infiltration	89.5% (14)	76.7% (12)	25.5% (4)
Metastasis	100% (3)	66.7% (2)	33.3% (1)

Table 5. Survival rate according to thymoma histology

Histology	≤ 3 years	≤ 5 years	≤10 years
Carcinoma	94.1% (14)	80.7% (12)	40.3% (6)
Cortical	96.4% (25)	69.4% (18)	30.8% (8)
Pred.cort.	87.5% (5)	70% (4)	35% (2)
Mixed/med.	100% (11)	90.9% (10)	45.5% (5)

symptoms (Osserman 0) and the AChR- antibody titer was negative at the time of operation, later she developed only mild unspecific weakness with increasing AChR- antibody titer, histology of the primary tumor was mixed thymoma.

4 patients did not respond to immunosuppressive therapy and were subsequently classified as azathioprine nonresponders and treated with the immunmodulating drug cyclosporine A. 3 of them responded well to this therapy, however 3 of them also developed a recurrence of thymoma. It could well be that the patients did not respond well to the treatment with azathioprine because of remaining tumor tissue. It remains unclear whether cyclosporine A did induce tumor growth of already existing thymoma cells or if tumor growth started independently from cyclosprine A therapy.

Causes of death could be subdivided into three groups: 1)thymoma associated (5 patients), 2) myasthenia gravis associated (2 patients), 3) non myasthenia or thymoma related (7 patients).

No significant correlation was found between age at the time of operation, sex, thymoma histology, tumor invasion or infiltration, postoperative adjuvant therapy and the recurrence of thymomas. The survival rate according to Kaplan-Meier was 95.8% after 3 years, 90.4% after 5 years, and 81.9% after 10 years. Thymoma histology and grade of tumor invasion did not significantly influence the long term survival rate during the first 10 years after thymmectomy.

It was also interesting that postoperative adjuvant therapy (radiation/ chemotherapy) did not influence significantly long term survival compared to those patients without adjuvant therapy.

REMISSION RATE OF MG

After thymomectomy in 36 patients with severe MG long term immunosuppression with azathioprine alone or in combination with cortisone was started within 2 weeks after the operation. Myasthenic symptoms were only mild in 16 patients but showed exacerbation of MG within 1 month, subsequently immunosuppression had to be started. Only 8 patients had such a mild MG that immunosuppressive therapy had not to be started within the first year after thymomectomy. After at least 1 year immunosuppressive therapy in 14 patients therapy was stoped, 6 of the patients developed a myasthenic relapse after 2 (3 x), 3, 4, 5 years. Myasthenic symptoms did not change significantly in the other 9 patients after discontinuation of azathioprine.

After thymomectomy 32 patients had to be treated with cortisone. In 15 patients cortisone therapy was only required once, mostly after thymomectomy. 17 patients had to be treated with 2 or more courses of cortisone treatment, 8 patients took cortisone as a long term medication.

No significant correlation could be found between the early and late course of MG after thymomectomy with sex, different age groups, HLA type, thymoma histology.

In patients with recurrence of tumor there was no significant difference in the course of MG in the early phase after the operation (<1.5 years). In the group of 10 patients with metastasis the MG score was significantly (p=0,011) higher (=worse) between 1,5 to 6 years, compared to patients (n=33) without recurrence.

DISCUSSION

Long term prognosis of patients with thymoma associated MG is not as good as in e.g. MG associated with LFH in the thymus. However it is difficult to say which factors mainly influence the long term survival rate and quality of life. Neither tumor histology, grade of infiltration, histology of the thymic remnant, postoperative adjuvant therapy, sex, age, HLA type significantly influenced the recurrence of tumor and survival rate. Only the primary finding of metastatic pleura implants led to an shortened survival expectancy. Whereas the grade of tumor infiltration and invasion correlated well with the thymoma subtype, the recurrence of tumor did not.

It is important to mention that none of the patients pretreated before the operation with cortisone developed recurrence of tumor, and even in the group pretreated with azathioprine the risk was much lower. It should be discussed whether it would be better to pretreat all thymoma patients with larger thymomas with cortisone and/or azathioprine to reduce tumor size and minimize the risk of tumor recurrence because it is possible that glucocorticoids have a specific effect on thymoma growth (8). It is thought that this cortisone effect is mediated by a lympholytic effect, but if this would be the case no long term effect would be verifiable (3). On the other hand it should be discussed whether MG patients with thymoma which do not respond to azathioprine therapy or develop severe side effects to this immunosuppressive drug (e.g. severe lymphopenia or leucopenia) should be treated with cyclosporine A or not, because it can not be excluded that this drug induces tumor regrowth. In vitro experiments can help to answer some of these open questions (e.g. induction/ inhibition of thymoma lymphocyte or epithelial tumorcell growth by immunosuppressive or immunomodulating drugs).

The role of postoperative radiation remains open. Some patients clearly profit from this therapy, in others tumor recurrence can not be prevented. Previous radiation therapy may preclude further surgical or radiation therapy (3). Chemotherapy as a first line therapy might be beneficial in patients with incomplete thymomectomy and/or distant disease although till now little is known about chemosensitivity of different thymoma subtypes. Further data from prospective studies are needed to improve long term prognosis of patients with this rare malignancy often combined with paraneoplastic disorders.

REFERENCES

1. Kirchner T, Müller-Hermelink HK. New appproaches to the diagnosis of thymic epithelial tumors. Progress in Surgical Pathology. vol 10. ed: Fenoglio-Preiser CM, Wolff M. Rilke F. Philadelphia, Field and Wood, (1989) :167–186
2. Kirchner T, Schalke B, Buchwald J, Ritter M, Marx A, Müller-Hermelink HK. Well differentiated thymic carcinoma. Am J Surg Pathol (1992) 16:1153–1169
3. Loehrer PJ, Bonomi P, Goldman S, Reddy S, Faber P, Jensik R, Dainauskas JR. Remission of invasive thymoma due to chemotherapy.CHEST (1985) vol.87: 377–380

4. Masaoka A, Nagaoka Y, Maeda M, Monden Y, Seike Y. Study on the ratio of lymphocytes to epithelial cells in thymoma. Cancer (1977); 40:1222–1228
5. Osserman KE. Myasthenia gravis. Grune & Stratton, New York (1958):66–89
6. Perlo VP, Arnason B, Poskanzer D, Castleman B, Schwab RS, Osserman KE, Papatestis A, Alpert L, Kark A. The role thymectomy in the treatment of myasthenia gravis. Ann NY Acad Sci (1971) :308–333
7. Schalke B, Mertens HG, Lindner H, Kirchner T, Marx A, Müller-Hermelink HK, Andreas-Zietz A, Albert E. Myasthenia gravis: Immungenetik, Thymusmorphologie und klinischer Verlauf. In: Kunze, Arlt, Thayssen (ed), Neuromuskuläre Erkrankungen. G Fischer,Stuttgart (1992) :157–164
8. Tandan R, Taylor R, DiConstanzo DP, Sharma K,fries T, Roberts J. Metastasizing thymoma and myasthenia gravis.Favorable response to glucocorticoids after failed chemotherapy and radiation therapy.Cancer, vol 65 (1990) 1286–1290

45

THYMOMA AND MYASTHENIA GRAVIS

Incidence of Tumor Recurrences in 126 Patients

A. Evoli,[1] A. P. Batocchi,[1] M. T. Palmisani,[1] L. Lauriola,[2] G. B. Doglietto,[3] and P. Tonali[1]

[1]Institute of Neurology, Catholic University
[2]Institute of Pathology, Catholic University
[3]Institute of Surgery, Catholic University
L.go F. Vito 1, 00168 Roma, Italy

INTRODUCTION

The prognosis of thymoma appears to be correlated mainly with the extent of the tumor, the radicality of surgical exeresis[1,2] and, as it has recently been reported, with the histological type.[3] Association with myasthenia gravis (MG) does not adversely affect patients' survival.[4]

Extrathoracic metastases are very uncommon; on the contrary, local recurrences have been reported by several authors.[1,2,5–7]

The post-operative management of patients with thymoma, the surveillance of recurrences and their treatment are not yet codified.

Here we report our experience of diagnosis and treatment of thymoma recurrences in a series of patients in whom this tumor was associated with MG.

PATIENTS AND METHODS

We investigated recurrences of thymoma in myasthenic patients who had undergone thymectomy for thymoma during the last 23 years. Only patients with at least 2 years of clinical follow-up from the time of the first operation were included in this study.

Our series is made up of 126 patients (64 males and 62 females) with age at thymomectomy ranging from 15 to 70 years.

Surgical approach was by postero-lateral thoracotomy in 5 cases; median sternotomy followed by extended thymomectomy was performed in all the other patients. Extended thymomectomy included complete resection of the thymoma together with the thymic

Epithelial Tumors of the Thymus, edited by Marx and Müller-Hermelink.
Plenum Press, New York, 1997

gland and the pery-thymic fat tissue; when necessary, it was associated with resection of pleura, pericardium, lung, phrenic nerve and pleural implants.

Tumor extent at surgery was evaluated retrospectively according to Masaoka[8] staging using careful review of the written operative records, histological findings and personal interview with the individual surgeon. A capsulated thymoma (stage I) was present in 57 cases, while 69 patients had an invasive tumor in stages II, III and IVa.

Mediastinal irradiation at doses ranging 40–50 Gy was generally performed after removal of an invasive thymoma; no patient received chemotherapy at the time of the first operation.

Post-operative follow-up was performed with mediastinal CT scan every 1–2 years.

In patients who complained of thymoma relapses, histology of both the first tumor and recurrences was reviewed according to Marino and Muller-Hermelink classification.[9,10]

Patients in whom recurrence consisted of multiple pleural implants received chemotherapy based on a combination of prednisolone, doxorubicin, cyclophosphamide and cysplatin.[11]

RESULTS

We observed tumor relapses only in patients with invasive thymoma. Recurrences were found in 12 patients out of 126 (9.5%). One patient suffered of thymoma relapse twice.

Clinical characteristics of these 12 patients at the time of the first operation are shown in table 1.

They were 4 females and 8 males with age at surgery ranging from 27 to 48 years. At thymomectomy, 3 patients had no signs of MG; one patient had purely ocular myasthenia and 8 had generalized disease. MG patients received anticholinesterases (ACHE) associated in most cases with corticosteroids (CS). With respect to the tumor extent, 4 patients had a tumor with invasion through the capsule or into mediastinal pleura (stage II); 5 had a thymoma infiltrating surrounding tissues (stage III); 3 had an intrathoracic disseminated

Table 1. Clinico-pathological features at thymomectomy

Case	Sex/age	MG	MG Therapy	Masaoka stage	Surgical approach	Adjuvant therapy	Histology
1	F/42	No	None	II	Lateral thoracotomy	None	Cortical thymoma
2	M/48	Yes	ACHE	III	Median sternotomy	RT	Cortical thymoma
3	M/43	Yes	ACHE	III	Median sternotomy	RT	Cortical thymoma
4	M/36	Yes	ACHE, CS	III	Median sternotomy	RT	WDTC
5	F/38	Yes	ACHE, CS	II	Median sternotomy	RT	Cortical thymoma
6	F/37	No	None	II	Lateral thoracotomy	None	Cortical thymoma
7	M/27	Yes	ACHE, CS	IVa	Median sternotomy	RT	WDTC
8	M/42	Yes	ACHE, CS	II	Median sternotomy	None	Cortical thymoma
9	M/33	No	None	IVa	Median sternotomy	RT	WDTC
10	M/43	Yes	ACHE, CS	III	Median sternotomy	RT	WDTC
11	M/32	Yes	ACHE, CS	IVa	Median sternotomy	RT	WDTC
12	F/34	Yes	ACHE, CS	III	Median sternotomy	RT	Cortical thymoma

RT=radiotherapy
ACHE=anticholinesterase drugs, CS= Corticosteroids
WDTC= well differentiated thymic carcinoma

tumor (stage IV a). Surgical approach was by postero-lateral thoracotomy in 2 cases and by median sternotomy in all the other patients. Postoperative radiotherapy was performed in all patients but 3. With respect to histological findings, 7 cases had a cortical thymoma often with small foci of epidermoid differentiation and 6 had a well differentiated thymic carcinoma.

Thymoma recurrences were only intrathoracic. Their histology was the same as at the first operation.

The time interval between thymomectomy and the radiological detection of recurrences showed quite a broad range. Although more than 50% of relapses were detected within 5 years of the first operation, we also observed later recurrences, up to 16 years after thymomectomy. These data are shown in figure 1.

MG symptoms were not uniformly affected. With respect to the 9 patients with MG at thymomectomy, when recurrence was detected we found a mild deterioration of the disease in 6 and no change in MG severity in the other 3. In the 3 patients without MG at thymomectomy, the onset of MG was: when thymoma recurrence was detected (2 years after the first operation) in the first patient; 1 year before recurrence detection (3 years after thymomectomy) in the second patient; at the time of the 2nd recurrence detection (10 years after the first operation) in the third patient.

Four patients had 1 or 2 recurrences confined to the anterior mediastinum; in the others, multiples nodules were present on the pleura or on pleura and pericardium, with lung infiltration in one case. One patient was treated only with radiotherapy; she died after 4 years of thymoma recurrences. Two patients both with multiple pleural nodules refused any treatment; one of them died of unrelated causes after 2 years, the other is still alive after 5 years. Patients with 1–2 mediastinal masses underwent complete surgical resection; those with multiple recurrences were treated with subtotal surgery associated with chemotherapy or with chemotherapy alone. All of them are alive and tumor free at the last CT scan. Immunosuppressive drugs for the treatment of MG were associated in most cases. In patients who did not undergo surgery, histological diagnosis was made by needle biopsy.

The characteristics of thymoma recurrences, their treatment and evolution are summarized in table 2.

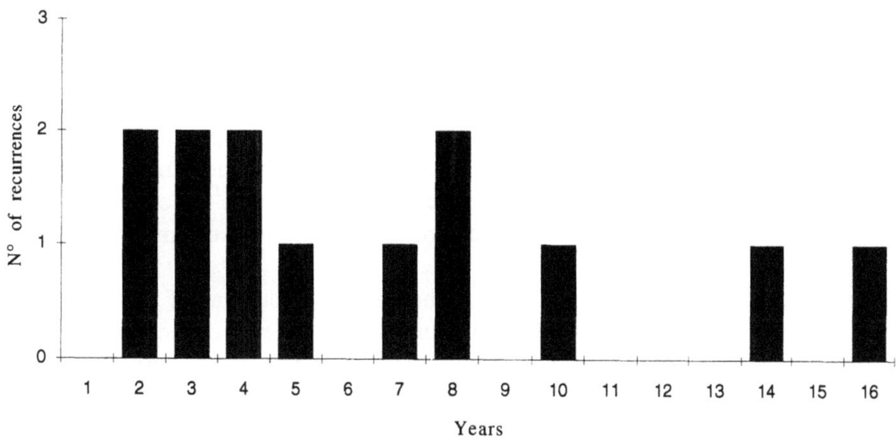

Figure 1. Interval from surgery.

Table 2. Thymoma recurrences: treatment and evolution

Case	Years from surgery	Recurrences number	Site	Treatment	MG treatment	Evolution (follow-up)
1	2	One	Mediastinum	Radiotherapy	ACHE, CS	Died (4 years)
2	7	Multiple	Pleura	None	ACHE	Died (2 years)
3	14	One	Mediastinum	Surgery	ACHE, CS	Alive (7 years)
4	4	Two	Pleura	Surgery	ACHE, CS	Alive (8 years)
5	8	Multiple	Pleura	Surgery, chemotherapy	ACHE, CS	Alive (3 years)
6	8	One	Mediastinum	Surgery		
	10	One	Mediastinum	Surgery, radiotherapy	ACHE, CS	Alive (7 years)
7	5	Multiple	Pleura	Surgery, chemotherapy	ACHE,CS,Aza	Alive (1 year)
8	16	Multiple	Pleura/Pericardium	None	ACHE, CS	Alive (5 years)
9	4	Multiple	Pleura	Chemotherapy	ACHE, CS	Alive (2 years)
10	3	Multiple	Pleura	Surgery, chemotherapy	ACHE	Alive (1 year)
11	2	Multiple	Pleura	Chemotherapy	ACHE, CS	Alive (5 years)
12	2	Multiple	Pleura/Lung	Chemotherapy	ACHE, CS	Alive (1 year)

ACHE= anticholinesterase drugs, CS= corticosteroids, AZA= azathioprine

DISCUSSION

It has been reported that both the extent of the tumor and histology are significant in predicting thymoma relapses and, though correlated, they act as independent factors.[12] With reference to the histologic classification of thymoma proposed by Marino and Muller-Hermelink, histological types related to thymic cortical cells show an aggressive behaviour[12,13] and an histologic pattern of epidermoid differentiation is strongly predictive of invasiveness and relapse. [10,12]

Our data confirm these reports as all our patients who complained of recurrences had either cortical thymomas or well differentiated thymic carcinomas. Moreover, cortical thymomas in these cases often showed small epidermoid foci thus exhibiting an increased grade of malignancy.[10]

The origins of recurrences are likely to be either tumor remnants due to incomplete surgical resection or pleural seedings possibly undetected at the initial operation or due to surgical manipulation.[5,6]

As the radicality of thymoma exeresis is one of the most important factors in preventing recurrences, surgical approach must ensure adequate exposure. In this respect median longitudinal sternotomy appears to be the technique of choice.[13] We can not exclude that recurrences in the 2 patients operated on through lateral thoracotomy are due to thymoma remnants.

Although most authors recommend radiotherapy after removal of an invasive thymoma on account of the radiosensitivity of this tumor,[1,2,4,14] the role of mediastinal irradiation as adjuvant therapy is to be further assessed. In fact, some authors found no significant differences in the incidence of thymoma relapses in patients who had received post-operative irradiation and in those who had not.[7]

Chemotherapy has been less used as adjuvant therapy. Recently it has been proposed for patients with disseminated thymoma.[15]

Surveillance of recurrences requires a prolonged or even life-long follow-up on account of both slow growth and late relapse of thymoma. In addition to our experience, other authors have reported detection of recurrences many years after the first operation.[1,5,6,16] So far we have performed periodic CT scans of the mediastinum only after removal of an invasive thymoma. As recurrence of encapsulated thymomas has occasionally been reported,[17,18] surveillance should perhaps be extended also to patients with thymoma in stage I.

With respect to the treatment of thymoma recurrences, reoperation with radical excision, when feasible, proved both effective and safe.[1,5,6] In our experience, chemotherapy also produced good results. Lastly, we can not exclude that, as reported by other authors,[19] immunosuppressive drugs used for the tretment of MG, may have therapeutic effects also on thymoma recurrences.

REFERENCES

1. Urgesi A, Monetti U, Rossi G, Ricardi U, Maggi G, Sannazzari GL: Aggressive treatment of intrathoracic recurrences of thymoma. Radiother Oncol 1992, 24: 221–225
2. Wilkins EW Jr, Grillo HC, Scannel JG, Moncure AC, Mathisen DJ: Role of staging in prognosis and management of thymoma. Ann Thorac Surg 1991, 51: 888–892
3. Quintanilla-Martinez L, Wilkins EW Jr, Ferry JA, Harris NL: Thymoma. Morphologic subclassification correlates with invasiveness and immunohistologic features: a study of 122 cases. Hum Pathol 1993, 24: 958–969
4. Cooper JD: Current therapy for thymoma. Chest 1993, 103 (Suppl): 334S-336S
5. Ohmi M, Ohuchi M: Recurrent thymoma in patients with myasthenia gravis. Ann Thorac Surg 1990, 50: 243–247
6. Kirschner PA: Reoperation for thymoma; report of 23 cases. Ann Thorac Surg 1990, 49: 550–555
7. Maggi G, Casadio C, Cavallo A, Cianci R, Molinatti M, Ruffini: Thymoma: results of 241 operated cases. Ann Thorac Surg 1991, 51: 152–156
8. Masaoka A, Monden Y, Nakahara K, Tanioka T: Follow-up study of thymomas with special reference to their clinical stages. Cancer 1981, 48: 2485–2492
9. Marino M, Muller-Hermelink HK: Thymoma and thymic carcinoma. Relation of thymoma epithelial cells to the cortical and medullary differentiation of the thymus. Virchows Arch Pathol Anat 1985, 407: 119–149
10. Kirchner T, Schalke B, Buchwald J, Ritter M, Marx A, Muller- Hermelink HK: Well-differentiated thymic carcinoma. An organotypical low-grade carcinoma with relationship to cortical thymoma. Am J surg Pathol 1992, 16: 1153–1169
11. Hu E, Levine J: Chemotherapy of malignant thymoma. Cancer 1986, 57: 1101–1104
12. Quintanilla-Martinez L, Wilkins EW Jr, Choi N, Efird J, Hug E, Harris NL: Thymoma. Histologic subclassification is an independent prognostic factor. Cancer 1994, 74: 606–617
13. Blossom GB, Ernstoff RM, Howells GA, Bendick PJ, Glover JL: Thymectomy for myasthenia gravis. Arch Surg 1993,128: 855- 862
14. Nakahara K, Ohno K, Hashimoto J, Maeda H, Miyoshi S, Sakurai M, Monden Y, Kawashima Y: Thymoma: results with complete resection and adjuvant postoperative irradiation in 141 consecutive patients. J Thorac Cardiovasc Surg 1988, 95: 1041- 1047
15. Wakata N, Fujioka T, Nishina M, Kawamura Y, Kobayashi M, Kinoshita M: Myasthenia gravis and invasive thymoma. A 20- year experience. Eur Neurol 1993, 33:115–120
16. Gotti G, Paladini P, Haid MM, Biagi G, Di Bisceglie M, Cioni R, Ciacci G: Late recurrence of thymoma and myasthenia gravis. Scand J Thorac Cardiovasc Surg 1995, 29: 37–38
17. Fechner RE: Recurrence of noninvasive thymomas. Report of four cases and review of literature. Cancer 1969, 23: 1423- 1427
18. Masunaga A, Sugawara I, Yoshitake T, Nakamura H, Itoyama S, Shimoyama N, Ishidate T: A case of encapsulated noninvasive thymoma (stage I) with myasthenia gravis showing metastasis after a 2-year dormancy. Surg Today 1995, 25: 369–372
19. Kumagai M, Kondou T, Handa M, Shiraishi Y, Fujimura S, Nakata T: Treatment of invasive thymoma with myasthenia gravis: a case report responsive to azathioprine and metylprednisolone. Kyobu-Geka 1990, 43: 321–235

THYMOMA—PROGNOSTIC FACTORS AND OUTCOME

K. Friström,* A. Cervin, J. P. Enoksson, M. Albertsson, and L. Johansson

Departments of Oncology and Pathology
University Hospital
S-221 85 Lund, Sweden

ABSTRACT

Thymomas are common mediastinal lesions, especially in association with myasthenia gravis. Here we report a material of 67 patients treated for thymoma. The incidence of myasthenia gravis was 43%. There was no difference in relapse-free survival for patients with or without myasthenia gravis, nor taken into concideration autoimmune diseases in general. Twenty-seven per cent had no symptoms of their tumor and this group fared better regarding relapse-free survival during a follow-up of nine years. There was no significant difference regarding survival neither for age, nor sex, however a significant difference was noted in relation to stage I-IV. Eighty-two per cent were macroscopically radically resected and 28% had some kind of further treatment, and in the latter group survival was significantly lower.

The patients are followed up to ten years. Twenty-one patients have passed away. Forty-five patients are alive with no evidence of disease. One patient is alive with disease.

Thymomas are often malignant (about 25%), but they rarely metastasize. Their malignant potential is demonstrated by a direct invasion of the lung, pericardium, blood vessels, and lymphatics.

1. INTRODUCTION

Thymomas comprise about 20% of all mediastinal tumors and cysts and they are the most common anterior mediastinal tumor. They may occur at any age, but are rare before the age of 20. They occur with equal frequency in both sexes. The natural history of a patient with thymoma is unpredictable, partly because of the difficulty of distinguishing his-

* Corresponding author: Kristina Friström, Departments of Oncology and Pathology, Lund University Hospital. Phone + 46 46 17 75 20; fax + 46 46 13 99 57.

Epithelial Tumors of the Thymus, edited by Marx and Müller-Hermelink.
Plenum Press, New York, 1997

tologically between malignant and benign thymomas and partly because of the effects of associated diseases such as Myasthenia gravis (MG) on the prognosis[1]. Thymomas express their malignant potential by invading surrounding tissues and by developing local recurrences and implants in the chest. Until now, the preferred method of assessing malignant potential has been evaluation by the surgeon. Two different classification systems have been described, where the Müller-Hermelink system seems to be most closely correlated with prognosis[2]. In this article we have retrospectively analyzed a patient material with thymoma treated at the University Hospital Lund, Sweden. Clinicopathological features, complicating diseases and therapy were analyzed in order to find prognostic factors.

2. PATIENTS AND METHODS

The group was comprised of 67 patients, 41 women with a mean age of 62 years (SD=13) and 26 men with a mean age of 52 years (SD=13).

Staging

The classification suggested by Masaoka et al.[3] was used.

Stage I: Macroscopically, completely encapsulated and microscopically, now capsular invasion.
Stage II: Macroscopic invasion into surrounding fatty tissue or mediastinal pleura, or microscopic invasion into capsule.
Stage III: Macroscopic invasion into a neighbouring organ, i.e. pericardium, great vessels, or lung.
Stage IVa: Pleural or pericardial dissemination.
Stage IVb: Lymphogenous or hematogenous metastases.

There were 41 stage I patients, 13 stage II patients, 11 stage III patients and two stage IV patients.

Staging was carried out on the basis of the surgeon´s description and histopathological investigation. Presurgery staging included computerized tomography in 53 cases, pulmonary radiography in 59 cases and mediastinoscopy in two cases.

In two patients there were distant metastases on diagnosis. Further diagnostic procedures included bronchoscopy (n=12), cytology (n=9), transthoracic needle aspiration (n=1)and sputum cytology (n=2).

Classification of pathology was according to Marino and Müller-Hermelink[2], modified by Kirchner and Müller-Hermelink[4,5]. There were two medullary thymomas, 3 predominantly medullary mixed thymomas, 10 mixed common thymomas, 6 predominantly cortical mixed thymomas, 31 cortical thymomas and 15 well differentiated carcinomas.

There was an overrepresentation of mixed thymomas in stage I, (11 cases of 15, p=0,02). Cortical thymomas also had a greater representation in the lower stages, 24 cases in stage I and 8 cases in stage II (p= 0,16), while well-differentiated thymic carcinomas were more heavily represented in stages II and IV, (7 cases of 14, p=0,12). (Table 1). There were no significant gender differences regarding the incidence of the various histological types.

Table 1. Pathological classification and stage

	Medullary, predominantly medullary and mixed thymomas	Cortical and predominantly cortical thymomas	Well differentiated carcinomas
Stage I	11	24	6
Stage II	3	8	2
Stage III	–	5	6
Stage IV	1	0	1

3. RESULTS

3.1 Diagnosis

In this group of patients, 18 had no symptoms, and the thymomas were discovered en passant at routine pulmonary radiography examination or in the course of surgery for heart disease. Twenty-eight patients had symptoms of Myasthenia gravis at time of diagnosis. Local symptoms such as cough, dyspnea and retrosternal pain were seen in 18 patients. Thirty-two patients had a medical history of less than four months and 35 had a medical history of more than four months. There was a significant correlation between survival and length of medical history (p=0,05). (Fig. 1).

When a classification of the material according to Müller-Hermelink was done, no significant correlation to survival was seen (p=0,23).

3.2 Treatment

The most effective treatment for thymoma is its complete removal, and in this material, primary surgery was the first treatment of choice. In 55 cases surgery was macroscopically radical, but in twelve cases this could not be achieved. Within the group of macroscopically radically operated, a significantly improved relapse-free survival was observed (p=0,04), (Fig 2). There was also a significant difference in the rate of relapse-free survival which could be noticed in the different stages (p=0,02), (Fig 3).

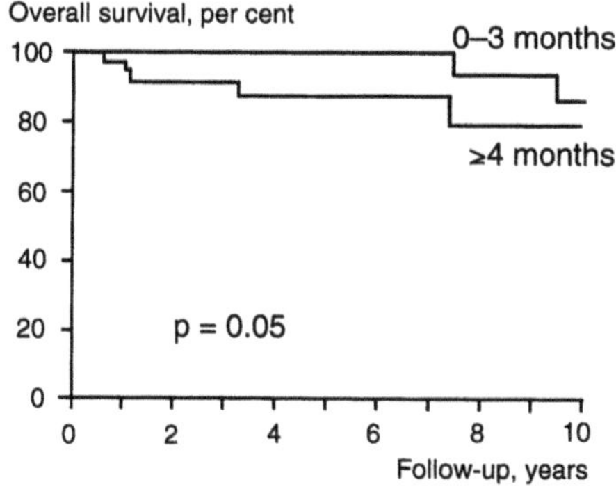

Figure 1. Survival in relation to length of medical history.

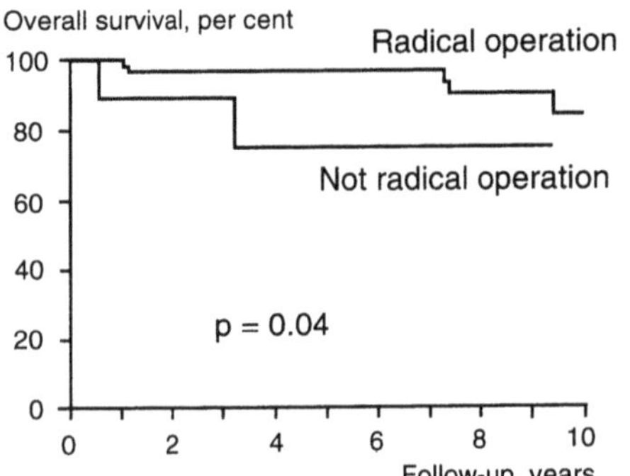

Figure 2. Relapse-free survival in relation to radical or not radical operation.

3.2.1 Chemotherapy and Radiotherapy. Nineteen patients recieved further treatment with chemotherapy (n=1), radiotherapy (n=15) or both (n=3). Fourty-eight patients recieved no further treatment, and this group had a significantly better survival (p=0,02), (Fig 4).

3.3 Autoimmune Disorders

Myasthenia gravis was reported in 28 (16 women and 12 men) of the 67 patients. The survival of patients with myasthenia gravis did not differ significantly from that of patients without myasthenia gravis (p=0,41). Other autoimmune diseases included SLE (n=1), polymyalgia rheumatica, RA (n=1), ankylosing spondylitis (n=1), collagenosis (n=1), autoimmune thyreoiditis (n=5). There was no evidence in this group either, that an autoimmune disorder as such had a negativ effect on survival (p=0,13). Thirty-three of the 67 patients had some kind of autoimmune disease, and autoimmune disease was especially common in the group with cortical thymomas. Three of the 33 patients proved to have a mixed thymoma, 23 had cortical or predominantly cortical thymoma. (p=0,04). Myasthenia gravis was also overrepresented in, and significantly correlated to the group whith cortical thymoma. (p=0,05).

3.4 Recurrence

Four patients had only a local recurrence, one patient had only metastases and six patients both local recurrence and metastases. Time to local recurrence varied between 15

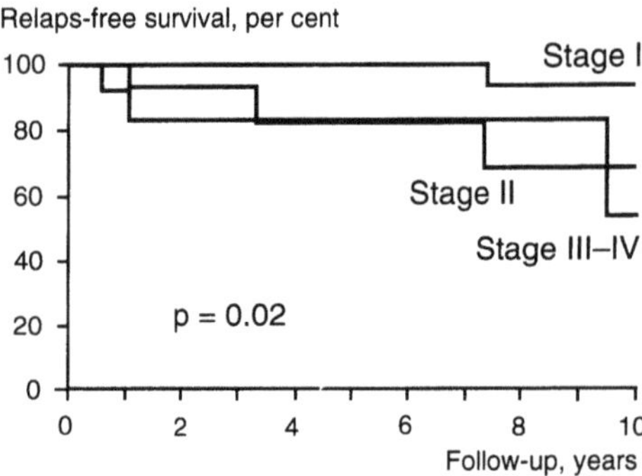

Figure 3. Relapse-free survival in relation to clinical staging.

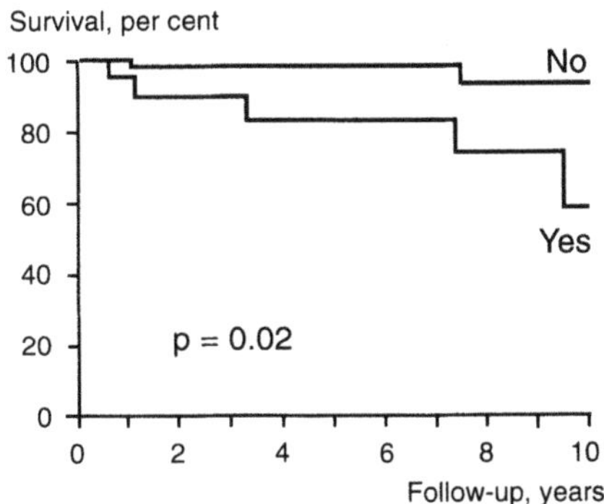

Figure 4. Survival in relation to complementary therapy.

and 143 months. Two patients had metastases at diagnosis and for the other four patients with metastases, these were discovered from 13 to 39 months after diagnosis.

With regards to location, there were two cases which only had metastases in the lungs, two cases with metastases in the pleura and one case with metastases in both pleura and lung. One patient had a metastasis in a rib. The two patients with lung metastases recieved regimens including cisplatin; one case in combination with vepesid, and one case in combination with corticosteroids. In both cases there was complete remission (CR) of the tumor; however in the case treated with cisplatin and vepesid there was a relapse seven months after CR. One patient recieved cyclophosphamide and his condition was initially stable, but then deterioated rapidly; and the condition of one patient treated with corticosteroids only also deterioated during treatment. One patient with a local recurrence, who was given a regimen including cisplatin, responded with partial remission (PR). The remaining patients were treated with surgery or radiotherapy.

3.5 Other Malignancies

Other malignancies were seen in eleven of the 67 patients. They included thyroid cancer (2 patients), mammary carcinoma (2 patients), pancreatic cancer (1 patient), non-Hodgkin´s lymphoma (1 patient), Merkel cell carcinoma (1 patient), prostatic cancer (1 patient), colonic cancer (1 patient), gastric cancer (1 patient). No difference in survival was seen for the group who developed a different malignancy (p=0.49).

3.6 Follow-up

Fourty-five patients are alive with no evidence of disease and one patient is alive with disease. Twenty-one patients have passed away. Of these, thirteen died of intercurrent diseases (coronary heart infarction n=5), four died of secondary malignancies (pancreatic cancer, colonic cancer, prostatic cancer, mammary carcinoma), one died of pulmonary disease, one comitted suicide after being informed that he had a recurrent disease with poor prognosis, one died of gastrointestinal bleeding, and one of bilateral pneumonia after lengthy treatment with corticosteroids and intermittent high-dose cisplatin. At autopsy he had no sign of disease. One patient died of his metastases, one of a local recurrence and one from both local recurrence and metastases. Four deaths were disease-related, two from myasthenia gravis, one patient with distant metastases died in toxic hepatitis and myasthenia gravis, and one with a local recurrence after ten years died of pneumonia and bilaterally pulmonary embolism. Four of the diseased underwent autopsy.

4. DISCUSSION

Thymomas are slow growing tumors and in up to 75% of cases are located in the anterior mediastinum. They present in adulthood and have no sex predilection[6]. At the time of operation, local invasion or distant metastases are observed in 30 to 70% of the cases. Extrathoracic metastases are observed in less than 10% of patients[7]. Distant metastases may result from hematogenous or lymphatic dissemination.

The majority present with symptoms related to one of the associated syndroms, the most common of which is myasthenia gravis.

Myasthenia gravis is reported in 10 to 50% of patient with thymomas. the incidence of thymoma in patients with myasthenia gravis ranges from 8 to 15%. Nearly 60% of patients with thymoma have disorders related to immunological phenomena. There is reportedly no difference in survival rate between patients with or without MG during the first years postoperatively, but at ten years the survival rate of MG patients is lower than that of patients without MG[3]. However, this could not be confirmed in our study were 28 of the 67 patients had MG. No significant difference in survival in patients with or without MG was seen (p=0,41). This holds true for the group of other autoimmune diseases as well. We could not find any dfference in survival here either (p=0,13).

So far, the degree of invasiveness has been considered the most important prognostic factor. The 5 and 10-year survival rates are approximately 98% and 75% respectively for stage I disease, 90% and 70% for stage II disease, 70% and 60% for stage III disease and 50% and 0% for stage IV disease. This was confirmed in our study were a significant correlation was found between stage and survival (p=0.02).

Furthermore, a significant correlation was found between survival and macroscopically radical operation (p=0,04).

In this material an overrepresentation of cortical thymomas was seen in stage I and of well differentiated carcinoma in stage IV. This is in concordance with the results earlier reported[18,19]. In our material there were few medullary thymomas.

Operative treatment alone is successfull in nearly all cases of non-invasive thymoma, whereas a relapse rate of 38 to 100 % has been observed after radical surgery for invasive thymoma. The most definitive procedure for exstirpation of this tumor is extended thymectomy, which involves removal of the thymus gland perithymic tissue, mediastinal fat, and all non-vital adjacent structures involved by the tumor. Subtotal thymectomy is not a correct procedure for controlling this type of tumor. The recurrence/persistence rate after radiation therapy is 73 % in patients who undergo mediastinoscopy and /or exploratory thoracotomy with biopsy, 53 % after subtotal thymectomy, and 8 % after extended thymectomy[8,9].

Although surgical extirpation remains the mainstay of therapy for invasive thymoma, adjunctive irradiation and chemotherapy are widely advocated. The recommended dose for radiotherapy is 40 to 60 Gy, given in 20 to 30 fractions[10,11,12]. There is no clear relationship between radiation dose and local control of disease[7]. Local recurrence has been observed in 20 to 30 % of patients with invasive thymomas after radiotherapy[9].

Nineteen of the patients had some form of supplementary therapy. However, this group fared worse in terms of survival than the group with no further treatments (p=0.02).

This could be due to bias in treatment, since more advanced cases are most likely to recieve radiotherapy or chemotherapy in addition to surgery.

The available data on systemic treatment of invasive thymoma are limited. Cisplatin has a documented efficacy with a response rate of more than 50 % and even long-standing complete remission. A response rate of 61% has been demonstrated for ifosfamid (18 patients of which 9 CR and 2 PR). Experience with other single agents; nitrogen mustard, maytansine, chlorambucil and doxorubicin have been tested without convincing effect. Also corticosteroids have been tested with tumor effects, even complete remission[13,14].

Combination chemotherapy has been used in invasive thymoma with a variety of different treatment programs. In a report of 66 patients treated with regimens including platinum, 22 (33%) achieved CR and 28 (42%) PR[15,16]. The median duration of response was 11 months. In another report on 52 patients with platinum-free regimens, 20 (37%) achieved CR and 15 (28%) PR[13,14,17]. The median duration of response in this case was 15 months.

5. CONCLUSION

Malignant thymoma is an aggressive mediastinal tumor which spreads by local invasion and distant metastases. Its histological features are similar to those of benign tumors. So far the degree of invasion is the most accurate prognostic parameter. In our study a significant correlation to survival was also found versus radical surgery, duration of symptoms, staging and additional therapy. Classification according to Marino and Müller Hermelink showed a significant correlation between the cortical type of thymomas and myasthenia gravis/autoimmune disease. The classification did not correlate to survival. The incidence of myasthenia gravis or secondary malignancies was not significantly related to survival.

REFERENCES

1. Lattes R.; Thymoma and other types of tumor of the thymus, an analysis of 107 cases.; Cancer 15:1224–1260,1962.
2. Marino M, Müller-Hermelink HK; Thymoma and thymic carcinoma. Relation of thymoma epithelial cells to the cortical and medullary differentiation of the thymus. ; Virchows Arch A Pathol Anat Histopathol. 407:119–49, 1985.
3. Masaoka et al.; Follow-up study of thymomas with specal reference to their clinical stages.; Cancer 48: 2485–2492, 1981.
4. Kirchner T, Müller-Hermelink HK; New approaches to the diagnosis of thymic epithelial tumors.; Prog Surg Pathol 10:167–189, 1989.
5. Kirchner T et al.; Well differentiated thymic carcinoma: an organotypical low-grade carcinoma with relationship to cortical thymoma. Am J Surg Pathol. 16:1153–1169, 1992
6. Ryback L P.; Metastatic thymoma to the head and neck.; Laryngoscope 98:418–421, 1988.
7. Batata M.A. et al.; Thymomas: Clinicopathological Features, Therapy and prognosis.; Cancer, 34:389–396, 1974.
8. Wick M R et al.; Primary Thymic Carcinomas.; Am J. Surg. Pathol, &:229–242,1982.
9. Monden Y et al.; Recurrence of thymoma: Clinicopathological features, Therapy and Prognosis.; The Annals of Thoracic Surgery, 39,2,165–169,185.
10. Arrigada R et al.; Invasive carcinoma of thymus. A multicenter retrospective review of 56 cases.; Eur. J. Cancer 20:69–74,1984.
11. Uematsu M et al.; A proposal of treatment of invasive thymoma.; Cancer 58:1979–1984, 1986.

12. Arakawa a et al.; Radiation therapy of invasive thymoma.; Int. J. Radiat. Oncol. Biol. Phys. 18:529–534, 1990.
13. Daugaard G et al.; Combination therapy for malignant thymoma.; Ann Intern. Med. 998:189–190,1983.
14. Daugaard G.; the effect of chemotherapy in the treatment of malignant thymoma.; In Sarrzin, Vrousos, Vincent (eds.): Thymic Tumors, Karger Basel 1989, pp 112–119.
15. Loehrer Pj et al.; Chemotherapy for advanced thymoma. Preliminary results of an intergroup study.; Ann. Intern. Med. 113:520–524, 1990.
16. Fornasiero A et al.; Chemotherapy of invasive thymoma.; J. Clin. Oncol. 8:1419–1423, 1990.
17. Ewans W.K. et al.; Combination chemotherapy in invasive thymoma. Role of COPP.; Cancer 46:1523–1527, 1980.
18. Tseng-Tong Kuo et al.; Thymoma: a study of the pathology classification of 71 cases with evaluation of the Müller-Hermelink system; Human Pathology vol. 24 7:766–778, 1993.
19. Quintanilla-Martinez L. et al.; Thymoma - morphologic sub classification correlates with invasiveness and immunohistologic features: a study of 122 cases; Human Pathology vol. 24 9:958–969,1993.

MANAGEMENT OF THYMECTOMISED MYASTHENIC PATIENTS

W. A. Nix,[1] H. Große-Höötmann,[1] T. Kirchner,[2] and A. Marx[3]

[1]Department of Neurology
University Clinic, 55101 Mainz
[2]Department of Pathology
University of Erlangen
Department of Pathology
University of Würzburg, Germany

SUMMARY

This prospective study followed-up fifty-six thymectomised patients with thymoma- and non thymoma-associated generalized myasthenia gravis for at least 2 years. To study the effect of thymectomy, no immunosuppression was given until needed after surgery. Forty-one percent patients with thymitis went into spontaneous remission, 37% after additional immunosuppression. Only 11% of patients with thymoma or an atrophic thymus went into spontaneous remission. This group proved difficult to be treated as within the remaining 89% over 40% improved only partially in their symptoms with immunosuppression. Within all groups it was possible to withhold without adverse effects immunosuppression until there was a definite clinical need for therapy. Early diagnosis of spontaneous remission improves considerably the quality of life, especially in young patients.

INTRODUCTION

Pharmacological and surgical treatment of myasthenic patients has profoundly improved their prognosis. In spite of the general acceptance of thymectomy as a therapeutic tool, there is still some debate on the extent of its therapeutic contribution (8). This especially in regard to the indication of thymectomy in different age ranges. Less when myasthenia is associated with thymoma and more when there is an unspecific radiological chest examination. An other matter of debate is the question when to start immunosuppression. A decision is often based on personal experiences and the idea that immunosuppression is always needed anyway. Some advocate immunosupression before surgery, others at vary-

Epithelial Tumors of the Thymus, edited by Marx and Müller-Hermelink.
Plenum Press, New York, 1997

ing times after surgery. All studies dealing with this aspect of therapy are done retrospectively (1,2,4,5,10,15). The lack of a common histopathological classification for the thymus does not allow to correlate in these studies histology with therapeutic outcome. A further problem of these retrospective studies is the lack of communication of the exact regime and time pattern of immunosuppression before and after surgery. Therefore, the aim of this study was to monitor the outcome of myasthenic patients and to conduct therapy under defined criteria (13).

METHODS

Fifty-six patients with myasthenia, who gave consent to thymectomy, were prospectively followed-up for at least two years. All patients had generalized myasthenia, some a thymoma others a normal CT or MRT study of the chest. To monitor the disease course, the patients were examined at the beginning of the study and at each office visit thereafter. Score points were used to classify disease severity. For defined symptoms points were assigned and added up to a score. In case of pure ocular symptoms one score point was give. No cases with pure ocular myasthenia entered the study. Only those patients underwent thymectomy who had generalized symptoms. Mere ocular symptoms initiated detailed studies including single fiber myography of the extensor digitorum communis (EDC) muscle. In case of positive jitter findings in the EDC the criteria for a generalized myasthenia were fulfilled. Mere clinical bulbar symptoms were also scored with one point. In case of additional or only generalized symptoms two points were given. The criteria were fulfilled with the complaint of situations with difficulties to raise and hold the head in sitting or prone position during the day, mild facial weakness or fatigue at mild exercise. Four points were given after the report of problems to work with arms raised, climbing stairs or with a limited walking distance. Respiratory difficulties were scores with the addition of 4 points to the sum-score. When the diagnosis of myasthenia was established most of the patients received anticholinesterase therapy. In the majority of cases this gave control over their symptoms, allowed surgery and a save recovery from anesthesia. None of the patients had due to this regime any postoperative problems. Only about ten percent of the patients needed corticosteroids prior to surgery in addition to esterase inhibitors and another ten percent had only subclincial symptoms and needed therefore no medication. In about 90% of patients it was possible to avoid corticosteroid medication or immunosuppression before surgery. This was important as this pharmacological intervention quickly influences thymus histology, especially the extent of the inflammatory components within hypertrophic tissue. So preoperative therapy can influence the histology and the classification of the thymus.

After surgery, performed as a maximum thymectomy(6), medication was left unchanged. Patients with progressive symptoms were put on immunosuppressive therapy. According to the acuity and physical disability of the symptoms azathioprine alone was used or in combination with corticosteroids which were tapered off within three to four month after initiation of therapy. Patients with only anticholinesterase therapy were soon asked after surgery to slowly decrease medication and to stop it if they felt no further need for it. All patients were seen before surgery and after discharge from hospital regularly as out-patients, at first each month and after ½ year at about 4 month intervals always by one of the authors (WAN). This allowed constant evaluation of patients, a stable doctor-patient relationship and standardized guidelines for therapeutic decisions. Following the first half year after thymectomy patients could be divided in groups. One group consistet of patients who went into remission without any medication, others went into remission under immunosuppressive therapy, a third group improved under immunosuppresive and anticholinesterase inhibitor medication. Those who remained unchanged in spite of medication or even worsened were put in the last group.

The removed thymus was kept in ice under sterile conditions and shipped to Würzburg were it was, a few hours later, submitted to histological and immunohistochemical studies. This allowed consistent evaluation and classification of the thymus (7,12). Histology divided the patients in three groups, those with thymoma-, atrophy- and hyperplasia associated myasthenia.

RESULTS

In twenty-four myasthenic patients the thymus was diagnosed showing thymitis, the patients median age was 36.2 years, 75% were female (Tab. 1). Thymitis could be differentiated as being low, medium or high. The seven patients with a high degree of thymitis were all women with a median age of 37,7 years. The group with medium degree thymitis included 4 women and 1 man and had a median age of 32,8. The low degree thymitis group was the largest group containing 12 patients. This group represented 50% of all patients with thymitis, the male to female relation was 5 to 7 and their median age 38,1 years.

In nine patients (6 men, 3 women) the thymus was classified as atrophic. Patients age ranged from 46 to 77 year with a median age of 65,7.

Twenty three patients had a thymoma, the median age of this group with 13 men and 10 women was 55,1 years. Thirteen patients (9 men, 4 women) had a cortical thymoma, five patients (1 man, 4 women) a mixed thymoma, 3 patients (1 man, 2 women) thymic carcinoma, in two men a thymolipoma was found.

Within the thymitis group 41% of the patients went into remission, 37% remitted under immunosuppression with azathioprine. Thirteen percent improved under medication,

Table 1. Therapeutic outcome in thymectomised myasthenic patients with different thymus histology. The numbers (n) of patients and their age (age) are listed to gether with their response after thymectomy. Four different outcome groups are formed: (R) Patients who went into spontaneous remission without any medication, (PR) patients who needed additional immunosuppression and went into pharmacological remission, (I) patient who improved under thymectomy and immunosuppression, (U/W) patients who were left (U) unchanged or (W) worsened under treatment

Thymitis	n	Age median	R number	PR number	I number	U/W number
low	12	38,1	5	3	2	1
medium	5	32,8	2	3		
high	7	37,7	3	2	1	1
	24	36,2	10	8	3	2
	24=100%		41%	37%	13%	9%
Atrophies	9	65,7	1	3	3	1
	9=100%		11%	34%	34%	11%
Thymomas	23	55,1	3	10	3	6
	23=100%		13%	44%	17%	26%

only two patients had no positive response and, rather compliance induced, no improvement under medication. The results prove young women with thymitis to have a very high likelihood to go into remission after thymectomy.

This is different with patients having an atrophied thymus. Spontaneous remission played in this group no major role, but 68% of the patients who are under immunosuppression will go into pharmacological remission or experience improvement of symptoms.

Myasthenic symptoms of patients with a thymoma were far more difficult to threat than in those with thymitis. Some even worsened after thymectomy in spite of pharmacological intervention. Only 13% went in spontaneous remission after thymectomy, in 44% immunosuppression led to pharmacological remission.

The follow-up of patients, especially those with thymitis, proved that there is no immediate need for immunosupression after thymectomy. Monitoring the patients myasthenic symptoms over about 3–4 month disclosed the need for treatment. The retarded initiation of immunosuppression after a postoperative observation period had no negative influence on the disease course and did not prolong the time of remission.

In 87% of patients with a thymoma and 89% of patients with an atrophic thymus immunosuppression was necessary. Within the thymoma group the numbers for different thymomas are so small that in this study it is not possible to draw conclusions from subgroups. As an overall statement the study shows that the low rate of spontaneous remission in thymoma and atrophy should be taken as an indicator for an early implementation of pharmacotherapy.

DISCUSSION

A questionnaire send to American neurologists, who take a special interest in myasthenic patients, disclosed a broad acceptance for thymectomy in myasthenia gravis (8). The spectrum of individual opinions was very broad and only three neurologist out of fifty-six approved thymectomy without objections. All felt that thymectomy is indicated under certain circumstances. Recent studies on the natural course of myasthenia are lacking and due to ethical considerations not possible. Old studies date back to times, where diagnostic and therapeutic possibility were lacking today's precision and efficacy (4,5,16). Studies from that time have shown that myasthenia worsens usually within the first 3–5 years after diagnosis. Symptoms then remain on a plateau and improves after that phase (11,16). Increasing duration of the disease state increases the likelihood of remission (5,15,16). Studies performed before the era of immunosuppression report a spontaneous remission rate of 10–15% within the first 10 year which increases to over 20% in the following 10 years (5,16). Oosterhuis found in his series of thymectomised patients a remission rate of 35% as opposed to 33% in non thymectomised patients with acetylcholinesterase inhibitor therapy only. He sees a benefical effect of thymectomy in the fact that thymectomised patients are easier to treat and have less deterioration and relapses of symptoms than non thymectomised myasthenics. Recently published studies are all done retrospectively and it is not quit clear what actually induced remission (1,2,9,10). Very different forms of pharmacological interventions that led to remission are lumped together with spontaneous remissions which all together have a cumulative remission rates between 46 and 59% in nonthymomatous patients (1,2,3,9,17). These studies have as a further uncertainty the problem that thymus histology and the surgical intervention has not been performed in a standardized manner and this does not allow to compare the results in-between these studies. Our prospective study shows in thymitis patients a remission rate after thymectomy within the first half year of 41%. Thirty-seven percent went into remission after additional implementation of immunosuppression. This is an overall remission rate of 78%. Of special interest are the patients who went into spontaneous remission following thymectomy. This are to a large extent young people, especially women. For them the implementation of immunosuppression during their reproductive period has a profound effect on family planning. Thymitis associated myasthenia is by now a disease with a very good prognosis under proper treatment. The beneficial achievement of handling and treatment should be quickly implemented in routine patient care to improve the patients quality of life.

Thymectomy in young age groups is widely accepted. Heterogeneous are the opinions on the upper age for thymectomy (14). We feel that thymectomy should be performed routinely up to 65 years of age in late-onset myasthenia if there is no major other co-morbidity. Between the age of 55 and 65 year we had two patients with atrophy and 3 with thymitis, all needed after thymectomy immunosuppression. Old age should not be in itself a limiting factor for thymectomy.

Within our 56 patients there are 43% who had a thymitis, 9% with an atrophic thymus and 41% with a thymoma. The prevalence of thymoma in myasthenic patients was found in larger studies to be between 11 and 26% (5,15). Increasing age is a high risk factor for a thymoma. Our large group of thymoma associated myasthenia is not what one would expect. It reflects the situation of a specialized clinic, as ours, which has a recruiting bias toward the more complicated cases. Therefore, our numbers do not reflect the distribution of thymus alteration in the population.

In atrophy and thymoma associated myasthenia thymectomy has a different effect on myasthenic symptoms. Surgical intervention has only little effect on spontaneous remission (1,2). In case of thymoma thymectomy is performed in the first place to remove the tumor and to start according to histology and staging additional treatment. All patients are in average of older age and in the majority men compared with those having thymitis. They also have in association with their higher age very often different additional co-morbidities. In spite of proper treatment symptom control is difficult to achieve in about 50% of the patients. It has been seen also by others (1,18). This emphasizes the need for an early and stringent therapeutic approach. Correct diagnosis of the type of thymoma is of great importance. In our limited number of thymomas we saw with maximal thymectomy no recurrence in cortical and mixed thymomas but with thymic carcinoma. In two cases of recurrence of a tumor, which was at the time of the first thymectomy diagnosed as mixed thymoma, it proved now to be a thymic carcinoma. On reevaluation of the old pathology slides signs of carcinoma were already present at that time.

Of interest are the two cases of thymolipoma, a tumor which is only seldom seen with myasthenia (19). In both cases, which were men and are followed up for over 5 years, thymectomy led to different results. One patient needed corticosteroids and azathioprine to go into pharmacological remission which is maintained until today with azathioprine alone. Tapering off azathioprine initiated a myasthenic relapse and proved the need for further medication. The other patient went into spontaneous remmission.

REFERENCES

1. Durelli L, Maggi G, Casadio C, Ferri R, Rendine S, Bergamini L. Actuarial analysis of the occurrence of remission following thymectomy for myasthenia gravis in 400 patients. J Neurol Neurosurg Psychiatry 1991; 54:406–11.
2. Evoli A, Batocchi AP, Provenzano C, Ricci E, Tonali P. Thymectomy in the treatment of myasthenia gravis: report of 247 patients. J Neurol 1988; 235(5):272–6.

3. Fujii N, Itoyama Y, Machi M, Goto I. Analysis of Prognostic Factors in Thymectomized Patients with Myasthenia Gravis - Correlation Between Thymic Lymphoid Cell Subsets and Postoperative Clinical Course. J Neurol Sci 1991; 105(2):143–9.
4. Genkins G, Kornfeld P, Papatestas AE, Bender AN, Matta RJ. Clinical experience in more than 2000 patients with myasthenia gravis. Ann N Y Acad Sci 1987; 505(Review):500–13.
5. Grob D, Arsura EL, Brunner NG, Namba T. The course of myasthenia gravis and therapies affecting outcome. Ann N Y Acad Sci 1987; 505. P 472–99(Review).
6. Jaretzki A3, Penn AS, Younger DS *et al.* "Maximal" thymectomy for myasthenia gravis. Results. J Thorac Cardiovasc Surg 1988; 95:747–57.
7. Kirchner Th, Schalke B, Melms A, von Kügelgen T, Müller-Hermelink H K. Immunohistological patterns of non-neoplastic changes in the thymus in myasthenia gravis. Virchows Arch [Cell Pathol] 1986; 52:237–57.
8. Lanska DJ. Indications for thymectomy in myasthenia gravis. Neurology 1990; 40:1828–9.
9. Lindberg G, Andersen O, Larsson S, Oden A. Remission rate after thymectomy in myasthenia gravis when the bias of immunosupressive therapy is eliminated. Acta Neurol Scand 1992; 86:323–8.
10. Maggi G, Giaccone G, Donadio M *et al.* Thymomas. A review of 169 cases, with particular reference to results of surgical treatment. Cancer 1986; 58(3):765–76.
11. Mantegazza R, Beghi E, Pareyson D *et al.* A multicenter follow-up study of 1152 patients with myasthenia gravis in Italy. J Neurol 1990; 6:339–44.
12. Müller-Hermelink HK, Marino M, Palestro G. Pathology of thymic epithelial tumors. Vol. 75. Berlin: Springer, 1986: 207–68. (Müller-Hermelink HK Ed; The Human Thymus: Histopathology and Pathology. Current Topics in Pathology).
13. Nix WA, Große-Höötmann H, Kirchner T, Marx A. Remission rate after thymectomy in myasthenia gravis. Neurology 1995; 45:A352–253.
14. Olanow CW, Lane.R JM, Roses AD. Thymectomy in late-onset myasthenia gravis. Arch Neurol 1982; 39:82–3.
15. Oosterhuis HJ. Long-term effects of treatment in 374 patients with myasthenia gravis. Monogr Allergy. 1988; 25:75–85.
16. Oosterhuis HJGH. The Natural Course of Myasthenia Gravis - A Long Term Follow Up Study. J Neurol Neurosurg Psychiatry 1989; 52(10):1121–7.
17. Paletto AE, Maggi G. Thymectomy in the treatment of myasthenia gravis: results in 320 patients. Int Surg 1982; 67:13–6.
18. Palmisani MP, Evoli A, Batocchi AP, Provenzano C, Tonali P. Myasthenia gravis associated with thymoma: Clinical characteristics and long-term outcome. Eur Neurol 1993; 34:78–82.
19. Pan CH, Chiang CY, Chen SS. Thymolipoma in patients with myasthenia gravis: report of two cases and review. Acta Neurol Scand 1988; 78(1):16–21.

MANAGEMENT OF THYMECTOMIZED MYASTHENIC PATIENTS

L. Fornádi, R. Horváth, and A. Szobor

Neurological Department
Jahn Ferenc-Teaching Hospital
Budapest, Köves str. 2-4. 1204 Hungary

INTRODUCTION

Up to now the exstirpation of thymus gland stands in the central position of the immuno-therapeutic strategy of myasthenia gravis promising alone the chance of total and definitive recovery in some cases. FIGURE 1. The current antigen-specific therapeutical approaches inducing autoimmune unresponsiveness to acetylcholin receptor are still in experimental phase.(ref. 1) They certainly need a rather long period until one or more of them will be applied in humans. This is the reason why the therapeutic centers elaborated new management for the therapy-resistant patients.(ref. 2,3,4,5). FIGURE 2. In some dubious cases the diagnosis of myasthenia gravis and the indication of thymectomy are difficult and need a long-lasting observation. The benefit from maintaining anticholinesterase therapy, the significant respond to plasma-exchange in crisis, the secondary generalization of ocular symptoms and the electrodiagnostic tests becoming positive after some years all strengthen the indication for thymectomy. FIGURE 3. As you can see on the third figure the indication of immunotherapies other than thymectomy has pro- and contra-arguments. We used to apply these methods at thymectomy unresponders, elderly X-ray unresponders, pregnants in crisis-prone state and in anticholinesterase resistance or intolerance. The crisis tendency is the major reason for applying these expensive therapies, but decreasing the drug doses and making rare the myasthenic relapses in the interest of improving life-quality are not negligible standpoints, either. FIGURE 4. In some severe cases both the plasma-exchange and the high-dose intravenous methylprednisolon infusion as well as the repeated high-dose intravenous immunoglobulin therapy may unfortunately fail.(ref. 6,7,8) All these observations induced us preparing new effectual therapeutic pattern. The role of our combined methods in the therapeutic strategy of myasthenia gravis is shown on the fourth figure. They all serve the preparation for surgery or can be considered supplementary therapies after surgery, because the results of even total or maximal

Epithelial Tumors of the Thymus, edited by Marx and Müller-Hermelink.
Plenum Press, New York, 1997

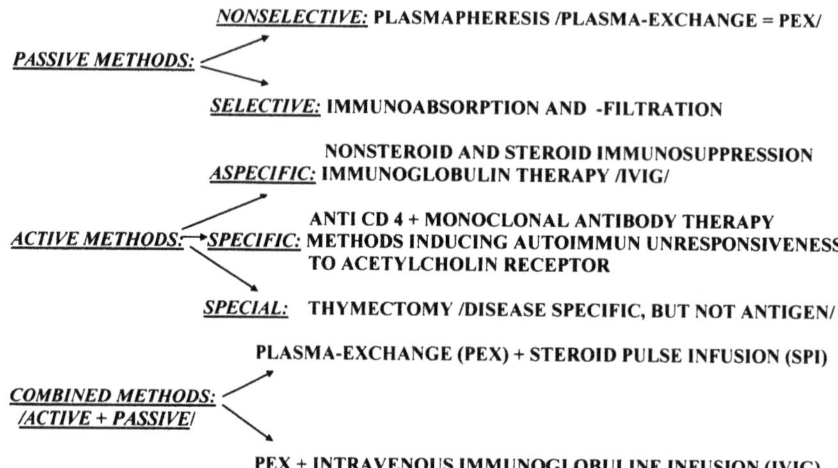

Figure 1. Classification of the current immuntherapies in myasthenia.

thymectomy may not be satisfactory and patients may require further active treatments. These so-called active therapies are able to solve the refractory crises and to make possible the indication of thymectomy also in formerly inoperable cases.(ref. 9,10) The therapies mentioned before proved to be essential not only for the quick solution of crises, but also for prevention of their rather frequent complications. It should not be forgotten that the myasthenic or cholinergic forms of respiratory crisis, as well as the alternating, so-called oscillating forms represent a very difficult problem for intensive therapy. During the controlled respiration the active therapies make possible the utilisation of "synaptic resting process", and the decrease of the anticholinesterase drug-demand.(ref. 11)

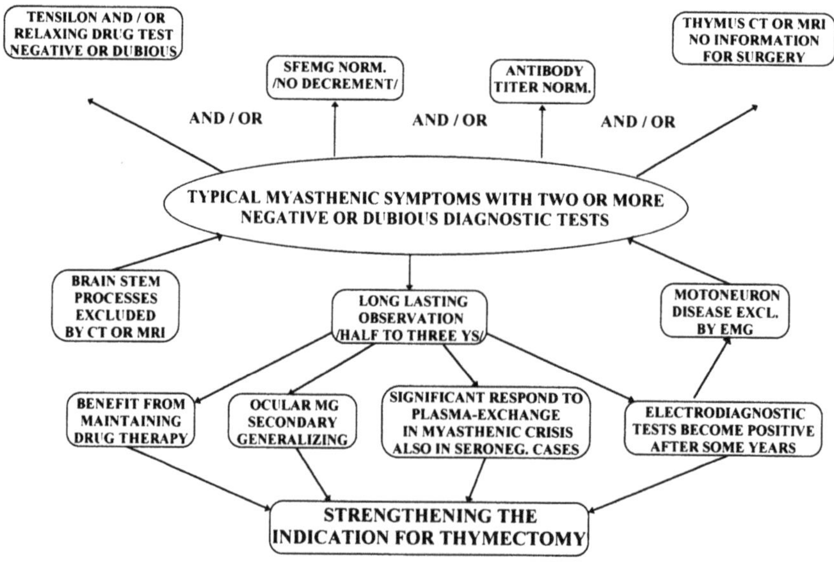

Figure 2. The diagnosis and the indication of thymectomy in dubious cases of myasthenia gravis.

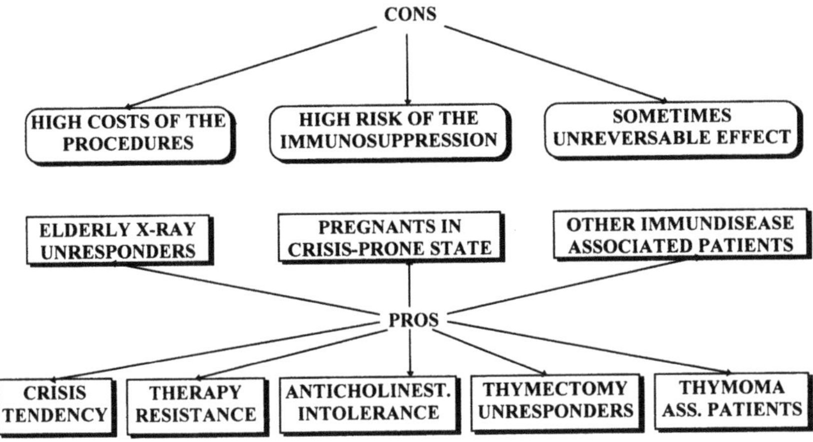

Figure 3. Indication of the current immuntherapies of myasthenia gravis.

CASUISTICS AND METHODS

FIGURE 5. The diagnosis, therapy and follow up of the patients have been based on more than fourty years experiences of one of us. We surveyed about one thousand and seven hundred cases of myasthenia gravis. The prevalence of them in Hungary is about sixty patients in a year. Our therapeutic workshop performed about three hundred plasma-exchange procedures yearly. Out of the thousand and seven hundred cases almost eight hundred passed thymectomy and about one hundred and fifty of them were thymoma exstirpation. We observed total recovery after thymectomy at about thirty five percent, while fifteen percent was totally unresponder to thymectomy. The longest postoperative survival after thymoma exstirpation was 25 years. The postthymectomy crises in the first five years

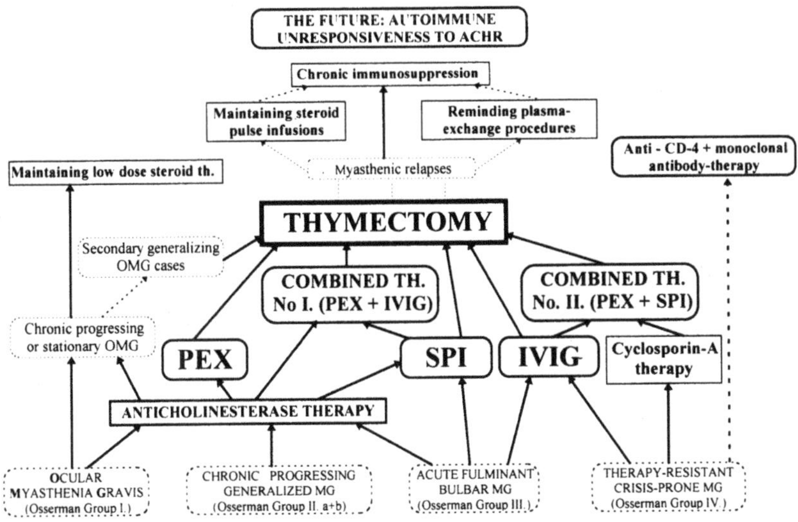

Figure 4. Therapeutic strategy for myasthenia gravis. Abbreviations: PEX = plasma-exchange; SPI = steroid "pulse" infusion; IVIG = iv. immunoglobulin.

1. PRESENT PATIENT NUMBER: 1700 FOR OVER 45 YEARS	/PREVALENCE: 60 PATIENT / YEAR /IN HUNGARY/
2. CRISIS-PRONE CASES / YEAR: ABOUT 30	3. THERAPY RESISTANT CASES / YEAR: ABOUT 20
4. BURNT-OUT CASES: 15 % OF ALL	5. OTHER IMMUNDISEASE ASSOCIATIONS: 10 %
6. SEC. GENERALIZED OCULAR MG CASES 40 %	7. PLASMA-EXCHANGE PROCEDURES / YEAR: ABOUT 300
8. THYMECTOMY: 785.	9. EXSTIRPATION OF THYMOMA: 148 /OUT OF THEM/
10. TOTAL RECOVERY AFTER THYMECTOMY : AB. 35%	11. TOTAL UNRESPONSIVENESS TO THYMECTOMY: 15%
12. THE SHORTEST IMPROVEMENT AFTER IT: HALF A YR	13. THE LONGEST IMPROVEMENT AFTER IT: 10-15 YS
14. THYMOMA - POSTOPERATIVE LIFETIME: HALF - 25 YS	15. POSTTHYMECTOMY CRISES IN THE 1ST 5 YS: 8 %

16. POSTTHYMECTOMY ANTICHOLINESTERASE	-RESISTANCE:	5 %
	-INTOLERANCE:	5 %
17. MORTALITY BEFORE OUR NEW IMMUNTHERAPEUTIC METHODS		15-20 / YR
MORTALITY SINCE OUR NEW IMMUNTHERAPEUTIC METHODS		3-5 / YR

Figure 5. Data of our myasthenic patient material.

after surgery appeared in eight to ten percent. The mortality of the not-thymectomized crisis-prone cases decreased from fifteen-twenty to three-five patients every year since the introduction of our new immunotherapeutic manner. FIGURE 6. Our therapeutic protocol in myasthenia gravis can be observed on the sixth figure. The application of nonsteroid immunosuppressive therapy has great importance not only in the postapheresis rebound prevention but in making rare the too frequent myasthenic relapses and in the solution of the therapy resistance.(ref. 14) In our practice we prefer Azathioprin because of the less complications caused by it, even in longer application. The long-lasting low-dose steroid therapy has more drawback than the intermittently applied mega-dose steroid infusion therapy. In particular its alternate combination with plasma-exchange is able to solve the refractory myasthenic or cholinergic crisis. The use of steroid mega-doses is limited for the arteficially respirated cases, because patients in precrisis state have no tolerance to their side-effects, especially the transitory muscled denervating effect. The unique benefit of the combination of plasma-exchange with steroid pulse therapy is the safe control of

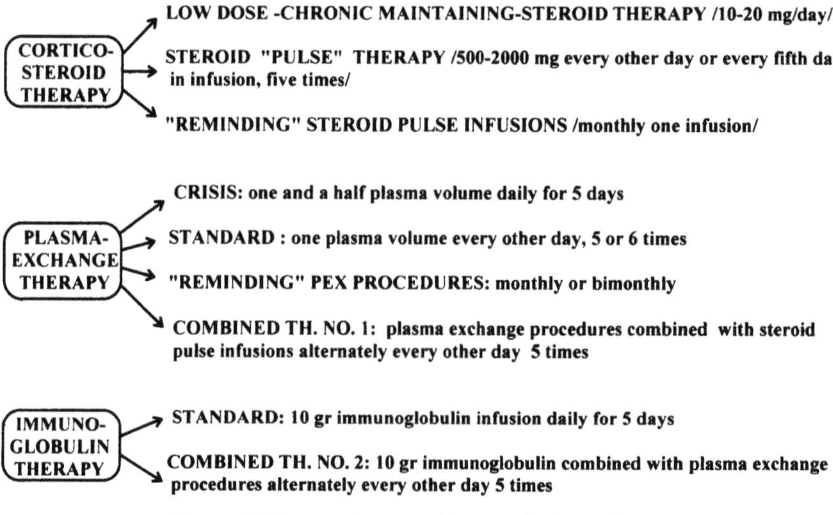

Figure 6. Therapeutic protocol in myasthenia gravis.

CONTRAS:

1. ONLY HIGH DOSES AND REPEATED PROCEDURES ARE EFFECTIVE
2. THE RECOMMENDED DOSAGE (0,4 G/KGBW) MAKES HIGH COSTS
3. IN HIGH DOSES THEY CAN CAUSE SOMETIMES SEVERE COMPLICATIONS

PROS:

1. THE HALF OF THE RECOMMENDED DOSE IS EFFECTIVE IN COMBINATION WITH PEX
2. THE COUNTER-INDICATIONS CAN BE ELIMINATED BY LOWER DOSES
3. THE INTERCURRENT INFECTION IS NOT AN EXCLUDING FACTOR DURING RESPIRATORY CRISES (CONTRASTED WITH PLASMA-EXCHANGE)
4. ELDERLY AND/OR WEAKENED IMMUNDEFENSING PATIENTS TOLERATE THIS METHOD WELL (BECAUSE THE REMOVED IgG IS ALTERNATELY REPLACED DURING THE PROCEDURE)
5. THE SERONEGATIVE MYASTHENIC FORMS ALSO RESPOND TO IT WELL
6. THE OTHER IMMUN-DISEASE ASSOCIATED CASES CAN BE IMPROVED SOONER BY THIS MANNER
7. PREGNANTS IN CRISIS-PRONE STATE HAVE A SAFE AND NOT FETAL-INJURING TREATMENT
8. ANTICHOLINESTERASE UNRESPONDERS AND CHOLINERG INTOLERANTS HAVE ANOTHER CHOICE FOR IMPROVING
9. THE RISK OF PLASMA-EXCHANGE DEPENDENCY DECREASES
10. THE MYASTHENIC RELAPSES BECOME LESS FREQUENT AND THE REMISSION OF SYMPTOMS CAN BE PROLONGED FOR A LONGER PERIOD

Figure 7. Arguments for intravenous immunoglobuline therapy in myasthenia gravis.

plasma-exchange procedures on the transitory myasthenic state-worsening caused by the application of steroid mega-doses. Furthermore their consecutive alternation always prevents the rebound phenomenon after plasma-exchange procedures. FIGURE 7. The immunoglobuline therapy in grave myasthenic exacerbations might be a safe alternative of plasma-exchange, but only high doses and repeated procedures are beneficial, and they make high costs in the recommended doses. Moreover they have sometimes severe complications in high doses. (ref. 15) But the arguments for application of the immunoglobuline therapy, especially in combination with plasma-exchange, are strong in numbers. First af all in combination the half of the recommended dose is effective, thus the counter-indications can be eliminated by the lower doses. The intercurrent infection during the respiratory crises doesn't exclude the application of this therapeutic combination in contrast with plasma-exchange alone, which decreases the immundefence in itself. Elderly and/or weakened immundefensing patients tolerate this method well, because the removed IgG-s are alternately replaced during the procedure assuring the continuity of the normal immun-defence. The seronegative forms also respond well to this manner. The other immundisease associated myasthenic patients can be improved sooner by this method. The pregnants in crisis-prone state have a safe and not fetal-injuring treatment. The anticholinesterase unresponders and cholinerg drug intolerants have another choice for improving. The risk of plasma-exchange dependency decreases with the help of IgG-s. The myasthenic relapses become less frequent and the remission of symptoms can be prolonged for a longer period.

RESULTS

FIGURE 8. This diagram illustrates the results of our combined therapies evaluating the patients' condition on the basis of Kurtzke's disability status scale (DSS) system adapted for myasthenia gravis by Szobor.(ref. 16) Both of the "pulse" steroid infusion (PSI)-plasma-exchange combination and the alternate application of intravenous immunoglobuline therapy with plasma-exchange have sightly improved the patients' condition within two weeks, even in refractory cases. Further on there was no difference between these methods considering the duration of the therapeutic effect.

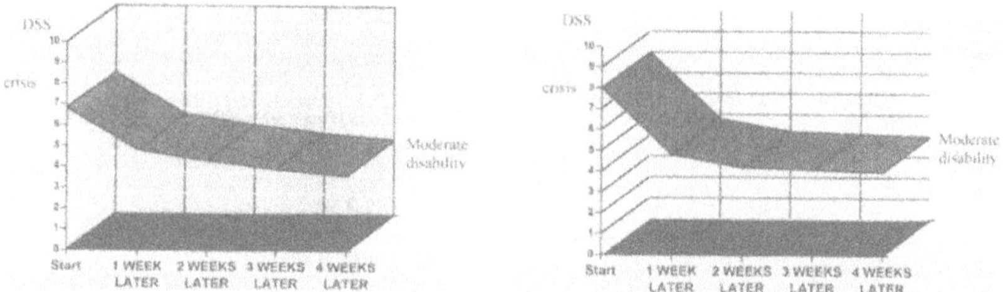

Figure 8. The effect of combined immunoactive therapies in myasthenia. (a) IVIG + PEX. n = 50; mean age: 42 years; f = 32; m = 18; DSS = disability status scale; IVIG = iv. immunoglobuline; PEX = plasma-exchange. (b) PSI + PEX. n = 50; mean age: 47 years; f = 24; m = 26; DSS = disability status scale. PSI = pulsus steroid infusion; PEX = plasma-exchange.

DISCUSSION

Both the clinical observation and the laboratory or pathological findings have a great importance for the indication of immunotherapies.(ref. 12) For instance there was significant thymic hyperplasy only in twenty percent of our seronegative cases. The thymectomy of the other eighty percent required consideration, although a part of the seronegative cases responded well to thymectomy also in absence of significant thymic hyperplasy. On the other hand, both the plasma-exchange and immunoglobuline therapy were very effective in most of the seronegative cases, thus the role of elimination of immunoactive agents other than anti-acetylcholin receptor antibody may be supposed.(ref. 13) After many symptomfree and medicineless years of the postthymectomy period the disease may be activated by a somatic or psychic effect influencing the immune system. In such cases the course of the disease may become foudroyant and malignant. After the failure of all possible ace therapy in the refractory crisis-prone cases we have started to adopt the combined alternate therapies, namely the intravenous immunoglobuline and plasma-exchange combination, as well as the steroid mega-dose, so-called "pulse" infusion combined with plasma-exchange.

FIGURE 9. Our last figure elucidates some crucial standpoints in the pre- and post-thymectomy management of myasthenia gravis, which can help us improving the efficacy of our work. The early recognition and diagnosis of myasthenia gravis enables the choice of total recovery by the adequate timing of thymectomy. We have to adapt the therapeutic plan for the various forms of the disease or for the present condition of the patients. The disease process can be influenced by the selection of the adequate immunotherapy in the concrete case considering the individual susceptibility, other former diseases or immun-disease associations. The tendency of recovery can be improved by the previously cured associating disease. The adequate timing of the therapy has great importance in the crisis prevention and the preparation for thymectomy. The adequate dosage and extension of the therapy can assure the lasting and sometimes total recovery. The adequate duration of the therapy prevents the too frequent relapses. The therapeutic combinations increase the efficacy even in refractory cases. Intensive Care Unit with the potential of immediate application of plasma-exchange and a permanent connection with thymus surgery are essential in every Myasthenia Center. Finally we would like to emphasize the importance of post-thymectomy follow-up, care and consultation in the interest of preventing the myasthenic relapses because of the negative influence of other diseases or surgery, pregnancy, psychic

1. EARLY RECOGNITION AND DIAGNOSIS OF MYASTHENIA GRAVIS ENABLES THE CHOICE OF TOTAL RECOVERY BY THE ADEQUATE TIMING OF THYMECTOMY.
2. ADAPTATION OF THE THERAPEUTIC PLAN TO THE VARIOUS DISEASE FORMS OR TO THE PRESENT CONDITION OF THE PATIENT IS ESSENTIAL.
3. THE DISEASE PROCESS CAN BE INFLUENCED BY THE SELECTION OF THE ADEQUATE IMMUNOTHERAPY IN THE CONCRETE CASE CONSIDERING THE INDIVIDUAL SUSCEPTIBILITY, OTHER PRIOR DISEASES OR IMMUN-DISEASE ASSOCIATIONS.
4. TENDENCY OF THE RECOVERY CAN BE IMPROVED BY THE PREVIOUSLY CURED ASSOCIATING DISEASE.
5. ADEQUATE TIMING OF THE THERAPY HAS GREAT IMPORTANCE IN THE CRISIS PREVENTION AND PREPARATION FOR THYMECTOMY.
6. ADEQUAT DOSAGE AND EXTENSION OF THE THERAPY CAN ASSURE THE LASTING AND SOMETIMES TOTAL RECOVERY.
7. ADEQUATE DURATION OF THE THERAPY PREVENTS THE FREQUENT RELAPSES.
8. THERAPEUTIC COMBINATIONS INCREASE THE EFFICACY EVEN IN REFRACTORY CASES.
9. INTENSIV CARE UNIT WITH THE POTENTIAL OF IMMEDIATE APPLICATION OF PEX AND A PERMANENT CONNECTION WITH THYMUS SURGERY ARE ESSENTIAL IN EVERY MYASTHENIA CENTER.
10. POSTTHYMECTOMY FOLLOW-UP, CARE AND CONSULTATION IS IMPORTANT IN THE INTEREST OF PREVENTING THE MYASTHENIC RELAPSES BECAUSE OF THE NEGATIV INFLUENCE OF OTHER DISEASES OR SURGERY, PREGNANCY, PSYCHIC STRESS ETC.

Figure 9. Some crucial standpoints in the pre- and post-thymectomy management of myasthenia gravis.

stress etc. Thus our myasthenic patients' condition can be improved in this way, bettering their life-quality and elongating their life-time.

REFERENCES

1. Drachman D.B., K.R. McIntosh, J. Reim, L. Balcer. 1993. Strategies for treatment of myasthenia gravis. Ann.N.Y.Acad.Sci. 681: 515–528.
2. Åhlberg R., Q. Yi, R. Pirskanen, G. Matell, C. Swerup, P. Rieber, G. Riethmüller, G. Holm, A.K. Lefvert. 1993. Clinical improvement of myasthenia gravis by treatment with a chimeric anti-CD-4 monoclonal antibody. Ann.N.Y.Acad.Sci. 681:552–555.
3. Arsura E., N.G. Brunner, T. Namba, D. Grob. 1985. High-dose intravenous methylprednisolone in myasthenia gravis. Arch. Neurol. 42:1149–1153.
4. Devathasen G., Y.K. Kuch, P.N. Chong. 1984. High-dose intravenous gammaglobulin for myasthenia gravis. Lancet. 2:809.
5. Fateh-Moghadam A., M. Wock, U. Besinger, R.G. Geursen. 1984. High-dose intravenous gammaglobulin for myasthenia gravis. Lancet. 2:848.
6. Fornádi L., R. Horváth, A. Szobor. 1991. Treatment with plasma-exchange. Experiences over ten years. Acta Med. Hung. 48:137–144.
7. Kornfeld P., S. Fox, K. Maier, M. Mahjoub. 1992. Ten years experience with therapeutic apheresis in a community hospital. J. Clin. Apher. 7:63–68.
8. Fornádi L., R. Horváth, Z. Bárdosi, A. Szobor. 1994. Myasthenia gravis: effect of immunoactive therapies. Acta Med. Hung. 50:83–92.
9. Szobor A. 1990. Myasthenia gravis. pp. 120–143, 147–152, 154–189. Akadémiai kiadó, Budapest.
10. Szobor A., J. Molnár. 1990. Myasthenia gravis: results of thymectomy in 550 patients. Orv. Hetil. 131:2519–2527.
11. Szobor A. 1977. Pathomechanismen myasthenischer Krisenzustände. In: Schulze A.F., K. Seidel, S. Göllnitz (eds): Akute Krisenzustände und Notsituationen in der Neurologie und Psychiatrie. S. 7–10. Hirzel, Leipzig.
12. Cornelio F., C. Antozzi, R. Mantegazza, P. Confalonieri, E. Berta, D. Peluchetti, A. Sghirlanzoni, F. Fiacchino. 1993. Immunosuppressive treatments . Their efficacy on myasthenia gravis patients' outcome and on the natural course of the disease. Ann. N.Y.Acad.Sci. 681:594–602.
13. Vincent A., Z. Li, A. Hart, R. Barrett-Jolley, T. Yamamoto, J. Burges, D. Wray, N. Byne, P. Molenaar, J. Newsom-Davis. 1993. Seronegative myasthenia gravis. Evidence for plasma factor/s) interfering with acetylcholin-receptor function. Ann.N.Y.Acad.Sci. 681:529–538.
14. Tindall R.S.A., J.T. Phillips, J.A. Rollins, L. Wells, K. Hall. 1993. A clinical therapeutic trial of Cyclosporine in myasthenia gravis. Ann.N.Y.Acad.Sci. 681: 539–551.

15. Tan E., M. Hajinazarian, W. Bay, J. Neff, J.R. Mendell. 1993. Acut renal failure resulting from intravenous immunoglobuline therapy. Arch. Neurol. 50:135–139.
16. Szobor A. 1976. Myasthenia gravis: A quantitative evaluation system. Disability Status Scale /DSS) applied for myasthenia gravis. Eur.Neurol. 14:439–446.

49

THERAPEUTIC OPTIONS IN LOCALLY ADVANCED THYMOMA*

Patrick J. Loehrer,[1] Mauro Antimi,[2] Andrew Turrisi,[3] and Giuseppe Giaccone[4]

[1]Indiana University Medical Center, Indiana University Hospital
550 North University Boulevard, #1730
Indianapolis, Indiana 46202-5265
[2]USL Rm 7, Ospedele San Eugenio, Onco-Ematologica/Servisio Oncologico
00144 Roma, Piazzale Omanesimo, 10, Rome, Italy
[3]Medical University of South Carolina, Department of Radiation Oncology
171 Ashley Avenue, Charleston, South Carolina 29403
[4]Department of Oncology, Free University Hospital
De Boelelaan 1117, Amsterdam, 1081 HV The Netherlands

Thymoma is the most common tumor of the anterior mediastinum. Most thymomas will present as a well encapsulated tumor which can be resected for cure in 80–90% of patients. Many of these patients have paraneoplastic syndromes such as myasthenia gravis, hypogammaglobulinemia, or pure red cell aplasia, which others may have symptom of local disease such as chest pain or superior vena caval obstruction. About one-third of patients present with asymptomatic mass on chest radiograph which ultimately prompts further evaluation.[1]

A cohort of patients may present with locally invasive or metastatic tumor. These patients have a worse outcome with local therapy and may be candidates for more aggressive therapeutic measures. This paper will focus on invasive thymoma and discuss the various therapeutic options for such patients.

BACKGROUND

Pathologic Staging

Several pathologic staging nomenclatures have been published to date. In 1978, Levine and Rosai first distinguished thymoma from thymic carcinoma.[2] Other classifications have been published with an attempt to look at cellular differentiation, tumor archi-

* Supported in part by National Cancer Institute Grant 2 R 35 CA 39844–11, The Walther Cancer Institute (Indianapolis IN), The General Clinical Research Center MO 1 RR 00750–10, and R10 CA 28171–04 from the Public Health Service.

Epithelial Tumors of the Thymus, edited by Marx and Müller-Hermelink.
Plenum Press, New York, 1997

Table I. Histological classifications

Study	No. of Patients	Subgroups	% Total	Comments
				10-year overall survival, %
Verley and Hollman[3]	200	Type I: spindle and oval cell	30	75
		Type II: lymphocyte-rich	30	75
		Type III: differentiated epithelial-rich	33	50
		Type IV: undifferentiated epithelial-rich (type IV equivalent to thymic carcinoma)	7	0
				15-year disease-specific survival, %
Lewis, et al[4]	283*	Predominantly lymphocytic (> 66% lymphocytes)	25	90
		Mixed lymphoepithelial (33-66% lymphocytes)	43	80
		Predominantly epithelial (< 33% lymphocytes)	25	50
		Spindle cell (predominantly epithelial cells with prominent fusiform cells)	6	100
				Subgroup with invasion, % invasive
Marino and Müller-Hermelink[5]	58*	Cortical	43	67
		Mixed: predominantly cortical	8	0
		Mixed: common	36	0
		Medullary	5	0
		Mixed: predominantly medullary	8	0

*Thymic carcinoma excluded

tecture, and ultrastructural characteristics.[3–5] Examples of these staging systems are shown in Table I. Both systems proposed by Verley/Holmand and by Lewis, et al, used a percentage of leukocytes and epithelial cells.[3] The level of invasion and treatment outcome was directly proportional to the predominance of epithelial cells in both of these staging systems.

Marino and Müller-Hermelink staging system was based upon recognition of cortical and medullary[5] epithelial cells. Cortical thymomas and lesions classified as mixed with cortical predominance were the only subtypes which displayed invasiveness in this staging system. Other authors have confirmed a greater percentage of invasiveness with cortical or predominately cortical thymoma while others have not.[6] The differences may be secondary to inter- and intra-observer availability.

Thymic carcinomas are considered a subset of thymic neoplasms which have more obvious malignant cytologic and histologic features. In addition, these tumors must fulfill the criteria of having an anterior mediastinal location in the absence of another obvious primary tumor site.

Clinical Staging

One of the most widely staging systems, developed by Masaoka, et al., separates tumors into encapsulated, invasive and metastatic lesions (Table II).[7] The TNM system is similar in design.[8] In these staging systems, stage II tumors demonstrate macroscopic invasion into the surrounding fatty tissue (or mediastinal pleura) or microscopic invasion into the tumor capsule. Stage III tumors have macroscopic invasion into the neighboring

Table II. Staging systems

Masaoka, et al.		
I	Macroscopically completely encapsulated and microscopically no capsular invasion	
II	1) Macroscopic invasion into surrounding fatty tissue, mediastinal pleura, or both	
	2) Microscopic invasion into capsule	
III	Macroscopic invasion into neighboring organ, such as pericardium, great vessels, lung, and so on	
IVA	Pleural or pericardial dissemination	
IVB	Lymphogenous or hematogenous metastasis	
TNM		
T Factor		
	T1	Macroscopically completely encapsulated and microscopically no capsular invasion
	T2	Macroscopically adhesion or invasion into surrounding fatty tissue or mediastinal pleura, or microscopic invasion into capsule
	T3	Invasion into neighboring organs, such as pericardium, great vessels, and lung
	T4	Pleural or pericardial dissemination
N Factor		
	N0	No lymph node metastasis
	N1	Metastasis to anterior mediastinal lymph nodes
	N2	Metastasis to intrathoracic lymph nodes except anterior mediastinal lymph nodes
	N3	Metastasis to extrathoracic lymph nodes
M Factor		
	M0	No hematogenous metastasis
	M1	Hematogenous metastasis

structures such as the lung, pericardium, or grave vessels whereas Stage IV tumors have distant metastases to the pleura, pericardial or distant dissemination.

Although there is general agreement regarding the staging system of thymoma, the lack of uniform treatment trials make prognostic correlates with these staging systems difficult. Clinical correlation have demonstrated a proportional decrease in the relapse free survival and overall survival with increasing invasiveness. For instance, in two series,[7,9] over 80% of patients with completely resected stage I or stage II disease survived 5–10 years. In contrast, the 5 and 10 year survival were 70% and 23%, respectively, for patients with stage III disease. In multiple series, the long term disease free survival approaches 100% for patients with completely resected stage I disease.[6,10]

In a series of 283 patients who were seen at the Mayo Clinic between 1941 and 1981, 32% had locally invasive disease at the time of diagnosis.[11] In addition, 6% had distant metastases to the lung or pleura. Adverse prognostic factors included: presentation with tumor related symptoms, large tumor size, predominant epithelial tumor and local invasion or metastases.

Radiotherapy

The principle role of radiotherapy for patients with thymoma is the primary treatment of bulky unresectable disease and in patients with resected, but invasive disease. Thymomas are felt to be relatively radiosensitive, perhaps partially explained by the large lymphocytic component of many tumors.

In one retrospective review of three hospital experiences, Curran et al, found recurrences in 20/78 (26%) patients who underwent resection for II or III thymoma and did not receive postoperative radiotherapy.[12] This contrasts with a thoracic failure rate of only 2/43 (5%) similarly staged patients who received adjuvant radiotherapy following complete resection of tumor. A multivariant analysis demonstrated that stage, extent of resection, and history of myasthenia gravis were correlated with disease-free status. Of note, histology was not an independent prognostic variable. This retrospective data suggests that routine use of adjuvant radiotherapy is indicated for patients with invasive disease.

Another therapeutic challenge are those patients with incomplete resection or unresectable disease. The optimal treatment of such patients is not well defined. In the Curran series (mentioned above) 4/20 (20%) of such patients developed recurrent disease.[12] In a large retrospective review by Koh, et al, a 35% local relapse rate was noted in 255 patients managed with primary radiotherapy.[13] In summary, radiation therapy appears to play a role in decreasing the local recurrence rate but appears a less certain role in prolonging survival in patients with locally advanced thymoma. No prospective conducted trial using radiation therapy alone for this stage of disease has been performed with radiation therapy alone.

Chemotherapy

The experience with chemotherapy in patients with advanced disease is also limited. In numerous case reports and small patient series, it is clear that thymoma is a histologic subtype which is sensitive to chemotherapy. Only a few trials, however, have been designed to prospectively evaluate single agent or multiagent activity for chemotherapy.

Cisplatin, which is widely used as a component of combination therapy, produced only a 10% objective response rate as a single agent in 20 evaluable patients in a multi-institutional trial conducted by the Eastern Cooperative Oncology Group (ECOG).[14] Ifosfamide was noted to produce seven complete responses in 13 evaluable patients in a multi-institutional trial conducted in Europe.[15] The final prospective trial evaluating a single agent was with Interleukin-2. Interleukin-2 was found on a case report of have a durable complete remission in a heavily pretreated patient.[16] However, in a trial conducted at Indiana University in previously treated patients, none of 14 evaluable patients responded to Interleukin-2.[17]

Over the last several years, several prospective phase II trials of combination chemotherapy have been completed in patients with locally advanced or metastatic thymoma. In an intergroup trial coordinated by the Eastern Cooperative Oncology Group, cisplatin (50 mg/m2), doxorubicin (50 mg/m2), plus cyclophosphamide (500 mg/m2) or PAC were administered every three weeks to 30 patients with advanced disease.[18] Objective response were seen in 15 patients with the median survival being 38 months. The five-year survival was 32%.

The Eastern Cooperative Oncology Group also led an intergroup trial to evaluate combined modality therapy with PAC followed by radiation therapy.[19] Twenty-three patients with locally advanced and unresectable thymoma were treated with 2–4 cycles of PAC chemotherapy followed by 5400 cGy to the chest. Following chemotherapy 70% of patients had an objective response with a five-year survival of 52.5%.

In a slightly different regimen which also included vincristine (ADOC), Fornasiero, et al, reported a 90% objective response rate including a 47% complete response rate in 32 evaluable patients treated at a single institution.[20] The median survival time of these patients in this series, however, was only 15 months. More recently, Giaccone and colleagues reported a 56% objective response rate in 16 evaluable patients treated in a multi-institutional trial in Europe.[21] The median duration of response of 3.4 years and a five-year survival of 50% is quite similar to the experience with PAC chemotherapy.

In summary, thymoma appears to be a chemosensitive tumor. Cisplatin-based combination chemotherapy is associated with an approximate 30–50% five-year survival. This survival appears to be dependent on extent of disease. An intergroup trial evaluating etoposide, ifosfamide, and cisplatin is currently underway.

RECOMMENDATIONS

Based on the review of the literature, several recommendations for treatment can be made. In addition, several areas of future evaluation can be considered for patients with locally advanced or metastatic disease. In general, every effort should be made to render a patient disease-free including surgical resection of residual disease following primary chemotherapy. Progressive improvement in the therapeutic treatment in patients with advanced thymoma will depend on carefully designed multi-institutional trials in patients with this rare disease. Trials with combined modality therapy must also take into account the potential acute and long range complications including late cardiotoxicity which may be associated with radiation therapy and certain chemotherapeutic agents. Pathologic correlation is clearly indicated to evaluate those patients with high risk disease in whom more innovative and potentially more toxic therapy could be targeted. In contrast, a better understanding of patients with low risk disease may allow us to use simpler and less toxic therapy.

Thymoma is a unique malignancy with respect to its clinical presentation and multiplicity of treatment options. It is one of the few tumors in which treatment does afford prolonged disease-free survival. Therapeutic strategies to enhance the outcome of patients with locally advanced or minimally metastatic disease need to be considered in the context of these observations as published in this chapter.

REFERENCES

1. Loehrer PJ: Thymomas. Current experience and future directions in therapy. Drugs 45(4):477–487, 1993.
2. Levine GD and Rosai J: Thymic hyperplasia and neoplasia: A review of current concepts. Hum Pathol 9:494–515, 1978.
3. Verley JM and Hollman KH: Thymoma: A comparative study of clinical stages, histologic features, and survival in 200 cases. Cancer 55:1074–1086, 1985.
4. Lewis JE, Wick MR, Scheithauer BW, et al: Thymoma: A Clinicopathologic review. Cancer 60: 2727–2743, 1987.
5. Marino M and Müller-Hermelink HK: Thymoma and thymic carcinoma. Virchows Arch A Pathol Anat Histopathol 407:119–149, 1985.
6. Debono DJ and Loehrer PJ: Thymic neoplasms. Current Opinion in Oncology 8:112–119, 1996.
7. Masaoka A, Monden Y, Nakahara K, et al: Follow-up study of thymomas with special reference to their clinical stage. Cancer 48:2485–2492, 1981.
8. Yamakawa Y, Masaoka A, Hashimoto T, et al: A tentative tumor-node-metastasis classification of thymoma. Cancer 68:1984–1987, 1991.
9. Wilkins WE Jr and Castleman B: A continuing survey at the Massachusetts General Hospital. Ann Thorac Surg 28:252–2256, 1979.
10. Wilkins EW Jr, Grillo HC, Scannell JG, et al: Role of Staging in Prognosis and Management of Thymoma (J Maxwell Chamberlain Memorial Paper). Ann Thorac Surg 51:888–892, 1991.
11. Lewis JE, Wick MR, Scheithauer BW, et al: Thymoma. A clinicopathologic review. Cancer 60:2727–2743, 1987.

12. Curran WJ, Kornstein MJ, Brooks JJ, et al: Invasive thymoma: The role of mediastinal irradiation following complete or incomplete surgical resection. J Clin Oncol 6:1722–1727, 1988.
13. Koh W-J, Loehrer PJ, Thomas C: Thymoma: Radiation and chemotherapy. In Mediastinal Tumors: Update 1995. Edited by Wood DE, Thomas CR. New York: Springer-Verlag; 1995, 19–25.
14. Bonomi PD, Finkelstein D, Aisner S, et al: EST 2582 phase II trial of cisplatin in metastatic or recurrent thymoma. Am J Clin Oncol 16:342–345, 1993.
15. Harper PG, Highley M, Rankin E, et al: Ifosfamide monotherapy demonstrates high activity in malignant thymoma (abstract). Proc Am Soc Clin Oncol 10:300, 1991.
16. Berthaud P, le Chevalier T, Tursz T: Effective of Interleukin-2 in invasive lymphoepithelial thymoma (letter). Lancet 335:1590, 1990.
17. Gordon MS, Battiato LA, Gonin R, et al: A phase II trial of subcutaneously administered recombinant human interleukin-2 in patients with relapsed/refractory thymoma. J Immunother 1996 (in press).
18. Loehrer PJ, Kim K, Aisner SC, et al: Cisplatin plus doxorubicin plus cyclophosphamide in metastatic or recurrent thymoma: final results of an intergroup trial. J Clin Oncol 12:1164–1168, 1994.
19. Loehrer PJ, Kim K, Chen M, et al: Phase II trial of cisplatin (P), adriamycin (A), cyclophosphamide (C) plus radiotherapy in limited stage unresectable thymoma (abstract 1375). Proc Am Soc Clin Oncol 14:433, 1995.
20. Fornasiero A, Daniele O, Ghiotto C, et al: Chemotherapy of Invasive thymoma. J Clin Oncol 8:1419–1423, 1990.

50

THE ROLE OF RADIOTHERAPY IN TREATMENT OF THYMOMA

U. Oppitz,[1] D. Latz,[2] and M. Flentje[1]

[1]Department of Radiation Therapy
University of Würzburg
[2]Department of Clinical Radiology
University of Heidelberg

INTRODUCTION

Most thymomas are located in the anterior mediastinum. A small number is situated in the lateral cervical region and in some rare locations like the posterior mediastinum, the thyroid gland, within the pleura , or may spread out like a mesothelioma.

Thymomas have been shown to be relatively radiosensitive. In the past radiotherapy had been used predominantly for palliation. However, following early reports suggesting complete regressions in inoperable patients treated with external beam radiotherapy (Batata et al. 1972; Lattes 1962), interest in combined modality treatment developed. Modern megavoltage equipment and the institution of postoperative radiation treatment have had considerable impact in the local management of advanced thymoma and have been considered mandatory for patients with invasive thymomas (Rosenberg 1993).

STAGING

In earlier studies a thymoma has been considered "benign" or "malignant" on the basis of surgical assesment of tumor encapsulation or invasiveness (Koh et al. 1995). 1978 Bergh et al introduced a new clinical staging system which was modified by Masaoka et al. in 1981 (table 1). The latter systems which put more emphasis on the histologic evaluation were used or were slightly modified by other authors in the last 15 years. One of the more recent staging systems derived from the Masaoka system based on surgical and pathologic features has been described by the French Study Group on Thymic Tumours (GETT) (Cowen et al. 1995). It´s predominant criterion is the extent of surgery resection, more important than capsular invasion. Masaoka does not take into account the extent of surgical resection. This is an important prognostic factor relevant for the decision of adjuvant treatment.

Epithelial Tumors of the Thymus: Pathology, Biology, Treatment, edited by
Marx and Müller-Hermelink. Plenum Press, New York, 1997

Table 1. Clinicopathologic staging systems for thymoma

	Bergh et al. 1978
Stage I:	Intact capsule or growth within the capsule
Stage II:	Pericapsular growth into the mediastinal fat tissue
Stage III:	Invasive growth into the surrounding organs, intrathoracic metastases, or both
	Masaoka et al. 1981
Stage I:	Macroscopically completely encapsulated and microscopically no capsular invasion
Stage II:	1. Macroscopic invasion into surounding fatty tissue or mediastinal pleura, *or* 2. Microscopic invasion into capsule
Stage III:	Macroscopic invasion into neighboring organ, i.e. pericardium, great vessels, or lung
Stage IVa:	Pleural or pericardial dissemination
Stage IVb:	Lymphogenous or hematogenous metastasis
	GETT classification 1995
Stage I:	A. Encapsulated tumor, complete resection B. Potential capsular invasion, complete resection
Stage II:	Invasive tumor, complete resection
Stage III:	A. Invasive tumor, partial resection B. Invasive tumor, biopsy
Stage IV:	A. Supraclavicular or distant pleural invasion B. Distant metastases

SURGERY

The extent of the primary operation is the most significant prognostic factor in the treatment of thymoma. All published reports show higher overall survival rates and disease free survival (DSF) in totally resected cases compared to partial resection or biopsy only (Maggi et al. 1986, Curran et al. 1988). 5-year-survival range from 74–90 % in the case of total resection. Maggi et al. studied the results of 169 patients which received, except for 12 patients, no further treatment after complete or partial resection of the tumors. They were able to resect all patients with nonivasive thymoma completely and 58% of the patients with invasive tumor. The group of patients with invasive tumor and total resection showed a 5 year-survival-rate of 80% compared to 59% and 45%of patients with subtotal resection or biopsy only, respectively.

RADIATION THERAPY

Radiation therapy has been shown to be an effective adjuvant treatment for invasive thymomas. These are usually radioresponsive tumor and moderate radiation doses will be sufficient for achievement of local control. In general, thymomas are slow-growing and have a tendency to recur locally in correlation to their invasiveness. Because of the low incidence of thymomas no prospective clinical studies have been performed, but most institutions recommend postoperative irradiation of invasive tumors. A large number of retrospective studies have tried to clarify the indication for adjuvant radio- and chemotherapy.

However the rarity of the tumor, the above mentioned change in staging systems, the application of different adjuvant chemotherapy regimens over the past years and the often

Table 2. List of reviewed reports

Study	Number of pts	Reviewed time period	Staging system
Pollack et al. 1992	36	1962–87	Masaoka
Masaoka et al. 1980	96	1954–79	Masaoka
Verley et al. 1985	181	1955–82	Verley
Cowen et al. 1995	149	1979–90	GETT
Maggi et al. 1986	169	1956–84	none

retrospectively applied staging criterions make the comparison of results between different institutions difficult. Even single institutions have had difficulties comparing their treatment results, e.g. Park et al. 1994 divided their reviewed patients into three different groups to take the different chemotherapy regimen from 1951 to 1990 into account. Table 2 lists different studies and the number and timespan of the patients reviewed.

Noninvasive Stage I Thymomas

In all classifications in stage I the tumor does not infiltrate the capsule and can be resected completely (table 1). In most cases this stage did not require adjuvant treatment. Maggi et al. report 4 local recurrences in 106 stage I patients with surgery only (table 3).Verley finds 7 patients with local recurrence and 1 with a distant metastasis in 133 patients. Koh et al. 1995 cumulated the stage I patients from 11 different studies with no further treatment and find 14 recurrences in 434 cases. On the other hand Pollack reported 2/11 stage I patients with local recurrence (1 without adjuvant treatment and 1 with postoperative RT with a dose of 50 Gy). Cowen found no recurrences in 13 stage I patients who received postoperative radiotherapy (RT) in all and chemotherapy in 5 cases.

The risk of local recurrence in stage I disease after complete resection and without adjuvant therapy is about four percent. Most of the citated authors do not see justification for adjuvant treatment in this stage. Cowen et al. suggest RT in case of a large stage I tumor in case of suspicion of pleural or pericardial adhesion. Pollack et al. questioned if it is always possible to distinguish between stage I and II exspecially in a retrospective analysis to assess microscopic invasion into parathymic fat.

Table 3. Stage I thymomas with or without adjuvant therapy

Study	Number of pts	Therapy	Numbers failed
Pollack et al. 1992	11	S(4)S+RT(5)S+ CT(1)S+RT+CT(1)	1 Surgery only 1 Surgery + 50 Gy
Masaoka et al. 1980	37	S+preop.or postop.RT	2
Verley et al. 1985	133	Surgery	7 locally 1 distant
Cowen et al. 1995	13	Surgery+RT(50Gy)+CT(5/13)	0
Maggi et al. 1986	106	Surgery	4 locally

CT=Chemotherapy; RT=Radiotherapy; S=Surgery

Table 4. Totally resected invasive thymomas, Masaoka II-IVA and GETT stage II

Study	Number of pts	Therapy	Local recurrence	Staging
Pollack et al. 1992	10	S+RT(7) S only(3)	1 S+RT / 1 S only	both stage II
Masaoka et al. 1980	31	S only / S+RT	2 S+RT / 2 S only	13 Stage II 18 Stage III
Verley et al. 1985	21	S+RT 5000 rad	9	own staging
Cowen et al. 1995	46	S+RT 50 Gy+ CT (10/46)	1	GETT Stage II
Uetmatsu et al. 1996	23	S+55Gy EH-MRT	1	11 Masaoka II 12 Masaoka III
Arahaka et al. 1990	15	S+RT	2	Masaoka III+IV

EH-MRT=Entire hemithorax and postoperative mediastinal irradiation

Completely Resected Invasive Thymomas Masaoka II-IVA and GETT Stage II

In the Masaoka staging system the invasion of intrathoracic structures is the predominant criterion. It does not reflect the extent of surgery. In the following part the treatment-results after complete resection are reviewed. The rate of resectability in these stages ranges from 100% for Masaoka II to50–60 % for stage III and less then 20 % for stage IV A (Koh et al.)

Table 4 lists the results of seven different studies looking at patients with completely resected, invasive thymomas. In most cases patients were treated with postoperative RT (dose between 50 and 60 Gy) and rarely with adjuvant Chemotherapy. The recurrence rate ranges from 2% (Cowen et al) to 20% (Pollack et al.). In conflict to these data are the results of Verley et al., who find a 42% recurrence rate despite adjuvant radiation therapy up to a dose of 5000 rad. In contradiction to the other groups, these authors did not find differences between patients with complete and partially resected tumors. Curran et al. compared their data with the results of other studies and found a 28% intrathoracic failure rate for patients who did not receive RT compared to 5% failures in irradiated patients. Urgesi et al. and Nakahara et al. also support the indication for adjuvant RT in stage III completely resected invasive thymomas. They found no infield recurrences in 33 stage III patients and a 95% 15-year survival rate, respectively.

The data which would support adjuvant RT in Masaoka II are not as convincing as for stage III tumors. Some authors (Maggi, Urgesi) found only low recurrence rates in this stage. On the other hand Monden et al. found 2 recurrences in 7 patients with no further treatment compared to 2 recurrences in 25 postoperatively irradiated stage II patients. Cowen et al. do not differentiate Masaoka II-IVA and favor adjuvant RT with a dose of 50 Gy for completely resected, invasive thymoma irrespective of the depth of invasiveness. A just recently published study from Uetmatsu et al. compared entire hemithorax irradiation and postoperative mediastinal irradiation (EH-MRT) with mediastinal irradiation (MRT) alone. They saw only one true local recurrence but 6 out of 20 patients with MRT alone showed ipsilateral pleural dissemination or marginal recurrences compared to only one relapse in the EH-MRT group (23 patients).

Table 5. Incompletely resected thymomas Masaoka III-IVA and GETT stage III-IVA

Study	Subtotal/biopsy	Stages	Therapy	Recurrence
Uematsu et al.1986	1/9	6 GETT IIIB	RT 40–70 Gy	1 Stage IVA
		4 GETT IVA		1 Stage III B
Masaoka et al. 1981	11/9	12 Stage III	12 RT, 3 CT	4 réc. part. resect.
		8 Stage IVA	5 RT+CT	6 death biopsy only
Pollack et al. 1992	2/9	5 Stage III	50% of pts with	1 DOD with part.res.
		6 Stage IVA	50–60 Gy	All DOD with biop.
Mornex et al.1995	21/65	21 GETT IIIA	median RT-Dose	3/21 IIIA (14%)
		37 GETT IIIB	50 Gy	15/37 IIIB (41%)
		32 GETT IVA	59/90 CT	13/32 IVA(41%)

DOD=Dead of disease

Incompletely Resected Invasive Thymomas

Most of the patients in this category are Masaoka stage III and IV A or GETT Stages III and IVA, respectively. Because of different size of the residual tumors after partial resection or biopsy the results of different studies can not be compared easily, especially if postoperative treatment is different as to radiation dosage, chemotherapeutic regimen or combination of both. Koh et al. 1995 cumulated data of incompletely resected invasive thymomas treated with radical radiotherapy in 14 different institutions. The number of locally controlled tumors range from 100% to 37%. In table 5 results of 5 studies are given which emphasize the difficulties encountered in comparing treatments which changed over time with advances in vascular surgery, chemotherapy and radiation oncology. There is one important message in table 5: The local failure rate increases rapidly from partial resection to biopsy only. The extent of the residual tumor before the start of radiation therapy seems to have a significant impact on tumor control and survival (Koh et al.).

The Role of Radiation Therapy in Intrathoracic Recurrences

Urgesi et al. 1992 report a group of 21 patients (8 stage II, 10 stage III, 3 stage IVA) with recurrences in the mediastinum and/or in the pleura. The five patients who were irradiated postoperatively showed pleural relaps only. 11 patients were reoperated (5 total, 6 subtotal). All 21 patients were irradiated at the time of recurrence with a dose of 38–44 Gy and a 10–16 Gy boost for patients without repeated salvage surgery. The 7-year survival rate of the whole group was 70%. The results of the inoperable , only irradiated patients were not inferior to the surgery/RT-group.

OWN EXPERIENCE

At the Universities of Heidelberg and Würzburg 45 patients with invasive thymomas have been treated by postoperative radiotherapy between 1984 and 1994. Patient characteristics are shown in Table 6. Completeness of resection was estimated according to the impression of the surgeon and histopathologic evaluation. This collective is particular because of its high proportion of assumed R0 resections. Local control at 5 years has been 71 %. Local control is significantly correlated with the extent of surgical tumor removal (R0 : 22/25; R1 : 1/2; R2 : 9/18). Distant failure was observed in 11/ 45 patients, in 9 cases this was combined

Table 6. University of Heidelberg/Würzburg 1984–1994 treatment results of invasive thymomas. n = 45 (21 f, 24 m) median age 53 yrs

Masaoka	I	n = 1	
	II	n = 10	R0 n = 25
	III	n = 15	R1 n = 2
	IV	n = 19	R2 n = 18

Postoperative radiotherapy 30–70 Gy (med. 52 Gy)
16 patients received chemotherapy (mainly cisplatin based or CHOP) 11/19 Masaoka IV and 4/12 Masaoka III

with local recurrence. Estimated overall survival is 53 % at 5 years (Fig.1) 4 patients succumbed to complications of myasthenia gravis with no signs of thymoma progression.

RADIOTHERAPY TECHNIQUE AND DOSAGE

In the past, relatively simple techniques have been used for radiotherapy of thymic malignancies. Two anterior wedged fields have been recommended for smaller tumors of the anterior mediastinum. In order to include the entire thymus gland (possible extension from the 6th cervical vertebra to the level of the 7th ICR typical field sizes of 15 x 8 cm have been prescribed. In inoperable or partially resected tumors even larger field sizes using ap/pa opposing fields have been employed. In these cases a considerable rate of pneumonitis (up to 40 %) with at least temporary morbidity resulted (Penn & Hope-Stone 1972). Some cases of radiation myelitis have been described, if a spinal chord dose of 40 Gy (commonly with single doses larger than 2 Gy) was exceeded (Marks et al. 1978).

With the advent of CT-based 3-dimensional treatment planning more complex field configurations have reduced the risk of adverse reactions. In addition to the true tumor bed / macroscopic residuals at least the mediastinal pleura of the involved side and the adja-

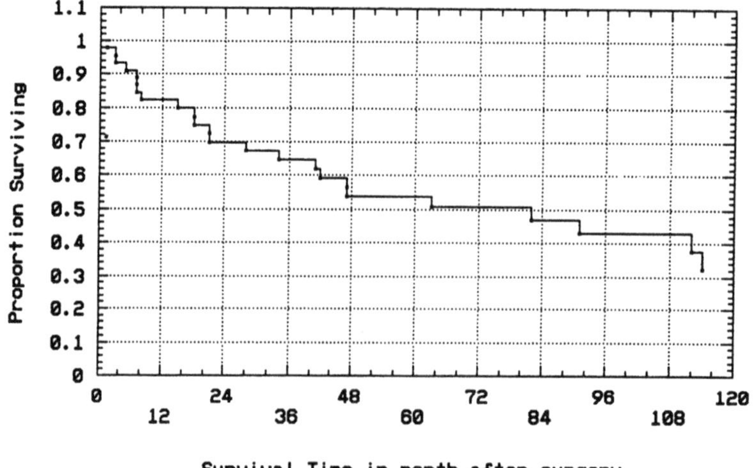

Figure 1. Invasive thymoma treated by surgery and irradiation Heidel-Würzburg, 1984–1994.

cent pericardium should be covered generously as pleural and pericardium dissemination is a common cause of failure. A typical example for treatment volume and irradiation used in our institution is shown in Fig. 2. With modern treatment technique side effects of adjuvant radiotherapy with a dose of about 50 Gy are usually moderate: pericarditis and pneumonitis with lung fibrosis occurred in less then 5% of the patients (Cowen et al. 1995).

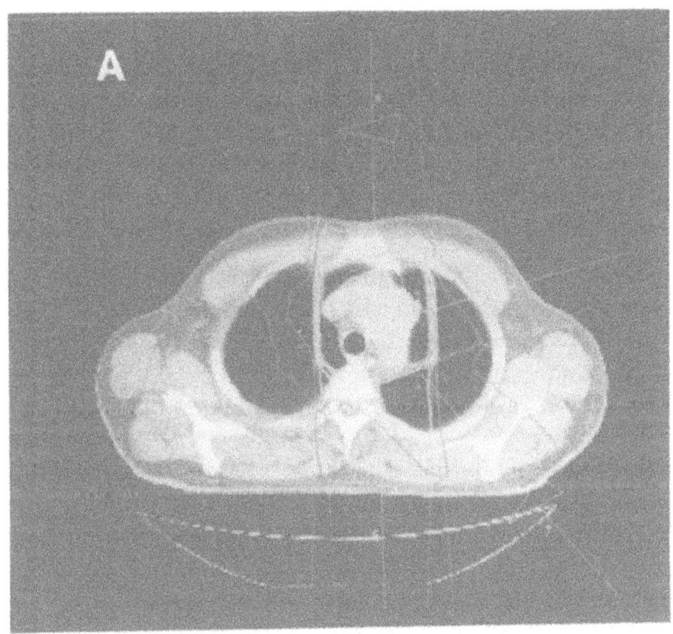

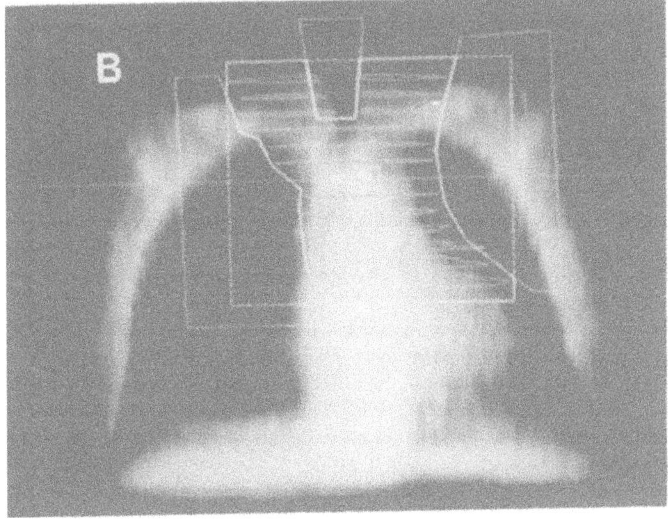

Figure 2. (A) CT-planned 4-field irradiation-technique. (B) Field 4, 0°.

Doses of 45 to 50 Gy in 5 to 6 weeks are recommended for irradiation of thymomas. In the past there has been no advantage for doses greater 50 Gy. This dose range will provide a high level of local control in the adjuvant situation. However , a recent analysis has questioned the ultimate efficacy of these "conventional" doses in large inoperable tumors (Cowen et al. 1995). In these patients doses up to 60 Gy using meticulous treatment planning and shrinking field techniques may be advocated. Hemi-thorax irradiation, as suggested by Uematsu et al. (1996) combined with mediastinal radiationtherapy seemed to reduce the intrathoracic relapses significantly in stage II thymomas but should be regarded with caution considering pulmonary toxicity.

CONCLUSIONS

Surgery is the primary treatment and the most important prognostic factor in the therapy of invasive and noninvasive thymoma. Introduction of the GETT-staging-system is recommended which combines surgical and pathological criteria and facilitates subgrouping of patients according to prognosis and possible benefit of adjunctive treatment.

Review of the literature and analysis of our own results at the Universities of Würzburg and Heidelberg suggest the following conclusions for the treatment of thymoma-patients.

- GETT stage I patients with completely resected tumors or with potentially capsular invasiveness do not need any adjuvant postoperative radiation- or chemotherapy.
- Completey resected invasive thymomas, GETT stage II, should be treated with postoperative adjuvant irradiation with 1.8 to 2.0 Gy per day and a total dose of 45–50 Gy. The inclusion of the supraclavicular fossae does not seem to improve the prognosis.
- Partially resected or biopsied tumors, GETT stage III A/Band IVA, should receive combined postoperative treatment with radio- and chemotherapy. The total radiation dose should be within the range of 50 to 56 Gy. Unfortunately a prospective randomized trial will require far too many patients and cannot possibly be conducted at a single insitution in a reasonable time frame.

There are only few data on the treatment of recurrent thymoma, but irradiation of intrathoracic relapse may result in tumor regression and longterm survival and seems to be superior to a second surgical intervention.

REFERENCES

Arakawa A., Yasunaga T., Saitoh Y.(1990):Radiation therapy of invasive carcinoma. Int.J.Radiat.Oncol.Biol.Phys 18:529–34

Batata, M.A.; Martini, N.; Nuvos, A.G. (1974): Thymomas : Clinicopathologic features, therapy and prognosis. Cancer 34 : 389–396

Bergh N.P., Gatzinsky P., Larsson S., Lundin P., Ridell B (1978): Tumors of the thymus and thymic region. I. Clinicopathological studies on thymomas. Ann. Thorac. Surg. 25:91–98

Cowen D., Richaud P., Mornex F., Bachelot T, Jung G.M., Mirabel X., Marchal C., Lagrange J.-L., ambert P, Chaplain G., N´Guyen T.D., Resbeut M. (1995): Thymoma: results of a multicentric retrospective series of 149 nonmetastatic irradiated patients and review of the literature. Radiother. Oncol. 34:9–16

Curran W.J., Kornstein M.J., Brooks J.J., Turrisi A.T. (1988): Invasive thymoma:the role of mediastinal irradiation following complete or incomplete surgical resection. J. Clin. Oncol. 6:1722–27

Koh W-J., Loehrer P., Thomas C.R. (1995) Thymoma:Radiation and chemotherapy. In:Wood D.E., Thomas C.R.(eds). Mediastinal tumors. Springer-Verlag, Heidelberg

Lattes, R. (1962): Thymomas and other tumors of the thymus. Cancer 15 : 1224–1231

Maggi G., Giaccone G., Donadio M., Ciuffreda L., Dalesio O., Leria G., Trifiletti G., Dasadio C., Palestro G., Mancuso M., Calciati A (1986): Thymomas. A review of 169 cases, with particular reference to results of surgical treatment. Cancer 58:765–76

Marks, R.D.; Wallace, K.M.; Pettit, H.S. (1978) Radiation therapy control of nine patients with malignant thymoma. Cancer 41: 117–119

Masaoka A., Monden Y., Nakahara K., Tanioka T. (1981): Follow-up study of thymomas with special reference to their clinical stages. Cancer 48:2485–92

Mornex F., Resbeut M., Richaud P., Jung G.M., Mirabel X., Marchal C., Lagrange J-L., Rambert P., Chaplain G., N'Guyen T.D. (1995): Radiotherapy and chemotherapy for invasive thymomas: a multicentric retrospective review of 90 cases. Int.J.Radiat.Oncol.Biol.Phys.32:651–59

Monden Y., Nakahara K., Iioka S (1985): Recurrence of thymoma: clinicopathological features, therapy, and prognosis. Ann. Thorac. Surg. 39:165–69

Nakahara K., Ohno K., Hashimoto J (1988): Thymoma: results with complete resection and adjuvant postoperative irradiation in 141 consecutive patients. J.Thorac Cardiovasc. Surg. 95:1041–47

Park H.S., Shin D.M., Lee J.S., Komati R., Pollack A., Putnam J.B., Cox J.D., Hong W.K. (1994): Thymoma: a retrospective study of 87 cases. Cancer 73:2491–98

Penn, C.R.H.; Hope-Stone, H.F. (1972): The role of radiotherapy in the management of malignant thymoma. Br.J.Surgery 59: 533–537

Pollack A., Komaki R., Cox J.D., Ro J.Y., Oswald M.J., Shin D.M., Putnam J.B. (1992): Thymoma: treatment and prognosis. Int.J.Radiat.Oncol.Biol.Phys.23:1037–43

Rosenberg, J.C. (1993): Neoplasmns of the mediastinum. in : deVita; T.; Hellman, S.; Rosenberg, S.A. Cancer. Principles and Practice of Oncology. 4th ed. J.C.Lippincott, Philadelphia. pp. 759–775

Uematsu M., Yoshida H., Kondo M., Itami J., Hatano K., Isobe K., Ito H., Kobayashi K., Yamaguchi Y., Kubo A. (1996): Entire hemithorax irradiation following complete resection in patients with stage II-III invasive thymoma. Int.J.Radiat.Oncol.Biol.Phys. 35:357–60

Urgesi A., Monetti U., Rossi G., Ricardi U., Casadio C. (1990): Role of radiation therapy in locally advanced thymoma. Radiother. Oncol. 19:273–80

Urgesi A., Monetti G., Ricardi U., Maggi G., Sannazzari G.L. (1992): Aggressive treatment of intrathorcic recurrences of thymoma. Radioth. Oncol. 24:221–25

Verley J.M., Hollmann K. (1985): Thymoma: a comparative study of clinical stages, histologic features, and survival in 200 cases. Cancer 55:1074–86

Walter E., Willich E., Hofmann W.J., Otto H.F., Webb W.R., De Geer G. (1992): Tumors of the thymus pp 110–193 In Walter E., Willich E. Webb W.R. (eds):The thymus.Springer-Verlag, Heidelberg

AUTHORS AND SPONSORS

Aarli, J. A.
Albertsson, M.
Antimi, M.
Antozzi, C.
Appiah-Boadu, S.
Arai, K.
Armengol, M.
Artuso, S.
Bartoccioni, E.
Baruzzi, G.
Batocchi, A.P.
Beltrami, C.A.
Benedetti, A.
Boaron, M.
Boerrigter, L.H.
Bouleksibat, M.
Bradl., M.
Brauch, H.
Cancellieri, A.
Cavazza, A.,
Cervin A.
Chi, J. G.
Chiarle, R.
Chilosi, M.
Chiusa, L.
Close, P.
Confalonieri, P.
Cornelio, F.
Di Loreto, C.
Diebold, J.
Doglietto, G. B.
Doglioni, C.
Dura, W.T.
Enoksson, M.
Espin, E.
Evoli, A.
Ezine, S.
Fellbaum, C.
Ferrari, G.
Ferro, M.T.
Finato, N.
Flentje, M.
Fornadi, L.
Fort, J.M.
Freiburg, A.
Friström, C.
Fujii, T.
Fujii, Y.
Fukayama, M.
Funata, N.
Furlan, G.
Gallucci, S.
Gardini, G.
Giaccone, G.
Gianelli, U.
Gilhus, N.E.
Gladkowska-Dura, M.J.
Greiner, A.
Grommisch, K.
Große-Höötemann, H.
Harris, N.L.
Hayashi, Y.
Hino, N.
Hishima, T.
Höfler, H.
Hofmann, W.
Horvath, R.
Jang, J. J.
Johansson, L.
Jong, D. de
Jung, A.
Jung, G.
Kääb, G.
Kahn, A.
Kawanami, S.
Kikuchi, M.
Kim, C. W.
Kirchner, Th.
Kiricuta, I. C.
Koike, M.
Kojima, K.
Kondo, K.
Kroczek, R.A.
Kuks, J.B.M.
Kuo, T.-T.
Kuwajima, G.
Lacava, N.
Lauriola, L.
Lee, S. S.
Lefvert, A.K.
Lestani, M.
Linington, C.
Lino, M.
Lo, S.K.L.
Loehrer, P. J.
Longoni, M.
Malcherek, G.
Mantegazza, R.
Marchini, C.
Martinon, C.
Marx, A.
Masaoka, A.
Matre, R.
Matsuda, H.
Melms, A.
Menestrina, F.
Mikoshiba, K.
Miquerol, L.
Miyoshi, T.
Molina T.
Moll, R.
Monden, Y.
Moran, C.A.
Morelli, L.
Mori, A.
Müller, C.
Müller-Hermelink, H.K.
Mygland, A.
Nathrath, W.
Nenninger, R.
Newsom-Davis, J.
Nishimaru, K.
Nix, W.A.
Novellino, L.
Okumura, M.
Oosterhuis, H.J.G.H.
Oppitz,U.
Oswald, E.
Otto, H.-F.

Palestro, G.
Pallini, V.
Palmisani, M. T.
Park, S.H.
Passarin, M.G.
Paulli, M.
Pedron, S.
Pescarona, E.
Peterson, S.
Pezzuoli, G.
Pizzolo, G.
Plum, J.
Poletti, V.
Ponseti, J.M.
Prampera, M.
Präuer, H.
Provenzano, C.
Puglisi, F.
Ranelletti, F.O.
Reindl, M.
Ribbains, G. de
Richel, D.J.
Riviera, A.P.
Rucco, V.
Santelmo, N.
Sarropoulos, A,
Sartini, M.
Scelsi, R.
Schalke, B
Schenkeveld, C.
Schmidt, A.
Schmitt, I.
Schneider, P.
Scholz, M.
Schömig, D.
Schultz, A
Scuderi, F.
Seo, J. S.
Seo, J.W.
Sgarzi, M.
Shimosato, Y.
Shiozawa, Y.
Shirakusa, T.
Skeie, G. O.
Sng, I.
Szobor, A.
Takeuchi, Y.
Tan, P.H.
Tezzon, F.
Tonali, P.
Toyka, K.V.
Tridente, G.
Turrisi, A.
Tzartos, S.
Uyama, T.
van't Veer, L.J.
Vandekerkhove, B.
VandeWalle, A.
Vanhecke, D.
Vincens, C.
Vincent, A.
Weichrich, G.
Weissert, R.
Wekerle, H.
Wilisch, A.
Willcox, N.
Willgeroth, K.
Yamakawa, Y.
Yoneda, S.
Zanoni, T.
Zelano, G.
Zivkovic, V.

INDEX

www.ingramcontent.com/pod-product-compliance
Ingram Content Group UK Ltd.
Pitfield, Milton Keynes, MK11 3LW, UK
UKHW061821260626
13402UKWH00046B/2190